CLINICAL TREATMENT MANUAL

FOR

OUTPATIENT PSYCHIATRY

EVIDENCE-BASED GUIDANCE FOR EVERYDAY CLINICAL PRACTICE

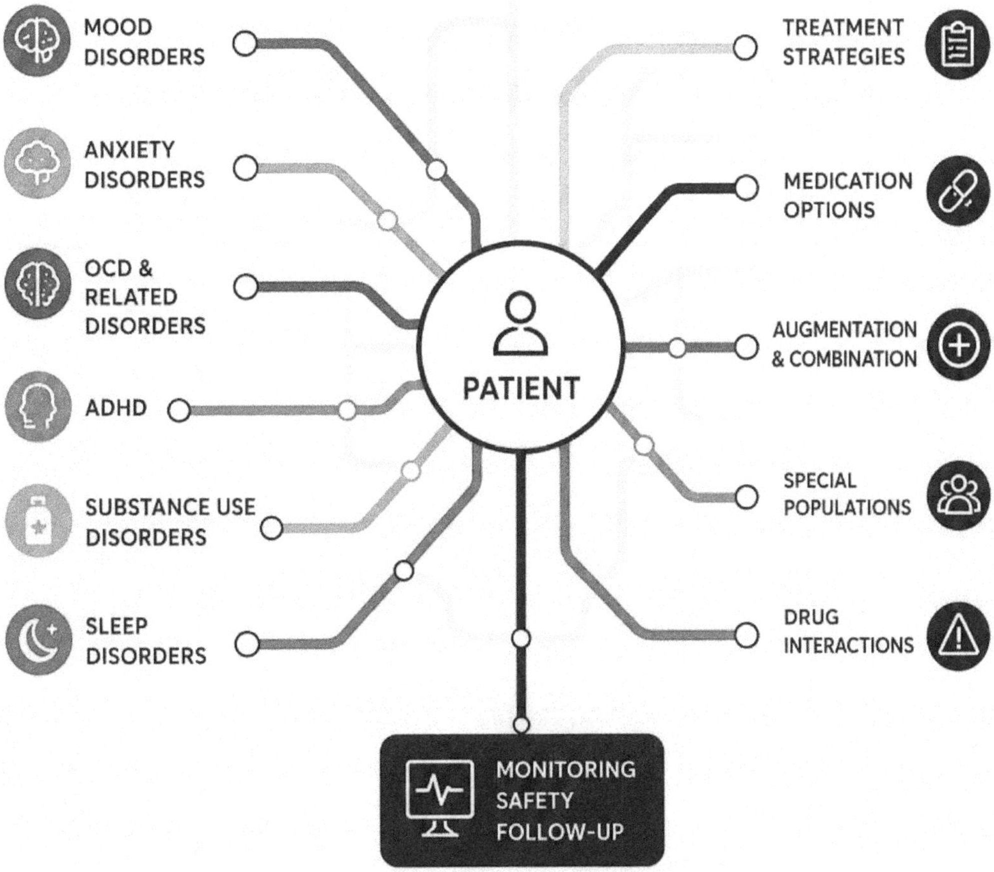

Marco Rabines, MD

NEUROSPARK PRESS

Clinical Treatment Manual for Outpatient Psychiatry

Evidence-Based Guidance for Everyday Clinical Practice

Marco Rabines, MD

Board-Certified Psychiatrist

FIRST EDITION — 2026

COPYRIGHT / DISCLAIMER / INSTITUTIONAL NOTICE

Clinical Treatment Manual for Outpatient Psychiatry

This manual is intended exclusively for educational, informational, and clinical reference purposes within outpatient psychiatric practice. The material contained herein is designed to support evidence-informed psychiatric evaluation, psychopharmacologic treatment planning, medication safety, and clinical decision-making. This manual does not replace individualized medical evaluation, independent clinical judgment, emergency medical assessment, institutional policy, specialist consultation, or applicable legal and regulatory requirements.

Recommendations contained throughout this manual are based on available clinical guidelines, peer-reviewed literature, expert consensus, and outpatient psychiatric practice standards available at the time of publication. Because psychiatric evidence, FDA labeling, medication safety data, regulatory standards, and clinical recommendations continue to evolve, clinicians remain responsible for independently verifying current prescribing information, laboratory monitoring requirements, contraindications, institutional policies, and applicable standards of care before implementing any clinical recommendation.

Medication selection, dosing, monitoring, emergency intervention, diagnostic formulation, and treatment planning must always be individualized according to patient-specific clinical presentation, medical comorbidity, psychiatric history, concurrent medications, physiologic status, and overall risk assessment. Clinical judgment remains essential in all patient-care situations.

This manual may include discussion of off-label medication use, augmentation strategies, investigational approaches, and complex psychopharmacologic interventions commonly encountered within psychiatric practice. Inclusion of such material does not constitute universal recommendation, guarantee of efficacy, or endorsement for all patient populations or clinical settings.

Psychiatric emergencies, medication toxicities, withdrawal syndromes, suicidality, severe agitation, intoxication states, and medically unstable conditions may require immediate emergency evaluation, hospitalization, consultation, or higher levels of care. Clinicians should activate emergency medical services (EMS) or appropriate emergency protocols whenever clinically indicated.

The author makes no warranties, express or implied, regarding the completeness, accuracy, reliability, or applicability of the material contained within this publication and assumes no responsibility or liability for adverse outcomes, injury, loss, or damages resulting from misuse, misinterpretation, or inappropriate application of the information presented.

This manual is not intended to establish a universal standard of care, replace institutional policy, or supersede local, state, federal, or international regulatory requirements. It is a clinical reference to be used alongside current FDA labeling, institutional protocols, and independent clinical judgment; all treatment decisions remain the responsibility of the treating clinician, who should verify current labeling before prescribing.

First Edition
2026

Marco Rabines, MD
Board-Certified Psychiatrist

Published by **NeuroSpark Press**
ISBN (Paperback): 979-8-9966648-1-8
Printed in the United States of America

DEDICATION

To God, to whom I owe everything and give thanks,

to my wife Giovanna and my daughter Isabela, my parents Nelly and Benjamin, and my brother Gustavo, for their unconditional love and support;

to my students and colleagues, from whom I learn each day;

and to my patients, to whom I owe my career and my mission in this life.

PREFACE

The Clinical Treatment Manual for Outpatient Psychiatry was written to meet a practical need: a concise, reliable, and clinically usable reference that supports real-world decision-making in the outpatient setting. It distills current psychiatric guidelines, regulatory labeling, and peer-reviewed evidence into structured, quick-reference guidance that clinicians can apply during a busy clinical day.

This manual is intended for practicing psychiatrists, psychiatric nurse practitioners, physician assistants, primary care clinicians who manage psychiatric conditions, and trainees in psychiatry and related fields. It assumes a working knowledge of psychiatric diagnosis and pharmacology and is designed to complement—not replace—clinical training, supervision, and individualized judgment.

The manual is organized around the conditions most commonly encountered in outpatient practice—mood, anxiety, obsessive-compulsive and related, trauma-related, neurodevelopmental, psychotic, neurocognitive, sleep-wake, and substance use disorders—framed by cross-cutting sections on initial evaluation and safety, treatment selection, medication options, augmentation and combination strategies, special populations, drug interactions, and ongoing monitoring. Appendices provide equivalency tables, conversion guides, dietary precautions, and patient-education handouts for rapid reference. Where a recommendation is labeled "Clinical consensus," it reflects expert opinion and prevailing practice rather than high-level trial or guideline evidence and should be weighed accordingly.

Recommendations throughout are grounded in the DSM-5-TR, major clinical practice guidelines, FDA labeling, and the primary literature, with sources cited within each section. Because psychiatric evidence, prescribing information, and safety data evolve continuously, the guidance here reflects standards available at the time of writing and should be verified against current sources before application.

How to Use This Manual

Each clinical section follows a consistent structure: a brief diagnostic orientation, evidence-based pharmacologic and non-pharmacologic options, practical treatment-selection guidance, and safety and monitoring considerations. Tables are used throughout to present dosing, monitoring, and comparative data in a scannable format.

The manual is intended for point-of-care consultation rather than cover-to-cover reading. Clinicians are encouraged to move directly to the relevant section, cross-referencing the drug-interaction, augmentation, and special-population material as needed for a given patient.

Throughout, the manual emphasizes safety-first prescribing, measurement-based care, and individualized clinical judgment. It does not establish a standard of care and does not substitute for emergency evaluation, specialist consultation, or institutional policy. Readers should review the disclaimer and institutional notice that accompany this edition.

LIST OF ABBREVIATIONS

The following abbreviations are used throughout this manual.

5-HT	Serotonin (5-hydroxytryptamine)
ADHD	Attention-Deficit/Hyperactivity Disorder
AIMS	Abnormal Involuntary Movement Scale
APA	American Psychiatric Association
AUD	Alcohol Use Disorder
BMI	Body Mass Index
BPD	Borderline Personality Disorder
BZD	Benzodiazepine
CBC	Complete Blood Count
CBT	Cognitive Behavioral Therapy
CGI	Clinical Global Impression scale
C-SSRS	Columbia–Suicide Severity Rating Scale
CYP	Cytochrome P450 (e.g., CYP2D6, CYP3A4)
DSM-5-TR	Diagnostic and Statistical Manual of Mental Disorders, Fifth Edition, Text Revision
ECG / EKG	Electrocardiogram
ECT	Electroconvulsive Therapy
eGFR	Estimated Glomerular Filtration Rate
EMS	Emergency Medical Services
ER / XR	Extended-Release (formulation)
FDA	U.S. Food and Drug Administration
FGA	First-Generation Antipsychotic
GAD	Generalized Anxiety Disorder
GAD-7	Generalized Anxiety Disorder 7-item scale
HAM-A	Hamilton Anxiety Rating Scale
HAM-D	Hamilton Depression Rating Scale
IR	Immediate-Release (formulation)
LAI	Long-Acting Injectable antipsychotic
LFT	Liver Function Test(s)
MADRS	Montgomery–Åsberg Depression Rating Scale
MAOI	Monoamine Oxidase Inhibitor
MBC	Measurement-Based Care

MDD	Major Depressive Disorder
MDE	Major Depressive Episode
NMS	Neuroleptic Malignant Syndrome
OCD	Obsessive-Compulsive Disorder
OSA	Obstructive Sleep Apnea
OUD	Opioid Use Disorder
PHQ-9	Patient Health Questionnaire 9-item
PMDD	Premenstrual Dysphoric Disorder
PTSD	Posttraumatic Stress Disorder
QTc	Corrected QT interval
REMS	Risk Evaluation and Mitigation Strategy
RLS	Restless Legs Syndrome
SGA	Second-Generation Antipsychotic
SI	Suicidal Ideation
SNRI	Serotonin–Norepinephrine Reuptake Inhibitor
SSRI	Selective Serotonin Reuptake Inhibitor
SUD	Substance Use Disorder
TCA	Tricyclic Antidepressant
TD	Tardive Dyskinesia
TMS	Transcranial Magnetic Stimulation
TSH	Thyroid-Stimulating Hormone
VNS	Vagus Nerve Stimulation
YMRS	Young Mania Rating Scale

TABLE OF CONTENTS

Clinical Treatment Manual for Outpatient Psychiatry

I. INSTITUTIONAL FOUNDATIONS

A. Institutional Purpose and Scope

This chapter establishes the institutional foundation for outpatient psychiatric evaluation, psychopharmacologic treatment, clinical monitoring, documentation standards, and patient safety procedures within the organization. The purpose of this manual is to support consistent, evidence-informed, and clinically responsible psychiatric care while preserving individualized clinical judgment and professional accountability.

This manual applies to clinicians practicing under the supervision of the Medical Director in the outpatient psychiatric setting. It is intended to function as a structured clinical framework and quality standard, not as a rigid legal rule, universal standard of care, or substitute for independent medical judgment.

Institutional Domain	Standard	Evidence Source
Purpose	Establish standardized outpatient psychiatric protocols for evaluation, pharmacologic treatment, monitoring, documentation, and safety management	Institutional policy; APA (2016); DSM-5-TR (APA, 2022)
Scope	Applies to clinicians practicing under Medical Director supervision in the outpatient setting	Institutional policy
Clinical function	Provides a shared framework for consistent, evidence-informed psychiatric practice	Institutional policy; Clinical consensus
Practice standard	Supports standardized care while preserving individualized clinical judgment	Institutional policy; Clinical consensus
Diagnostic framework	DSM-5-TR diagnostic criteria should guide diagnostic formulation and differential diagnosis when applicable	DSM-5-TR (APA, 2022)
Regulatory alignment	Medication use should consider FDA labeling, contraindications, warnings, and monitoring requirements	FDA labeling
Quality objective	Reduce unnecessary variability while supporting safe, clinically justified treatment decisions	Institutional policy; Clinical consensus

B. Clinical Judgment and Individualized Care

Psychiatric pharmacotherapy is grounded in scientific evidence derived from clinical trials, meta-analyses, regulatory guidance, and evidence-based practice guidelines. However, effective treatment also requires individualized clinical judgment. Patients may differ substantially in treatment response, tolerability, medical comorbidity, psychosocial context, adherence barriers, prior medication exposure, and personal treatment preferences.

Clinicians may reasonably deviate from standard recommendations when supported by patient-specific considerations, sound clinical reasoning, and appropriate documentation. When such deviations occur, the rationale should be clearly recorded in the medical record to support safety, continuity of care, and clinical accountability.

Clinical Principle	Clinical Application	Evidence Source
Evidence-informed care	Treatment decisions should consider high-quality evidence, major guidelines, FDA labeling, and patient-specific factors	FDA labeling; APA (2016); NICE NG222 (2022); Clinical consensus
Individual variability	Patients may respond differently to the same medication despite guideline-based recommendations	Clinical consensus
Prior treatment history	Previous medication efficacy, intolerance, dose, duration, adherence, and adverse effects should inform future treatment selection	APA (2016); Clinical consensus
Medical comorbidity	Treatment planning should incorporate medical conditions, metabolic risk, neurologic history, pregnancy status when relevant, and drug–drug interactions	APA (2016); Clinical consensus
Side-effect tolerability	Medication selection should consider patient-specific tolerability, functional impact, and safety risks	Clinical consensus
Psychosocial context	Social stressors, access barriers, adherence limitations, and environmental factors may influence treatment success	APA (2016); Clinical consensus
Patient preference	Shared decision-making and patient treatment preferences should be incorporated whenever clinically appropriate	NICE NG222 (2022); Clinical consensus
Clinical deviation	Deviation from first-line recommendations should include a documented rationale	Institutional policy
Clinical accountability	This manual supports, but does not replace, independent medical judgment	Institutional policy

C. Scope, Limitations, and Referral Boundaries

This manual is designed for outpatient community psychiatric practice and routine psychopharmacologic management. It does not replace comprehensive medical evaluation, emergency medical assessment, institutional policy, specialist consultation, or applicable legal and regulatory requirements.

Clinical decisions should always consider the specific needs, risks, comorbidities, physiologic status, psychosocial circumstances, and safety concerns of each patient. Referral to a higher level of care, emergency services, specialty consultation, or interventional psychiatry should be considered whenever clinically indicated.

While treatments such as electroconvulsive therapy (ECT), ketamine/esketamine-based therapies, transcranial magnetic stimulation (TMS), vagus nerve stimulation (VNS), and other neuromodulation approaches may be appropriate in selected treatment-resistant conditions, comprehensive procedural protocols for these interventions fall outside the primary scope of this manual. These treatments may require specialized training, procedural infrastructure, anesthesia support, REMS compliance, advanced monitoring systems, or dedicated interventional psychiatric programs.

Scope / Limitation	Clinical Application	Evidence Source
Outpatient focus	Designed primarily for outpatient psychiatric evaluation and medication management	Institutional policy
Not a rigid legal standard	Recommendations should not be interpreted as inflexible legal requirements	Institutional policy
Independent judgment	Clinicians remain responsible for individualized treatment decisions	Institutional policy; Clinical consensus
Medical evaluation	Psychiatric assessment should incorporate relevant medical, neurologic, substance use, and psychosocial factors	APA (2016); Clinical consensus
Emergency escalation	Acute psychiatric risk, medical instability, intoxication, severe withdrawal, or dangerousness may require emergency referral	Institutional policy; Clinical consensus
Higher level of care	Inpatient, intensive outpatient, partial hospitalization, emergency evaluation, or specialty services should be considered when clinically indicated	Clinical consensus
Interventional psychiatry	ECT, ketamine/esketamine, TMS, VNS, and related procedures require separate specialty protocols	Clinical consensus
Evolving evidence	Recommendations may change as new safety data, regulatory updates, or guideline revisions emerge	FDA labeling; Institutional policy

D. Conditions Outside the Scope of This Manual

This manual is designed to support the clinical management of psychiatric conditions most commonly encountered in outpatient ambulatory practice. Several diagnostic categories are not addressed or are only partially covered, either because they typically require inpatient stabilization, subspecialty referral, or higher levels of care, or because they fall outside the scope of routine outpatient psychiatric practice in this setting.

Conditions outside the scope of this manual include: catatonia, anorexia nervosa (moderate to severe), factitious disorder, and paraphilic disorders. These presentations require inpatient evaluation, multidisciplinary management, or subspecialty expertise beyond the outpatient setting.

Conditions that may occasionally present in outpatient practice but are not covered in detail in this manual include: bulimia nervosa, binge eating disorder, dissociative disorders, somatic symptom disorder, personality disorders beyond stabilization and basic management, and gender dysphoria. Clinicians encountering these presentations are encouraged to pursue subspecialty consultation or referral as clinically indicated.

E. Evidence Hierarchy and Guideline Interpretation

Clinical recommendations in this manual are based on a structured hierarchy of evidence intended to support safe, consistent, and evidence-informed outpatient psychiatric practice. Whenever available, treatment decisions should prioritize regulatory guidance, major clinical practice guidelines, randomized trials, meta-analyses, systematic reviews, and high-quality peer-reviewed literature. In areas where higher-level evidence is limited or unavailable, expert consensus and individualized clinical judgment may be necessary.

Guideline citations are intended primarily to support treatment role, level of recommendation, safety considerations, or overall clinical strategy. They may not correspond to every dose range, clinical nuance, or patient-specific adjustment listed in individual tables. Dose ranges presented throughout this manual reflect commonly used adult psychiatric prescribing ranges derived from FDA labeling, major clinical references, guideline-supported practice patterns, and routine outpatient psychopharmacology practice.

Certain treatments discussed in international guidelines may not carry identical FDA-approved indications in the United States. Clinicians should therefore interpret recommendations within the context of local regulatory standards, medication availability, institutional policies, and patient-specific clinical considerations.

Evidence Level	Clinical Application	Evidence Source
FDA labeling and regulatory guidance	Primary reference for approved indications, dosing, contraindications, boxed warnings, REMS requirements, and medication-specific monitoring	FDA labeling
DSM-5-TR	Primary diagnostic framework for psychiatric diagnosis and differential diagnosis	DSM-5-TR (APA, 2022)
Major clinical practice guidelines	Core framework for evidence-based psychiatric treatment recommendations	APA (2016); APA (2020); NICE NG222 (2022); VA/DoD (2023)
Randomized controlled trials	Used to evaluate efficacy, safety, and comparative treatment outcomes	High-quality clinical literature
Meta-analyses and systematic reviews	Support synthesis of broader evidence and consistency across studies	High-quality clinical literature
Consensus expert recommendations	May guide treatment decisions when higher-level evidence is insufficient or unavailable	Clinical consensus

Evidence Level	Clinical Application	Evidence Source
Off-label prescribing evidence	Off-label use may be appropriate when supported by scientific literature, clinical rationale, informed consent, and patient-specific risk–benefit assessment	Clinical consensus; FDA labeling when medication-specific
Institutional policy	Defines local workflow, documentation, review, supervision, and safety standards	Institutional policy
Individualized clinical judgment	Final treatment decisions should incorporate patient-specific clinical factors and professional judgment	Institutional policy; Clinical consensus

Note on “Clinical Consensus”

The term **Clinical consensus** throughout this manual refers to broadly accepted expert practice patterns used when high-quality guideline-based evidence, randomized controlled data, or formal regulatory guidance are limited, unavailable, or not sufficiently specific to the clinical scenario. These recommendations are informed by standard psychiatric practice, psychopharmacologic principles, safety considerations, and accumulated clinical experience rather than definitive guideline mandates.

F. Minimum Documentation and Safety Standards

Consistent documentation is essential to support patient safety, continuity of care, regulatory compliance, and appropriate clinical decision-making. Documentation should be clinically meaningful, reproducible across providers, and sufficient to justify diagnosis, treatment selection, medication changes, risk assessment, follow-up planning, and deviations from standard recommendations.

The following elements represent minimum documentation expectations for outpatient psychiatric encounters unless otherwise clinically justified.

Documentation Element	Minimum Clinical Requirement	Evidence Source
Diagnostic formulation	Document DSM-5-TR diagnosis and relevant differential considerations when appropriate	DSM-5-TR (APA, 2022); APA (2016)
Presenting problem	Document chief complaint, symptom course, severity, functional impairment, and relevant context	APA (2016)

Documentation Element	Minimum Clinical Requirement	Evidence Source
Psychiatric history	Document prior diagnoses, hospitalizations, suicide attempts, self-harm, psychotherapy, and medication trials	APA (2016)
Medical history	Document clinically relevant medical, neurologic, reproductive, hepatic, renal, cardiovascular, and metabolic history	APA (2016); Clinical consensus
Medication reconciliation	Review and document current psychiatric medications, non-psychiatric medications, OTC products, supplements, and substance use when relevant	APA (2016); Clinical consensus
Suicide risk assessment	Document suicide risk evaluation when clinically indicated, including risk factors, protective factors, access to means, and disposition rationale	VA/DoD (2023); Clinical consensus
Violence or safety risk	Document risk to others, impaired judgment, psychosis, severe agitation, intoxication, or other safety concerns when present	APA (2016); Clinical consensus
Treatment rationale	Record the clinical reasoning for medication initiation, discontinuation, dose adjustment, switch, or augmentation	Institutional policy; Clinical consensus
Risk–benefit discussion	Document relevant risks, anticipated benefits, alternatives, and clinical reasoning for significant treatment decisions	Clinical consensus; NICE NG222 (2022)
Informed consent	Document informed consent when clinically indicated, particularly for off-label, higher-risk, or complex interventions	FDA labeling; Clinical consensus
Side-effect assessment	Document medication tolerability and clinically relevant adverse effects	Clinical consensus; NICE NG222 (2022)

Documentation Element	Minimum Clinical Requirement	Evidence Source
Shared decision-making	Document patient preferences, concerns, treatment goals, and participation in treatment planning when applicable	NICE NG222 (2022); Clinical consensus
Follow-up planning	Specify follow-up interval, monitoring plan, safety instructions, and recommended clinical actions	Institutional policy
Deviation from standard approach	Document rationale when deviating from first-line, guideline-supported, or usual-care recommendations	Institutional policy

Medication-Specific Documentation and Monitoring Standards

Medication / Class	Required or Expected Monitoring	Evidence Source
Antipsychotics	Baseline and interval metabolic monitoring, including weight/BMI, glucose or HbA1c, and lipid assessment	ADA/APA Consensus (2004); APA (2020)
Lithium	Serum lithium level, renal function, and thyroid function should be documented at baseline and during ongoing treatment	FDA labeling; Clinical consensus
Valproate / divalproex	Liver function tests, CBC/platelets, and serum valproate level should be documented at baseline and periodically during treatment	FDA labeling; Clinical consensus
Clozapine	ANC monitoring is strongly recommended per FDA prescribing information (REMS eliminated June 13, 2025); document clearly in the record	FDA labeling (2025)
Stimulants	Cardiac history, blood pressure, heart rate, misuse risk, and relevant psychiatric comorbidity should be assessed before and during treatment	FDA labeling; Clinical consensus
QT-prolonging psychotropics	Baseline ECG should be considered when cardiac risk factors, high-risk combinations, electrolyte abnormalities, or dose-related risk are present	FDA labeling; Clinical consensus
Teratogenic or pregnancy-relevant medications	Pregnancy status, reproductive counseling, and risk–benefit discussion should be documented when clinically indicated	FDA labeling; Clinical consensus
Controlled substances	Misuse risk, dependence potential, PDMP review when applicable, safe prescribing rationale, follow-up plan, and urine drug/toxicology screening when clinically indicated, risk-based, or required by institutional policy should be documented	FDA labeling; Institutional policy; Clinical consensus

Institutional Safety Priorities

Safety Priority	Clinical Standard	Evidence Source
Suicide risk screening	Screen for suicidal ideation and acute safety concerns at baseline and each depression follow-up; complete full risk assessment when risk is endorsed or clinically suspected	VA/DoD (2023); Clinical consensus
Medication interaction review	Assess clinically significant drug–drug interactions before treatment initiation or modification	FDA labeling; Clinical consensus
OTC and supplement review	Review OTC medications, herbal products, supplements, energy products, and substances that may affect psychiatric treatment	APA (2016); Clinical consensus
Metabolic monitoring	Ensure appropriate metabolic monitoring for patients receiving antipsychotic treatment	ADA/APA Consensus (2004); APA (2020)
Controlled substance monitoring	Evaluate misuse risk, dependence potential, PDMP findings when applicable, safe prescribing rationale, and risk-based toxicology screening when clinically indicated or required by institutional policy	FDA labeling; Clinical consensus
Informed consent documentation	Document informed consent for clinically significant, higher-risk, or off-label treatment decisions	Clinical consensus; Institutional policy
Adverse effect monitoring	Monitor and document clinically significant medication side effects and safety concerns	Clinical consensus
Follow-up and continuity	Ensure appropriate follow-up intervals and continuity of care for high-risk or clinically unstable patients	Institutional policy
Emergency escalation	Refer to higher levels of care or emergency services when acute psychiatric or medical risk is identified	Institutional policy; Clinical consensus

G. Review Policy and Version Control

To maintain clinical relevance, regulatory alignment, and consistency with evolving evidence-based standards, this manual should undergo periodic institutional review and revision. Updates may occur as part of scheduled quality review processes or in response to significant regulatory, safety, formulary, or guideline changes affecting psychiatric practice.

All revisions should be formally documented to preserve version control, institutional accountability, and transparency regarding changes in clinical standards.

Review Component	Institutional Standard	Evidence Source
Scheduled review cycle	Manual should undergo formal review every two years, or earlier if major clinical, regulatory, or safety changes occur	Institutional policy

Review Component	Institutional Standard	Evidence Source
Regulatory updates	Major FDA approvals, labeling changes, boxed warnings, or REMS updates should prompt review when relevant to psychiatric practice	Institutional policy; FDA labeling
Guideline revisions	Significant updates to APA, NICE, VA/DoD, or other core references should trigger review consideration	Institutional policy
Safety communications	Major safety alerts, adverse effect data, or medication warnings should prompt reassessment of affected sections	Institutional policy; FDA labeling
Internal quality review	Procedural gaps, recurrent adverse events, audit findings, or documentation inconsistencies may require manual modification	Institutional policy
Version documentation	All revisions should include version number, revision date, description of changes, responsible party, and approval record	Institutional policy
Institutional oversight	Final approval and implementation authority remains under Medical Director supervision	Institutional policy

Version Control and Modification Log

Version	Date	Description of Changes	Author / Responsible Party	Approved: Medical Director Signature
1.0	April 4, 2026	Initial version of the manual; creation of baseline protocols for evaluation, safety assessment, documentation, and psychopharmacologic treatment	Medical Director / Responsible Party	Signed: ______ Date: ______

REFERENCES

American Diabetes Association, American Psychiatric Association, American Association of Clinical Endocrinologists, & North American Association for the Study of Obesity. (2004). Consensus development conference on antipsychotic drugs and obesity and diabetes. *Diabetes Care*, *27*(2), 596–601. https://doi.org/10.2337/diacare.27.2.596

American Psychiatric Association. (2016). *The American Psychiatric Association practice guidelines for the psychiatric evaluation of adults* (3rd ed.). American Psychiatric Association Publishing. https://doi.org/10.1176/appi.books.9780890426760

American Psychiatric Association. (2020). *The American Psychiatric Association practice guideline for the treatment of patients with schizophrenia* (3rd ed.). American Psychiatric Association Publishing. https://doi.org/10.1176/appi.books.9780890424841

American Psychiatric Association. (2022). *Diagnostic and statistical manual of mental disorders* (5th ed., text rev.; DSM-5-TR). American Psychiatric Association Publishing. https://doi.org/10.1176/appi.books.9780890425787

Department of Veterans Affairs & Department of Defense. (2023). *VA/DoD clinical practice guideline for assessment and management of patients at risk for suicide*. U.S. Department of Veterans Affairs and U.S. Department of Defense. https://www.healthquality.va.gov/guidelines/MH/srb/

Department of Veterans Affairs & Department of Defense. (2023). *VA/DoD clinical practice guideline for the management of major depressive disorder*. U.S. Department of Veterans Affairs and U.S. Department of Defense. https://www.healthquality.va.gov/guidelines/MH/mdd/

National Institute for Health and Care Excellence. (2022). *Depression in adults: Treatment and management* (NICE Guideline NG222). https://www.nice.org.uk/guidance/ng222

U.S. Food and Drug Administration. (1970, updated 2023). *Lithobid (lithium carbonate) prescribing information.* https://www.accessdata.fda.gov/drugsatfda_docs/label/2023/018557s110lbl.pdf

U.S. Food and Drug Administration. (1983, updated 2022). *Depakote (divalproex sodium) prescribing information.* https://www.accessdata.fda.gov/drugsatfda_docs/label/2022/018723s060lbl.pdf

U.S. Food and Drug Administration. (n.d.). *Drug approvals and databases.* https://www.fda.gov/drugs/development-approval-process-drugs/drug-approvals-and-databases

U.S. Food and Drug Administration. (n.d.). *Risk evaluation and mitigation strategies.* https://www.fda.gov/drugs/drug-safety-and-availability/risk-evaluation-and-mitigation-strategies-rems

II. INITIAL EVALUATION AND SAFETY PROTOCOL

A comprehensive psychiatric evaluation represents the foundation of safe, effective, and evidence-informed outpatient psychiatric care. Accurate diagnosis, identification of safety risks, assessment of psychosocial and medical factors, and establishment of an appropriate treatment plan depend on a structured and clinically thorough evaluation process. This chapter outlines the institutional standards for initial psychiatric assessment, suicide risk evaluation, crisis identification, informed consent, documentation requirements, and essential safety procedures intended to support high-quality, consistent, and patient-centered psychiatric practice.

1. OVERVIEW

Aspect	Detail	Evidence Source
Purpose	Establish a structured, comprehensive psychiatric evaluation to guide diagnosis, risk assessment, and treatment planning.	APA (2016); DSM-5-TR (APA, 2022)
Core components	Psychiatric history, medical history, substance use, mental status examination, and risk assessment.	APA (2016)
Clinical priority	Identify safety risks (suicide, violence, medical instability) and determine appropriate level of care.	Joint Commission (NPSG 15); APA (2016)
Measurement-Based care	Use validated scales (PHQ-9, GAD-7, C-SSRS, YMRS) to support clinical decision-making and track outcomes.	APA (2016); Clinical consensus
Documentation standard	Evaluation must be structured, complete, and reproducible across providers.	Institutional policy

Every new patient evaluation must include the following components:

A. Identifying Information

Age
Gender identity
Referral source
Living situation
Relationship status
Employment/education status
Insurance status (if relevant to care continuity)

B. Chief Complaint

Document verbatim when possible.

C. History of Present Illness (HPI)

Chronological and clinically structured assessment of:

- Onset
- Duration
- Symptom progression
- Severity
- Functional impairment (work, school, relationships)
- Precipitating factors
- Aggravating/relieving factors
- Prior episodes
- Prior treatments and response

For mood disorders, explicitly assess:

- Sleep pattern
- Energy
- Concentration
- Appetite
- Suicidal ideation
- Irritability
- Mixed symptoms (racing thoughts, decreased need for sleep)

D. Past Psychiatric History

- Prior psychiatric diagnoses
- Prior hospitalizations (voluntary/involuntary)
- Suicide attempts (method, lethality, medical severity)
- Self-harm behaviors
- Prior medication trials (dose, duration, response, adverse effects)
- History of treatment resistance
- Psychotherapy history and response
- History of trauma
- Legal history related to psychiatric symptoms (if relevant)

E. Substance Use History

Document use of:

- Alcohol (frequency, quantity, last use)
- Cannabis
- Stimulants

Opioids
Sedatives/benzodiazepines
Nicotine
Caffeine
OTC misuse
Energy drink consumption

Include:

History of withdrawal symptoms
Past treatment
Legal consequences
Blackouts
DUIs
Prior detox

Validated screening tools may be used when clinically indicated, including:

AUDIT-C for alcohol use screening (Bush et al., 1998)
Standardized screening instruments for substance use disorders (Sigmon & Dunn, 2010)

F. Medical History

Assess for:

Allergies
Cardiovascular disease
Hypertension
Diabetes
Thyroid disorders
Neurologic disorders
Hepatic or renal disease
Seizure history
Sleep apnea

G. Medication Reconciliation (Mandatory)

Document all current and recent:

Prescription medications
OTC medications
Herbal supplements
Vitamins
Energy products
Recent antibiotic use

Hormonal therapies
Contraceptives
Smoking and vaping status

Specifically ask about:

St. John's Wort
CBD products
Valerian
Ashwagandha
Kava

H. Psychosocial History

Document active stressors, including:

Living situation
Employment/education
Relationships
Social support
Financial status
Legal history
Cultural/spiritual factors
Access to care
Functional status

I. Family Psychiatric History

Document the presence or absence of:

Major depressive disorder
Bipolar disorder
Schizophrenia or psychotic disorders
Anxiety disorders
Substance use disorders
Suicide or suicide attempts
ADHD
Autism spectrum disorders

J. Mental Status Examination

Required components:

Appearance
Behavior
Speech

Mood
Affect
Thought process
Thought content
Perceptual disturbances
Cognition
Insight
Judgment

K. Risk Assessment Summary

Must clearly document:

Suicide risk level
Protective factors
Access to means
Safety planning
Disposition decision

L. Initial Diagnostic Impression

M. Initial Treatment Plan (Document baseline AIMS, and MMSE if pertinent)

2. Measurement-Based Care

Use the following tools when clinically appropriate:

Condition	Tool	Frequency
Depression	PHQ-9	Baseline + periodic follow-up; each visit when clinically active or changing treatment
Anxiety	GAD-7	Baseline + periodic follow-up; each visit when clinically active or changing treatment
Suicide risk	C-SSRS or structured assessment	Baseline + when indicated; safety screen at each depression follow-up
Bipolar symptoms	YMRS	When manic/hypomanic symptoms are suspected
Psychosis	Clinical assessment ± BPRS	As indicated
Extrapyramidal symptoms	AIMS	Baseline + periodically during antipsychotic treatment
Alcohol withdrawal	CIWA-Ar	As indicated

Condition	Tool	Frequency
Cognitive concerns	MMSE or MoCA	Baseline if suspected; repeat as indicated

3. Suicide Risk Assessment (Directive Section)

Suicide risk assessment should be documented using a structured clinical approach that includes risk factors, protective factors, access to lethal means, safety planning, and disposition rationale. (VA/DoD (2023); The Joint Commission (2023); Clinical consensus)

All new evaluations

- Medication changes
- Worsening symptoms
- Any expression of hopelessness
- Bipolar mixed states
- Postpartum mood changes

Core Risk Domains:

- Passive ideation
- Active ideation
- Plan
- Intent
- Access to means
- Prior attempts
- Substance use
- Agitation or mixed features

High-Risk Red Flags:

- Recent attempt
- Specific lethal plan
- Access to firearms
- Severe agitation
- Psychosis with command hallucinations
- Bipolar mixed episode
- Recent discharge from inpatient care

Protective Factors:

- Social support (family, friends, partner)
- Responsibilities/roles (children, pets, employment)
- Beliefs/values (religious or moral objections)

Coping skills (problem-solving, distress tolerance)
Hope/future orientation (plans, reasons for living)
Engagement in care (therapy, follow-up, medication adherence)
Access to resources (crisis services, safe housing)
Reduced access to means (secured medications, no firearms)
Lethal means restriction counseling when clinically indicated
Substance use stability
Clinical stability
Therapeutic alliance and reliable emergency contact
Legal/safety supports (court-ordered treatment, case management)

Safety planning should be collaborative and documented when suicide risk is present, but outpatient management remains clinically appropriate. This applies to patients whose suicide risk has been formally assessed as low to moderate and who can be safely supported in the community; higher-risk presentations warrant consideration of a higher level of care.

Evidence Source: (VA/DoD (2023); The Joint Commission (2023))

4. Baker Act Criteria (Florida)

Involuntary examination may be initiated when:

The person has a mental illness AND
The person refuses voluntary examination or is unable to determine the need for examination AND
Without treatment, the person is likely to suffer neglect or poses a substantial likelihood of serious harm to self or others.

Documentation must include:

Specific observed behaviors
Patient statements
Risk assessment findings
Rationale for involuntary action

Evidence Source: Florida Mental Health Act, Fla. Stat. § 394.463; Institutional policy

5. Crisis Pathways (Operational)

Situation	Recommended Action
Passive suicidal ideation without plan/intent, protective factors present, reliable follow-up, and verifiable support/containment	Outpatient safety plan with documented follow-up

Situation	Recommended Action
Passive suicidal ideation without plan/intent but limited protective factors, unreliable follow-up, no verifiable support, unsafe home environment, or clinician concern for poor containment	Consider urgent psychiatric evaluation, higher level of care, crisis stabilization, or Emergency Room referral
Active plan with intent, access to lethal means, psychosis with risk, severe mania, or mixed episode	Emergency Room Referral
Impaired judgment, inability to maintain safety, high impulsivity, severe postpartum symptoms, delirium/medical instability, or Clozapine-related complications	Hospitalization

6. Informed Consent and Off-Label Disclosure

Informed consent must include:

- Diagnosis
- Treatment rationale
- Risks (common and rare serious side effects)
- Alternative treatments
- Disclosure of off-label use (if applicable)

Documentation should state:

"Risks, benefits, and alternatives were discussed. Patient verbalized understanding."

Evidence Source: FDA labeling; Institutional policy; Clinical consensus

7. Follow-Up and Level of Care Determination

Case Type	Initial Follow-Up Interval
Antidepressants	2 – 4 weeks
High-risk outpatient cases	1 week or sooner when clinically indicated
Unstable bipolar or psychosis	1 week

Escalate the level of care if:

- Symptoms worsening
- Medication non-adherence with risk
- Recurrent crisis calls
- Substance relapses with instability

8. Essential Safety Checks before Prescribing

Medication Type	Recommended Safety Screening
Antidepressants	Screen for bipolar disorder (history of mania/hypomania)
Stimulants	Screen for cardiac history; measure blood pressure and heart rate
Antipsychotics	Baseline metabolic assessment (weight/BMI, fasting glucose or HbA1c, lipid panel)
QT-prolonging psychotropics	Consider baseline ECG in patients with cardiac risk factors
Lithium	Baseline BMP (renal function) + TSH
Valproate	Liver function tests (LFTs) + platelet count
Teratogenic medications	Pregnancy test when clinically indicated
Clozapine	Absolute neutrophil count (ANC) monitoring before and during treatment; REMS enrollment/ANC reporting to the REMS program discontinued June 13, 2025, but ANC monitoring remains recommended per FDA prescribing information

Clinical note

Some monitoring requirements are FDA-mandated, while others reflect guideline-based or consensus recommendations. The Clozapine REMS program was previously an FDA-mandated monitoring requirement but was eliminated in June 13, 2025; ANC monitoring is no longer required for dispensing but remains recommended per FDA prescribing information.

REFERENCES

American Psychiatric Association. (2016). *The American Psychiatric Association practice guidelines for the psychiatric evaluation of adults* (3rd ed.). American Psychiatric Association Publishing.

American Psychiatric Association. (2022). *Diagnostic and statistical manual of mental disorders* (5th ed., text rev.; DSM-5-TR). American Psychiatric Association Publishing. https://doi.org/10.1176/appi.books.9780890425787

American Diabetes Association, American Psychiatric Association, American Association of Clinical Endocrinologists, & North American Association for the Study of Obesity. (2004). *Consensus development conference on antipsychotic drugs and obesity and diabetes. Diabetes Care, 27*(2), 596–601. https://doi.org/10.2337/diacare.27.2.596

Bush, K., Kivlahan, D. R., McDonell, M. B., Fihn, S. D., & Bradley, K. A. (1998). The AUDIT Alcohol Consumption Questions (AUDIT-C): An effective brief screening test for problem drinking. *Archives of Internal Medicine, 158*(16), 1789–1795. https://doi.org/10.1001/archinte.158.16.1789

Department of Veterans Affairs & Department of Defense. (2023). *VA/DoD clinical practice guideline for the management of major depressive disorder (2022 guideline version).* U.S. Department of Veterans Affairs and Department of Defense. https://www.healthquality.va.gov/guidelines/MH/mdd/

National Institute for Health and Care Excellence. (2022). *Depression in adults: treatment and management (NICE Guideline NG222).* https://www.nice.org.uk/guidance/ng222

Sigmon, S. C., & Dunn, K. E. (2010). Screening and assessment tools in substance use disorders. *Current Psychiatry Reports, 12*, 344–351.

The Joint Commission. (2023). National Patient Safety Goals® effective January 2023 for the behavioral health care and human services program. https://www.jointcommission.org/

III. MOOD DISORDERS

SECTION INTRODUCTION

Mood disorders represent some of the most prevalent, disabling, and clinically significant conditions encountered in outpatient psychiatric practice. These disorders affect emotional regulation, cognition, motivation, sleep, appetite, energy, interpersonal functioning, occupational performance, and overall quality of life. The spectrum of mood disorders includes unipolar depressive disorders, bipolar disorders, and related affective presentations that may vary substantially in severity, chronicity, functional impairment, and suicide risk. Boxed warning (class): antidepressants carry an FDA boxed warning for an increased risk of suicidal thoughts and behaviors in patients aged 24 years and younger; monitor all patients for clinical worsening and emergent suicidality, especially early in treatment and after dose changes.

Major depressive disorder (MDD) is among the leading causes of disability worldwide and is estimated to affect approximately 15–20% of individuals during their lifetime. Bipolar disorders, although less prevalent, affect approximately 1–3% of the population and are associated with disproportionately high rates of hospitalization, psychosocial impairment, occupational dysfunction, substance use comorbidity, and suicide risk. Mood disorders collectively account for a substantial proportion of psychiatric morbidity encountered in both outpatient and acute-care psychiatric settings.

Major depressive disorder remains strongly associated with impaired functioning, reduced quality of life, increased medical morbidity, and elevated healthcare utilization. Bipolar disorders frequently involve recurrent mood episodes, impulsivity, financial and interpersonal consequences, psychosis, and significant diagnostic delay. Many patients with bipolar disorder are initially misdiagnosed with unipolar depression, which may contribute to inappropriate antidepressant monotherapy, mood destabilization, mixed symptoms, rapid cycling, or delayed initiation of mood-stabilizing treatment. Accurate differentiation between unipolar and bipolar depression is therefore essential, particularly prior to initiating antidepressant therapy.

Suicide risk represents a major clinical concern across the mood disorder spectrum. Mood disorders account for a substantial proportion of completed suicides worldwide, particularly in the presence of mixed features, psychosis, substance use disorders, severe anxiety, impulsivity, hopelessness, or treatment resistance. Patients with bipolar disorder demonstrate particularly elevated lifetime suicide risk compared to the general population. Comprehensive suicide risk assessment, safety planning, and ongoing monitoring therefore remain core components of psychiatric evaluation and longitudinal treatment planning.

Mood disorders rarely occur in isolation. Anxiety disorders, trauma-related disorders, substance use disorders, ADHD, personality pathology, chronic pain syndromes, insomnia, and medical illnesses commonly coexist and may significantly influence both diagnostic formulation and treatment response. Comprehensive psychiatric evaluation should therefore include assessment of longitudinal mood patterns, family psychiatric history, prior treatment response, suicidality, substance use, psychosocial stressors, and medical contributors that may mimic or worsen affective symptoms.

The clinical course of mood disorders is often recurrent and episodic, requiring ongoing monitoring, longitudinal reassessment, and individualized treatment planning. While pharmacotherapy remains a central component of treatment, effective management frequently requires integration of psychotherapy, psychosocial interventions, lifestyle modification, sleep regulation, substance use management, and collaborative care approaches. Treatment selection should incorporate evidence-based guidelines while also considering patient-specific variables including symptom profile, prior response, tolerability, comorbidities, metabolic risk, reproductive considerations, adherence patterns, and patient preference.

Particular attention should be given to the assessment of suicide risk, mixed features, psychotic symptoms, functional impairment, and treatment resistance, as these factors may substantially alter prognosis and level-of-care determination. Clinicians should also remain vigilant regarding antidepressant-induced activation, medication adherence difficulties, substance-related mood destabilization, and the potential impact of medical or neurologic disorders on psychiatric presentation.

The following sections provide a structured, evidence-informed framework for the evaluation and treatment of depressive and bipolar spectrum disorders within outpatient psychiatric practice. Recommendations are intended to support safe, consistent, and clinically individualized care while recognizing that treatment decisions ultimately require professional judgment and ongoing reassessment over time.

1.1 MAJOR DEPRESSIVE DISORDER (MDD)

A. OVERVIEW

Aspect	Clinical Notes	Evidence Source
Definition	Major depressive disorder is characterized by persistent depressed mood or loss of interest with associated cognitive, behavioral, and somatic symptoms.	DSM-5-TR (APA, 2022)
Common Clinical features	Depressed mood, anhedonia, sleep disturbance, appetite or weight change, fatigue, impaired concentration, guilt or worthlessness, psychomotor changes, and suicidal ideation	DSM-5-TR (APA, 2022)
Clinical importance	High morbidity, suicide risk, and functional impairment; requires early identification and treatment.	NICE (2022); VA/DoD (2022)
Treatment approach	Combination of pharmacotherapy, psychotherapy, and psychosocial interventions based on severity.	NICE (2022); VA/DoD (2022)

B. Diagnostic Considerations

Clinical Consideration	Clinical Notes	Evidence Source
Screen for bipolar disorder	Rule out bipolar spectrum disorder before initiating antidepressants	CANMAT (2024); Yatham et al. (2018)
Assess suicide risk	Suicide risk assessment is recommended during the initial depression evaluation	VA/DoD (2022); The Joint Commission (2023)
Evaluate substance use	Assess for possible substance-induced mood disorder	DSM-5-TR (APA, 2022)
Consider medical contributors	Thyroid dysfunction, anemia, and vitamin deficiencies may mimic depression	NICE (2022)
Assess mixed features	Evaluate for racing thoughts, decreased need for sleep, increased energy, irritability, agitation, or impulsivity during depressive episodes	DSM-5-TR (APA, 2022); CANMAT (2024)
Consider medication-induced depression	Corticosteroids, isotretinoin, interferon, hormonal agents, sedative-hypnotics, and other medications may contribute to depressive symptoms	DSM-5-TR (APA, 2022); Clinical consensus

C. Pharmacotherapy

Generic	Brand	Class	Dose Range	Clinical Notes	Evidence Source
Sertraline	Zoloft	SSRI	50–200 mg/day	Favorable safety; widely used	CANMAT (2024)

Generic	Brand	Class	Dose Range	Clinical Notes	Evidence Source
Escitalopram	Lexapro	SSRI	10–20 mg/day	Excellent tolerability	CANMAT (2024)
Fluoxetine	Prozac	SSRI	20–80 mg/day	Long half-life; activating	CANMAT (2024)
Paroxetine	Paxil	SSRI	20–50 mg/day (max 50 mg/day for MDD)	Sedating; withdrawal risk; avoid in pregnancy	FDA labeling
Venlafaxine XR	Effexor XR	SNRI	75–225 mg/day	Monitor BP; withdrawal risk	CANMAT (2024)
Desvenlafaxine	Pristiq	SNRI	50 mg/day	Minimal CYP interactions; no added benefit above 50 mg/day	CANMAT (2024)
Duloxetine	Cymbalta	SNRI	30–120 mg/day	Also useful for pain syndromes	CANMAT (2024); Clinical consensus
Levomilnacipran	Fetzima	SNRI	40–120 mg/day	Noradrenergic; activating	CANMAT (2024)
Bupropion XL	Wellbutrin XL	NDRI	150–450 mg/day	Activating; lower risk of weight gain and sexual dysfunction; avoid in seizure or eating disorders. Usual target 300 mg/day; maximum 450 mg/day (seizure-risk ceiling)	CANMAT (2024); Clinical consensus
Mirtazapine	Remeron	NaSSA	15–45 mg/day	Sedating; weight gain	CANMAT (2024); Clinical consensus
Dextromethorphan-Bupropion	Auvelity	NMDA modulator	45 mg/105 mg: one tablet once daily ×3 days, then twice daily	FDA-approved for MDD; less long-term comparative data than older first-line agents	FDA (2022); second-line per CANMAT (2024)

Generic	Brand	Class	Dose Range	Clinical Notes	Evidence Source
Vortioxetine	Trintellix	Multimodal	5–20 mg/day	Low weight-gain liability; possible cognitive benefit; nausea. Recommended start 10 mg/day (5 mg if higher doses not tolerated)	CANMAT (2024)
Vilazodone	Viibryd	Multimodal	Start 10 mg/day; therapeutic range 20–40 mg/day	Take with food; GI effects	CANMAT (2024); Clinical consensus
Gepirone	Exxua	5-HT1A agonist	18.2–72.6 mg/day	Novel selective 5-HT1A agonist; titrate (18.2→36.3→54.5→72.6 mg) and take with food. Obtain baseline and periodic ECG; do not initiate if QTc >450 ms. Reduce dose 50% with moderate CYP3A4 inhibitors; contraindicated with strong CYP3A4 inhibitors; 14-day MAOI washout. Lower sexual-dysfunction and weight-gain burden; place less established than first-line agents	FDA (2023)

Clinical note

First-line antidepressants have broadly comparable efficacy, with modest differences in efficacy and acceptability between agents (Cipriani et al., 2018); selection should be individualized based on tolerability, comorbidities, and prior response.

D. Practical Treatment Selection

Clinical Scenario	Preferred Agent	Rationale	Clinical Notes	Evidence Source
First episode, mild–moderate	SSRI, SNRI, bupropion, mirtazapine, or vortioxetine selected by symptom profile and tolerability	Multiple second-generation antidepressants are guideline-supported first-line options	Start low, titrate; monitor GI effects, activation, sedation, weight, BP, and sexual dysfunction	VA/DoD (2022); CANMAT (2024); NICE (2022)
Fatigue / low energy prominent	Bupropion or vortioxetine	Bupropion may be useful when low energy or hypersomnia are prominent; vortioxetine may help cognitive symptoms in selected patients	Avoid bupropion in seizure disorders or eating disorders; monitor activation/anxiety. Seizure risk is dose-dependent—do not exceed 450 mg/day	CANMAT (2024); VA/DoD (2022); Clinical consensus
Insomnia prominent	Mirtazapine at bedtime	Sedating profile may help insomnia and appetite loss in selected patients with MDD	Weight gain, increased appetite, and daytime sedation	CANMAT (2024); Clinical consensus
Cognitive complaints	Vortioxetine	May benefit subjective and objective cognitive symptoms in some patients with MDD	Nausea may occur, usually early/transient	CANMAT (2024)
Comorbid anxiety symptoms in MDD	SSRI or SNRI; consider escitalopram or sertraline when tolerability is prioritized; consider vortioxetine when cognitive symptoms or SSRI/SNRI tolerability concerns are prominent	SSRIs/SNRIs are commonly used across depressive and anxiety disorders; vortioxetine may help anxious depression and cognitive symptoms in selected patients	Paroxetine less preferred due to withdrawal, sedation, anticholinergic burden, and pregnancy concerns	NICE (2022); VA/DoD (2022); CANMAT (2024); Clinical consensus
Comorbid panic disorder	SSRI or SNRI; consider sertraline or escitalopram when tolerability is prioritized	SSRIs/SNRIs have stronger guideline support for panic symptoms than vortioxetine	Avoid highly activating starts; titrate gradually; paroxetine less preferred when tolerability is a concern	NICE (2022); VA/DoD (2022); Clinical consensus
Comorbid chronic pain / fibromyalgia	Duloxetine	Dual efficacy for depression and selected pain syndromes	Monitor BP, liver risk factors, and tolerability	VA/DoD (2022); NICE (2022); FDA labeling

Clinical Scenario	Preferred Agent	Rationale	Clinical Notes	Evidence Source
Sexual dysfunction concern	Bupropion; consider vortioxetine when SSRI/SNRI sexual adverse effects are problematic	Lower sexual side-effect burden than many SSRIs/SNRIs	Bupropion may worsen anxiety/insomnia in some patients	CANMAT (2024); VA/DoD (2022); Clinical consensus

E. Accepted Adjunctive Strategies

E.1 FDA-Approved Adjunctive Agents for MDD

Base Treatment	Add-On Agent	Dose Range	Clinical Notes	Evidence Source
SSRI / SNRI	Aripiprazole	2–15 mg/day	Risk of Akathisia; relatively lower metabolic burden	FDA (2007); CANMAT (2024)
SSRI / SNRI	Quetiapine XR	150–300 mg/day	Sedating; metabolic monitoring required. Initiate 50 mg on days 1–2, then 150 mg	FDA (2009); CANMAT (2024)
SSRI / SNRI	Brexpiprazole	0.5–3 mg/day	Adjunctive option; may be associated with less akathisia in clinical use. Start 0.5–1 mg/day, target 2 mg/day, maximum 3 mg/day	FDA (2015); CANMAT (2024)
SSRI / SNRI	Lumateperone	42 mg/day	FDA-approved option for MDD (2025); place in routine treatment algorithms remains less established than older, longer-validated adjunctive strategies such as aripiprazole, quetiapine XR, or brexpiprazole	FDA labeling; Clinical consensus

E.2 Evidence-Based Combinations Strategies

Base Treatment	Add-On Agent	Dose Range	Clinical Notes	Evidence Source
SSRI	Bupropion	150–450 mg/day	May help fatigue and sexual dysfunction	CANMAT (2024)
SSRI	Mirtazapine	15–45 mg/day	Sometimes used in selected treatment-resistant cases; not a routine first augmentation choice	CANMAT (2024)
SNRI	Bupropion	150–450 mg/day	Monitor blood pressure	CANMAT (2024)

Base Treatment	Add-On Agent	Dose Range	Clinical Notes	Evidence Source
Any antidepressant	Lithium	Serum level ~0.5–0.8 mEq/L (≥0.5 for an adequate trial)	Evidence-based augmentation strategy	CANMAT (2024)
Any antidepressant	Trazodone	25–100 mg HS	Used as a symptom-targeted adjunct for insomnia (sub-antidepressant dose)	Clinical consensus

F. Treatment Adjustment: Switch vs Augment

The following table provides a structured framework for clinical decision-making following an inadequate response to initial antidepressant therapy.

Clinical Scenario	Preferred Strategy	Rationale	Clinical Notes	Evidence Source
No meaningful improvement after an adequate trial	Switch	Minimal or no response favors changing antidepressant	Confirm dose, duration, adherence, diagnosis, bipolar screening	VA/DoD (2022); NICE (2022); CANMAT (2024)
Partial response with good tolerability	Augment may be preferred	Preserves benefit while targeting residual symptoms	Options: bupropion or SGA depending on symptoms	VA/DoD (2022); CANMAT (2024)
Poor tolerability or adverse effects	Switch	Side effects limit adherence and benefit	Choose agent with better tolerability profile	NICE (2022); VA/DoD (2022)
Residual insomnia, fatigue, or sexual dysfunction	Augment may be preferred or switch	If mood improving → augment; if side effects → switch	Bupropion (for fatigue/sexual), mirtazapine (for insomnia)	CANMAT (2024); Clinical consensus
Prior good response to another antidepressant	Switch	Past response is strong predictor	Consider family history and patient preference	VA/DoD (2022); NICE (2022)
Severe or recurrent illness with partial response and need for faster symptom control	Augment may be preferred	Faster symptom control may be required	Consider suicidality, functional decline	VA/DoD (2022); NICE (2022)

Clinical Scenario	Preferred Strategy	Rationale	Clinical Notes	Evidence Source
Failure of first antidepressant	Switch or augment	Both valid depending on response/tolerability	Use shared decision-making	NICE (2022); VA/DoD (2022); Rush et al. (2006)
Multiple failures (treatment-resistant)	Augment may be preferred / specialist approach	Higher complexity requires escalation	Reassess diagnosis, consider psychotherapy/interventions	VA/DoD (2022); NICE (2022); CANMAT (2024); Rush et al. (2006)
Psychotic depression	Special pathway	Requires different treatment approach	Antidepressant + antipsychotic or ECT	NICE (2022)
Suspected bipolar / mixed features	Reevaluate (do not augment AD blindly)	Antidepressants may worsen condition	Avoid AD monotherapy	VA/DoD (2022); NICE (2022); CANMAT (2024)

G. MAOI Washout Guidance

From	To	Washout Period	Clinical Notes	Evidence Source
Most antidepressants	MAOI	14 days	Risk of serotonin syndrome; fluoxetine requires longer washout	FDA prescribing information; Clinical consensus
Fluoxetine	MAOI	5 weeks	Long half-life increases carryover interaction risk	FDA prescribing information
MAOI	Serotonergic agent	14 days	Risk of serotonin syndrome	FDA prescribing information

H. Avoid or Use with Caution in MDD

Combination / Practice	Clinical Notes	Evidence Source
Dual SSRI therapy	No established efficacy advantage; increased adverse effects	CANMAT (2024)
SSRI + MAOI	Life-threatening serotonin syndrome	FDA prescribing information; Clinical consensus
Antidepressant monotherapy in bipolar disorder	Risk of manic switch or mood destabilization	Yatham et al. (2018); Keramatian et al. (2023)
Benzodiazepine monotherapy	Does not treat core depression; dependence risk	Clinical consensus; NICE (2022); FDA labeling

1.2 MDD WITH MIXED FEATURES.

A. OVERVIEW

Aspect	Detail	Evidence Source
Definition	Major depressive episode with ≥3 concurrent manic/hypomanic symptoms without meeting full criteria for mania/hypomania	DSM-5-TR (APA, 2022)
Core features	Depressed mood plus ≥3 of: elevated/expansive mood, grandiosity, increased energy or goal-directed activity, decreased need for sleep, racing thoughts, more talkative/pressured speech, or increased risk-taking. DSM-5-TR excludes irritability, agitation, and distractibility from the counted symptoms	DSM-5-TR (APA, 2022); Yatham et al. (2018); Keramatian et al. (2023)
Clinical importance	Increased risk of antidepressant-induced mood destabilization; higher suicide risk; diagnostic overlap with bipolar spectrum	Keramatian et al. (2023); VA/DoD (2022)
Treatment approach	Avoid antidepressant monotherapy; consider mood stabilizers or SGAs. Evidence is limited and largely extrapolated from bipolar disorder treatment frameworks.	Limited evidence; extrapolated from bipolar disorder guidelines (Yatham et al., 2018; Keramatian et al., 2023; VA/DoD, 2023)

B. Pharmacologic Options

Generic	Dose	Line / Role	Clinical Notes	When to Prefer
SGAs — First-line (monotherapy, without antidepressant)				
Cariprazine	1.5–3 mg/day	First-line	Partial D3/D2 agonist; targets depressive energy without directly using an antidepressant. May be activating early in treatment. Evidence extrapolated from bipolar disorder	Classic mixed symptoms; preferred option
Lurasidone	20–120 mg/day	First-line	Favorable metabolic profile. Take with ≥350 kcal; absorption is critical. Evidence extrapolated from bipolar disorder	Prominent anxiety; metabolic concern

Generic	Dose	Line / Role	Clinical Notes	When to Prefer
Quetiapine	300 mg/day	First-line	Sedating; metabolic risk and daytime sedation should be considered. Evidence extrapolated from bipolar disorder	Predominant severe insomnia
Mood Stabilizer — First-line (monotherapy or adjunctive)				
Lithium	Serum level 0.6–1.0 mEq/L	First-line	Gold-standard anti-suicidal agent. Requires monitoring of serum levels, renal function, and thyroid function. Provides protection against mood switching if an antidepressant is added	High suicide risk; foundation if adding an antidepressant
Antidepressants — Only in combination with MS/SGA, never as monotherapy				
Sertraline + MS/SGA	50–200 mg/day	Second-line	Only if partial response to SGA/MS. Add only on top of an established stabilizing agent. If mixed symptoms are active, taper gradually	Persistent depression with mild or controlled mixed symptoms
Bupropion + MS/SGA	150–450 mg/day	Second-line	Lower switch risk than some other antidepressants. Always use with MS or SGA coverage	Depression with fatigue; lower activating-switch concern
Patient already taking an antidepressant				
Prior AD + add MS/SGA	Agent-specific	Adjustment	Mild/moderate mixed symptoms: maintain AD and add SGA or lithium. Monitor clinical course	Mild mixed symptoms at presentation
Discontinue AD + optimize MS/SGA	Gradual taper	Urgent adjustment	Severe mixed symptoms, agitation, or high suicide risk. Taper gradually to avoid discontinuation syndrome	AD may be amplifying mixed symptoms
Contraindicated				

Generic	Dose	Line / Role	Clinical Notes	When to Prefer
AD monotherapy	—	Avoid	Risk of inducing manic switch, rapid cycling, or worsening mixed symptoms. Contraindicated in MDD with mixed features	Never as the only intervention

Clinical note

Antidepressant monotherapy may worsen mixed symptoms, agitation, or mood instability. Most recommendations are extrapolated from bipolar disorder treatment frameworks due to limited direct evidence. Yatham et al. (2018); Keramatian et al. (2023); DSM-5-TR (APA, 2022); VA/DoD (2022–2023).

2. ATYPICAL DEPRESSION

A. OVERVIEW

Aspect	Detail	Evidence Source
Definition & core features	Depressive presentation characterized by mood reactivity plus ≥2 of the following: hypersomnia, hyperphagia/weight gain, leaden paralysis, and marked interpersonal rejection sensitivity	DSM-5-TR (APA, 2022)
Clinical importance	May be associated with chronicity, functional impairment, and differential treatment response; important to distinguish from melancholic features and bipolar spectrum presentations	DSM-5-TR (APA, 2022); NICE (2022)
Treatment approach	SSRIs remain common first-line options; bupropion may be useful when hypersomnia and fatigue predominate; MAOIs may have a role in selected treatment-resistant cases	CANMAT (2024); Clinical consensus

B. Diagnostic Considerations

Clinical Consideration	Clinical Notes	Evidence Source
Confirm mood reactivity	Mood improves transiently in response to positive events	DSM-5-TR (APA, 2022)
Assess atypical features	At least 2 of: hypersomnia, hyperphagia, leaden paralysis, rejection sensitivity	DSM-5-TR (APA, 2022)
Rule out bipolar spectrum	Atypical features may overlap with bipolar II depression	Yatham et al. (2018)
Differentiate from melancholic features	Melancholic depression lacks mood reactivity	DSM-5-TR (APA, 2022)

Clinical Consideration	Clinical Notes	Evidence Source
Evaluate chronicity	Associated with earlier onset and chronic course	CANMAT (2024); Clinical consensus

C. Pharmacologic Options

Generic	Brand	Dose Range	Clinical Notes	Evidence Source
Phenelzine	Nardil	15–90 mg/day	First-line in treatment-resistant atypical depression. Requires strict tyramine-restricted diet (avoid aged cheeses, cured meats, fermented foods, certain wines and beers). Risk of hypertensive crisis if dietary restrictions not followed.	Quitkin et al. (1988); CANMAT (2024); Clinical consensus
Bupropion	Wellbutrin	150–450 mg/day	Activating; may help hypersomnia/fatigue	CANMAT (2024); Clinical consensus
Sertraline	Zoloft	50–200 mg/day	Standard SSRI option; well tolerated	CANMAT (2024)

3. PERSISTENT DEPRESSIVE DISORDER (DYSTHYMIA)

A. OVERVIEW

Aspect	Detail	Evidence Source
Definition	Chronic depressive symptoms lasting ≥2 years (≥1 year in children and adolescents) with no symptom-free period >2 months	DSM-5-TR (APA, 2022)
Core features	Persistent low mood, low energy, poor concentration, low self-esteem, hopelessness	DSM-5-TR (APA, 2022)
Clinical importance	Chronic functional impairment; high comorbidity with MDD ("double depression")	NICE (2022); VA/DoD (2022)
Treatment approach	SSRIs or SNRIs plus psychotherapy (CBT or interpersonal therapy); often requires long-term treatment	NICE (2022); VA/DoD (2022)

B. Pharmacologic Options

Clinical Recommendation	Clinical Notes	Evidence Source
Same pharmacologic options as MDD	SSRIs are commonly used first-line	CANMAT (2024); Clinical consensus

Clinical note

Long-term treatment and combined psychotherapy are often recommended due to the chronic course of illness.

4. BIPOLAR DISORDER

4.1 BIPOLAR I DISORDER ACUTE MANIA

A. OVERVIEW

Aspect	Detail	Evidence Source
Definition	Distinct period of abnormally elevated, expansive, or irritable mood with increased energy/activity lasting ≥1 week (or any duration if hospitalization required)	DSM-5-TR (APA, 2022)
Core features	Decreased need for sleep, grandiosity, pressured speech, flight of ideas, impulsivity, increased goal-directed activity	DSM-5-TR (APA, 2022)
Clinical importance	High risk of hospitalization, psychosis, financial/legal consequences, and harm to self/others	VA/DoD (2022); Yatham et al. (2018)
Treatment approach	First-line: mood stabilizers (lithium, valproate) and/or SGAs; combination therapy often required in severe cases	Yatham et al. (2018); Keramatian et al. (2023); VA/DoD (2022)

B. Diagnostic Considerations

Clinical Consideration	Clinical Notes	Evidence Source
Rule out substance-induced mania	Evaluate stimulants, corticosteroids, intoxication/withdrawal states	DSM-5-TR (APA, 2022)
Assess for psychotic features	Hallucinations or delusions indicate severe mania	DSM-5-TR (APA, 2022)
Evaluate need for hospitalization	Required if severe impairment, danger, or inability to care for self	VA/DoD (2022)
Identify mixed features	Presence of depressive symptoms alters treatment strategy	Yatham et al. (2018); Keramatian et al. (2023)
Assess suicide and risk behaviors	Impulsivity increases risk of harm despite elevated mood	VA/DoD (2022)

C. Pharmacologic Options

Generic	Brand	Dose Range	Clinical Notes	Evidence Source
Lithium	Lithobid	Serum level 0.8–1.2 mEq/L	Anti-suicide benefit	Yatham et al. (2018); Keramatian et al. (2023)
Valproate / Divalproex	Depakote	Serum level 50–125 µg/mL	Particularly useful in mixed states	Yatham et al. (2018); Keramatian et al. (2023)
Quetiapine	Seroquel	300–800 mg/day	Sedating antipsychotic	Yatham et al. (2018); Keramatian et al. (2023)
Risperidone	Risperdal	1–6 mg/day	Rapid antimanic onset	Yatham et al. (2018); Keramatian et al. (2023)
Aripiprazole	Abilify	10–30 mg/day	Risk of akathisia	Yatham et al. (2018); Keramatian et al. (2023)
Asenapine	Saphris	5–10 mg SL BID	Sublingual formulation	Yatham et al. (2018); Keramatian et al. (2023)
Cariprazine	Vraylar	3–6 mg/day	Active metabolites have prolonged half-life; risk of akathisia	Yatham et al. (2018); Keramatian et al. (2023)
Paliperidone	Invega	3–12 mg/day	Once-daily dosing	Yatham et al. (2018); Keramatian et al. (2023)
Olanzapine	Zyprexa	5–20 mg/day	Highly effective; high metabolic risk burden	Yatham et al. (2018); Keramatian et al. (2023)
Ziprasidone	Geodon	80–160 mg/day	Take with food (≥500 kcal) for adequate absorption; lower metabolic risk vs. other SGAs	Yatham et al. (2018); Keramatian et al. (2023)
Carbamazepine	Tegretol	400–1600 mg/day	Useful antimanic option in selected patients; monitor drug interactions, hyponatremia, and hepatic effects. Boxed warning: serious skin reactions (SJS/TEN) linked to HLA-B*1502 (and HLA-A*3101) — screen at-risk ancestries before starting; teratogenic (use reproductive-safety precautions)	Yatham et al. (2018); Keramatian et al. (2023)

Generic	Brand	Dose Range	Clinical Notes	Evidence Source
Iloperidone	Fanapt	12–24 mg/day (12 mg BID target)	FDA-approved for acute manic or mixed episodes (bipolar I); slow 7-day titration to limit orthostatic hypotension; QTc caution; halve dose in CYP2D6 poor metabolizers or with strong CYP2D6/3A4 inhibitors	FDA labeling (2024)
Milsaperidone	Bysanti	24 mg/day (12 mg BID)	Active metabolite of iloperidone; FDA-approved for acute manic or mixed episodes (bipolar I); 5-day titration (orthostasis); QTc caution; reduce dose in CYP2D6 poor metabolizers or with strong CYP2D6/3A4 inhibitors	FDA labeling (2026)

Clinical note

Short-term benzodiazepine adjuncts (e.g., clonazepam, lorazepam) may be used for acute agitation and insomnia during manic episodes. Not recommended as monotherapy or for long-term management. Yatham et al. (2018); VA/DoD (2022).

4.2 BIPOLAR I DEPRESSION

A. OVERVIEW

Aspect	Detail	Evidence Source
Definition	Major depressive episode occurring in the context of bipolar I disorder	DSM-5-TR (APA, 2022)
Core features	Depressed mood, anhedonia, fatigue, cognitive impairment, sleep/appetite disturbance, suicidal ideation	DSM-5-TR (APA, 2022)
Clinical importance	Major contributor to disability and suicide risk in bipolar disorder; often more persistent than manic episodes	VA/DoD (2022); Yatham et al. (2018)

Aspect	Detail	Evidence Source
Treatment approach	First-line options include quetiapine, lithium, lurasidone or lamotrigine; avoid antidepressant monotherapy.	Yatham et al. (2018); Keramatian et al. (2023); VA/DoD (2022)

B. Diagnostic Considerations

Clinical Consideration	Clinical Notes	Evidence Source
Differentiate from MDD	History of mania is diagnostic; avoid misclassification	DSM-5-TR (APA, 2022)
Avoid antidepressant monotherapy	Risk of mood switching or mixed states	Yatham et al. (2018); VA/DoD (2022)
Assess suicide risk	Elevated during depressive phases	VA/DoD (2022)
Evaluate mixed features	May worsen with antidepressants	Keramatian et al. (2023)
Review prior treatment response	Guides medication selection	VA/DoD (2022)

C. Pharmacological First Line

Generic	Brand	Dose Range	Clinical Notes	Evidence Source
Quetiapine	Seroquel	300 mg/day	Strong evidence for bipolar depression; somnolence and weight gain common. Target ~300 mg/day; 600 mg/day adds no efficacy and worsens tolerability.	Yatham et al. (2018); Keramatian et al. (2023)
Lithium	Lithobid	Serum level 0.6–1.0 mEq/L	Mood stabilization; anti-suicide benefit.	Yatham et al. (2018); Keramatian et al. (2023)
Lamotrigine	Lamictal	100–200 mg/day	Preferred for maintenance and relapse prevention; limited acute utility. Slow titration: 25 mg/day ×2 wk → 50 mg ×2 wk → 100 mg → ~200 mg/day target; halve every step with valproate (≈doubles levels), higher doses with enzyme inducers (e.g., carbamazepine). Stop for any rash with mucosal/systemic involvement (Stevens-Johnson syndrome; risk highest in first 8 weeks). Discontinue at the FIRST sign of any rash unless it is clearly attributable to a non-drug cause; do not wait for mucosal or systemic involvement	Yatham et al. (2018); Keramatian et al. (2023)
Lurasidone	Latuda	20–120 mg/day	May be used as monotherapy or adjunct to lithium/divalproex. Take with food (≥350 kcal)	Yatham et al. (2018); Keramatian et al. (2023)

Generic	Brand	Dose Range	Clinical Notes	Evidence Source
Lumateperone	Caplyta	42 mg/day	FDA-approved for bipolar I depression (monotherapy or adjunct to lithium/valproate); favorable metabolic profile. 42 mg/day is the standard adult dose. Reduce to 21 mg/day with moderate CYP3A4 inhibitors or moderate-to-severe (Child-Pugh B/C) hepatic impairment, and to 10.5 mg/day with strong CYP3A4 inhibitors; avoid CYP3A4 inducers	FDA labeling; Keramatian et al. (2023)

D. Pharmacological Second Line

Treatment	Dose Range	Clinical Notes	Evidence Source
Olanzapine + Fluoxetine (Symbyax)	6/25–12/50 mg/day	Effective combination but associated with substantial metabolic burden	Yatham et al. (2018); Keramatian et al. (2023)
Cariprazine	1.5–3 mg/day	Supported in updated bipolar treatment frameworks	Yatham et al. (2018); Keramatian et al. (2023)
Divalproex / Valproate	Serum level 50–125 µg/mL	Limited evidence for acute bipolar depression; more established for mania and maintenance	Yatham et al. (2018); Keramatian et al. (2023)
Adjunctive SSRI	Dosing per SSRI used	Adjunctive antidepressants are generally not preferred in bipolar I depression and should generally not be used as monotherapy; consider only in carefully selected non-mixed cases	Yatham et al. (2018); Keramatian et al. (2023)
Adjunctive Bupropion	150–450 mg/day	Only recommended as adjunctive treatment and generally not as monotherapy, in carefully selected non-mixed bipolar I depression due to switch risk	Yatham et al. (2018); Keramatian et al. (2023)
ECT	—	Considered for severe, psychotic, suicidal, or treatment-refractory depression	Yatham et al. (2018); Keramatian et al. (2023)

4.3. BIPOLAR DISORDER – EPISODES WITH MIXED FEATURES

A. OVERVIEW

Aspect	Detail	Evidence Source
Definition	Presence of simultaneous manic/hypomanic and depressive symptoms meeting full criteria for one pole, with subthreshold symptoms of the opposite pole present during the same episode	DSM-5-TR (APA, 2022)
Core features	Mood lability, irritability, agitation, insomnia, racing thoughts with concurrent depressive symptoms	DSM-5-TR (APA, 2022); Keramatian et al. (2023)
Clinical importance	Increased risk of suicide, poor treatment response, and diagnostic complexity	Keramatian et al. (2023); VA/DoD (2022)
Treatment approach	Favor mood stabilizers and SGAs; avoid antidepressant monotherapy in mixed states.	Yatham et al. (2018); Keramatian et al. (2023); VA/DoD (2022)

Clinical note

Recommendations are largely extrapolated from bipolar mixed-state treatment frameworks.

B. Diagnostic Considerations

Clinical Consideration	Clinical Notes	Evidence Source
Identify concurrent mood symptoms	Simultaneous manic and depressive features required	DSM-5-TR (APA, 2022)
Differentiate from pure mania/depression	Mixed states require different treatment approach	Keramatian et al. (2023)
Assess suicide risk	Higher than in pure mood episodes	Keramatian et al. (2023); VA/DoD (2022)
Avoid antidepressant monotherapy	May worsen agitation and instability	Yatham et al. (2018); Keramatian et al. (2023)
Evaluate diagnostic overlap	Consider bipolar spectrum conditions	Keramatian et al. (2023)

C. Pharmacological Options

Generic	Brand	Dose Range	Clinical Notes	Evidence Source
— Mood Stabilizers —				
Lithium	Lithobid	Serum level 0.8–1.2 mEq/L	Anti-suicide benefit; first-line in mixed states	Yatham et al. (2018); Keramatian et al. (2023)
Valproate / Divalproex	Depakote	Serum level 50–125 µg/mL	Particularly useful in mixed presentations	Yatham et al. (2018); Keramatian et al. (2023)
Carbamazepine	Tegretol	400–1600 mg/day	May be useful in selected mixed presentations; monitor drug interactions, hyponatremia, and hepatic effects. Boxed warning: serious skin reactions (SJS/TEN) linked to HLA-B*1502 (and HLA-A*3101) — screen at-risk ancestries before starting; teratogenic (use reproductive-safety precautions)	Yatham et al. (2018); Clinical consensus
— SGAs —				
Quetiapine	Seroquel	300–800 mg/day	Sedating; useful when insomnia and agitation predominate	Yatham et al. (2018); Keramatian et al. (2023)
Lurasidone	Latuda	20–120 mg/day	Take with food (≥350 kcal); useful when depressive component predominates	Yatham et al. (2018); Keramatian et al. (2023)

Generic	Brand	Dose Range	Clinical Notes	Evidence Source
Lumateperone	Caplyta	42 mg/day	FDA-approved for bipolar I and II depression; useful when depressive component predominates. 42 mg/day is the standard adult dose. Reduce to 21 mg/day with moderate CYP3A4 inhibitors or moderate-to-severe (Child-Pugh B/C) hepatic impairment, and to 10.5 mg/day with strong CYP3A4 inhibitors; avoid CYP3A4 inducers	FDA labeling; Keramatian et al. (2023)
Asenapine	Saphris	5–10 mg SL BID	Sublingual formulation	Yatham et al. (2018); Keramatian et al. (2023)
Aripiprazole	Abilify	10–30 mg/day	Risk of akathisia	Yatham et al. (2018); Keramatian et al. (2023)
Cariprazine	Vraylar	1.5–6 mg/day	Lower end (1.5–3 mg) when depressive component predominates; risk of akathisia	Yatham et al. (2018); Keramatian et al. (2023)
Olanzapine	Zyprexa	5–20 mg/day	Effective in mixed states; high metabolic risk burden	Yatham et al. (2018); Keramatian et al. (2023)
Iloperidone	Fanapt	12–24 mg/day	FDA-approved for acute manic or mixed episodes (bipolar I); target 12 mg BID with slow 7-day titration to limit orthostatic hypotension; QTc caution; halve dose in CYP2D6 poor metabolizers or with strong CYP2D6/3A4 inhibitors	FDA labeling (2024)

Clinical note

Antidepressant monotherapy should be avoided in bipolar mixed states due to risk of mood destabilization and cycle acceleration. If used, only as adjunct under mood stabilizer or SGA coverage in carefully selected non-mixed predominant cases.

5. BIPOLAR II DISORDER

A. OVERVIEW

Aspect	Detail	Evidence Source
Definition	At least one hypomanic episode and one major depressive episode; no history of full mania	DSM-5-TR (APA, 2022)
Core features	Episodic depression with periods of hypomania (elevated mood, increased productivity, reduced need for sleep)	DSM-5-TR (APA, 2022)
Clinical importance	Frequently misdiagnosed as unipolar depression; high suicide risk driven by depressive burden	Yatham et al. (2018); Keramatian et al. (2023); VA/DoD (2022)
Treatment approach	First-line: quetiapine, lithium, lamotrigine; cautious use of antidepressants, generally with a mood stabilizer	Yatham et al. (2018); Keramatian et al. (2023); VA/DoD (2022)

Clinical note

Bipolar II disorder is characterized by recurrent depressive episodes and hypomania without full manic episodes. Treatment typically focuses on bipolar depression and long-term mood stabilization.

B. Diagnostic Considerations

Clinical Consideration	Clinical Notes	Evidence Source
Differentiate from MDD	Hypomania is often underreported; requires detailed longitudinal history	DSM-5-TR (APA, 2022)
Assess antidepressant-induced hypomania	May reveal underlying bipolar spectrum disorder	Yatham et al. (2018); Keramatian et al. (2023)
Evaluate mixed features	May increase risk of mood instability and poor response to antidepressants	Keramatian et al. (2023)
Assess suicide risk	High risk driven by recurrent depressive episodes	VA/DoD (2022)
Evaluate functional impairment	Hypomania may appear adaptive but still contributes to illness burden	DSM-5-TR (APA, 2022)

5.1 BIPOLAR II DEPRESSION

A. OVERVIEW

Aspect	Detail	Evidence Source
Definition	Major depressive episode occurring in bipolar II disorder (history of hypomania without full mania)	DSM-5-TR (APA, 2022)
Core features	Persistent depressive symptoms with episodic hypomania; often misdiagnosed as unipolar depression	DSM-5-TR (APA, 2022); Yatham et al. (2018)
Clinical importance	High burden of illness driven by recurrent depression; increased suicide risk	VA/DoD (2022); Keramatian et al. (2023)
Treatment approach	First-line: quetiapine; alternatives include lithium or lamotrigine; antidepressants only in selected non-mixed cases	Yatham et al. (2018); Keramatian et al. (2023); VA/DoD (2022)

B. Pharmacologic Options

Generic	Brand	Dose Range	Clinical Notes	Evidence Source
— First Line —				
Quetiapine	Seroquel	300 mg/day	Strong evidence for bipolar II depression; somnolence and weight gain common. Target ~300 mg/day; 600 mg/day adds no added efficacy	Yatham et al. (2018); Keramatian et al. (2023)
Lurasidone	Latuda	20–120 mg/day	May be used as monotherapy or adjunct to lithium/divalproex; take with food (≥350 kcal)	Yatham et al. (2018); Keramatian et al. (2023)

Generic	Brand	Dose Range	Clinical Notes	Evidence Source
Lumateperone	Caplyta	42 mg/day	FDA-approved for bipolar II depression (monotherapy or adjunct); favorable metabolic and EPS profile. 42 mg/day is the standard adult dose. Reduce to 21 mg/day with moderate CYP3A4 inhibitors or moderate-to-severe (Child-Pugh B/C) hepatic impairment, and to 10.5 mg/day with strong CYP3A4 inhibitors; avoid CYP3A4 inducers	FDA labeling; Keramatian et al. (2023)
Lithium	Lithobid	Serum level 0.6–1.0 mEq/L	Mood stabilization; anti-suicide benefit	Yatham et al. (2018); Keramatian et al. (2023)
— Second Line —				
Lamotrigine	Lamictal	100–200 mg/day	Useful for depressive polarity. Slow titration: 25 mg/day ×2 wk → 50 mg ×2 wk → 100 mg → ~200 mg/day target; halve every step with valproate (≈doubles levels), higher doses with enzyme inducers (e.g., carbamazepine). Stop for any rash, especially with mucosal/systemic involvement (Stevens-Johnson syndrome; risk highest in first 8 weeks). Discontinue at the FIRST sign of any rash unless it is clearly attributable to a non-drug cause; do not wait for mucosal or systemic involvement	Yatham et al. (2018); Keramatian et al. (2023)

Generic	Brand	Dose Range	Clinical Notes	Evidence Source
Cariprazine	Vraylar	1.5–3 mg/day	Off-label in bipolar II depression; FDA-approved for bipolar I depression (2019); risk of akathisia	Keramatian et al. (2023); Clinical consensus
— Adjunctive Only (non-mixed cases under mood stabilizer coverage) —				
Bupropion	Wellbutrin	150–450 mg/day	Lower switch risk vs. other antidepressants; never as monotherapy	Yatham et al. (2018); Keramatian et al. (2023)
Sertraline	Zoloft	50–200 mg/day	Limited evidence; use cautiously in non-mixed bipolar II depression; never as monotherapy	Yatham et al. (2018); Keramatian et al. (2023)
Venlafaxine XR	Effexor XR	75–225 mg/day	Higher switch risk vs. SSRIs; use only in carefully selected non-mixed cases; never as monotherapy	Yatham et al. (2018); Keramatian et al. (2023)

Clinical note

Antidepressant monotherapy should be avoided in bipolar II depression due to risk of mood destabilization and hypomania induction. When used, antidepressants must be combined with a mood stabilizer or SGA in carefully selected non-mixed cases. Yatham et al. (2018); Keramatian et al. (2023); VA/DoD (2022).

5.2 BIPOLAR II HYPOMANIA

A. OVERVIEW

Aspect	Detail	Evidence Source
Definition	Period of elevated or irritable mood with increased activity lasting ≥4 days without marked functional impairment or hospitalization	DSM-5-TR (APA, 2022)
Core features	Increased energy, decreased need for sleep, increased productivity, impulsivity, but less severe than mania	DSM-5-TR (APA, 2022)
Clinical importance	May be perceived as functional but contributes to illness burden and diagnostic delay	Yatham et al. (2018); Keramatian et al. (2023)
Treatment approach	Often does not require acute pharmacologic treatment unless symptoms are impairing; mood stabilizers or SGAs may be considered if symptoms escalate	Clinical consensus; Yatham et al. (2018)

B. Pharmacologic Options

Generic	Brand	Dose Range	Clinical Notes	Evidence Source
Lithium	Lithobid	Serum level 0.6–1.0 mEq/L	Mood stabilization; first-line option	Yatham et al. (2018); Keramatian et al. (2023)
Valproate / Divalproex	Depakote	Serum level 50–125 µg/mL	Useful if symptoms escalate	Yatham et al. (2018); Keramatian et al. (2023)
Quetiapine	Seroquel	50–300 mg/day	Lower doses often sufficient in milder hypomanic presentations; sedating	Yatham et al. (2018); Keramatian et al. (2023)
Aripiprazole	Abilify	10–30 mg/day	Lower metabolic burden; risk of akathisia	Yatham et al. (2018); Keramatian et al. (2023)
Cariprazine	Vraylar	1.5–3 mg/day	Off-label in bipolar II hypomania; extrapolated from bipolar I mania data; risk of akathisia	Keramatian et al. (2023); Clinical consensus

Clinical note

Many hypomanic episodes in bipolar II do not require acute pharmacologic intervention. Treatment should focus on sleep regulation, stress reduction, and close monitoring. Escalation to mood stabilizers or SGAs is indicated if symptoms worsen or impair functioning. Yatham et al. (2018); Clinical consensus.

6. CYCLOTHYMIC DISORDER (BIPOLAR SPECTRUM DISORDER)

A. OVERVIEW

Aspect	Detail	Evidence Source
Definition	≥2 years (≥1 year in children/adolescents) of fluctuating hypomanic and depressive symptoms, present at least half the time with no symptom-free period >2 months, not meeting full criteria for hypomanic or major depressive episodes	DSM-5-TR (APA, 2022)
Core features	Chronic mood instability with alternating subthreshold hypomanic and depressive symptoms	DSM-5-TR (APA, 2022)
Clinical importance	Risk of progression to bipolar I or II; chronic interpersonal and occupational impairment	Yatham et al. (2018); Keramatian et al. (2023)
Treatment approach	Mood stabilizers and psychotherapy; avoid antidepressant monotherapy due to mood destabilization risk	Yatham et al. (2018); Keramatian et al. (2023)

B. Diagnostic Considerations

Clinical Consideration	Clinical Notes	Evidence Source
Differentiate from bipolar I/II	Symptoms do not meet full criteria for hypomanic or depressive episodes	DSM-5-TR (APA, 2022)
Assess chronicity	Symptoms must be present ≥2 years (≥1 year in youth), at least half the time, with no symptom-free period >2 months	DSM-5-TR (APA, 2022)
Evaluate mood instability patterns	Frequent mood fluctuations are characteristic	DSM-5-TR (APA, 2022)
Rule out substance-induced symptoms	Substance use may mimic mood instability	DSM-5-TR (APA, 2022)
Assess progression risk	May evolve into bipolar I or II disorder	Yatham et al. (2018); Keramatian et al. (2023)

C. Pharmacologic Options (Limited Evidence)

Generic	Brand	Dose Range	Clinical Notes	Evidence Source
Lithium	Lithobid	Serum level 0.6–1.0 mEq/L	Mood stabilization; first-line option in bipolar spectrum disorders	Yatham et al. (2018); Keramatian et al. (2023)

Generic	Brand	Dose Range	Clinical Notes	Evidence Source
Lamotrigine	Lamictal	100–200 mg/day	May help depressive polarity. Slow titration: 25 mg/day ×2 wk → 50 mg ×2 wk → 100 mg → ~200 mg/day target; halve every step with valproate (≈doubles levels), higher doses with enzyme inducers (e.g., carbamazepine). Stop for any rash, especially with mucosal/systemic involvement (Stevens-Johnson syndrome; risk highest in first 8 weeks). Discontinue at the FIRST sign of any rash unless it is clearly attributable to a non-drug cause; do not wait for mucosal or systemic involvement	Yatham et al. (2018); Keramatian et al. (2023)
Valproate / Divalproex	Depakote	Serum level 50–125 µg/mL	Mood-stabilizing option; extrapolated from bipolar spectrum data	Yatham et al. (2018); Keramatian et al. (2023)
Oxcarbazepine	Trileptal	600–2400 mg/day	Selected-use option only; evidence is less established than for core bipolar agents	Limited evidence; Clinical consensus
Quetiapine	Seroquel	50–300 mg/day	Low doses may help mood stabilization and sleep; extrapolated from bipolar spectrum data	Yatham et al. (2018); Clinical consensus

Generic	Brand	Dose Range	Clinical Notes	Evidence Source
Topiramate	Topamax	Variable; not standard bipolar dosing framework	Not a core evidence-based mood stabilizer; not recommended for cyclothymia	Limited evidence; Clinical consensus

Clinical note

Pharmacologic evidence for cyclothymic disorder is limited and largely extrapolated from bipolar I and II treatment frameworks. Psychotherapy (CBT, interpersonal therapy) is a cornerstone of treatment. Antidepressant monotherapy should be avoided due to risk of mood destabilization. Yatham et al. (2018); Keramatian et al. (2023)

7. ADJUSTMENT DISORDER

A. OVERVIEW

Aspect	Detail	Evidence Source
Definition	Emotional or behavioral symptoms within 3 months of an identifiable stressor, not meeting criteria for another disorder, and not persisting >6 months after the stressor (or its consequences) resolves	DSM-5-TR (APA, 2022)
Core features	Low mood, anxiety, distress disproportionate to stressor, functional impairment	DSM-5-TR (APA, 2022)
Clinical importance	Must differentiate from MDD; typically time-limited; risk of progression if stressor persists	NICE (2022)
Treatment approach	Psychotherapy first-line; short-term pharmacotherapy if severe symptoms	NICE (2022); VA/DoD (2022)

Clinical note

Pharmacologic recommendations are symptom-targeted and extrapolated from depression/anxiety treatment guidelines; psychotherapy remains first-line.

B. Diagnostic Considerations

Clinical Consideration	Clinical Notes	Evidence Source
Differentiate from MDD	Symptoms must not meet full criteria for major depressive episode	DSM-5-TR (APA, 2022)
Identify precipitating stressor	Symptoms must occur within 3 months of identifiable stressor	DSM-5-TR (APA, 2022)

Clinical Consideration	Clinical Notes	Evidence Source
Assess proportionality of response	Distress must be disproportionate to stressor but contextually linked	DSM-5-TR (APA, 2022)
Evaluate functional impairment	Symptoms must cause clinically significant impairment	DSM-5-TR (APA, 2022)
Rule out normal stress response	Must exceed expected cultural or contextual reaction	DSM-5-TR (APA, 2022)

C. Symptom-Targeted Pharmacologic Options (If Needed)

Generic	Brand	Dose Range	Clinical Notes	Evidence Source
Sertraline	Zoloft	50–150 mg/day	May help depressive or anxiety symptoms in selected cases when medication is needed	Clinical consensus; extrapolated from NICE (2022)
Escitalopram	Lexapro	10–20 mg/day	Often well tolerated	Clinical consensus; extrapolated from NICE (2022)
Bupropion	Wellbutrin	150–300 mg/day	Useful when fatigue and low motivation predominate	Clinical consensus
Buspirone	Buspar	15–60 mg/day	For anxiety-predominant presentations; non-sedating, non-habit forming	Clinical consensus
Hydroxyzine	Vistaril	25–50 mg TID/PRN	Short-term anxiety and insomnia management; non-habit forming	Clinical consensus
Trazodone	Desyrel	25–100 mg HS	Used mainly for insomnia. Counsel about priapism: although rare, a sustained or painful erection lasting more than 4 hours is a urological emergency requiring immediate care	Clinical consensus; extrapolated from NICE (2022)

Clinical note

The primary treatment for adjustment disorder is psychotherapy and resolution or management of the precipitating stressor. Pharmacologic treatment is not routine and, when used, should be symptom-targeted and short-term.

8. PREMENSTRUAL DYSPHORIC DISORDER (PMDD)

A. OVERVIEW

Aspect	Detail	Evidence Source
Definition	≥5 symptoms in the final premenstrual (luteal) week, including ≥1 core mood symptom (affective lability, irritability/anger, depressed mood/hopelessness, or anxiety/tension), improving within days after menses onset; confirmed by ≥2 cycles of prospective daily ratings	DSM-5-TR (APA, 2022)
Core features	Mood lability, irritability, depression, anxiety, somatic symptoms (e.g., bloating, breast tenderness)	DSM-5-TR (APA, 2022)
Clinical importance	Significant functional impairment; strong hormonal component; often underdiagnosed	ACOG (2023)
Treatment approach	SSRIs (continuous or luteal dosing); hormonal therapy if needed	ACOG (2023)

B. Diagnostic Considerations

Clinical Consideration	Clinical Notes	Evidence Source
Confirm cyclic pattern	Symptoms occur during luteal phase and remit after menses	DSM-5-TR (APA, 2022); ACOG (2023)
Use prospective symptom tracking	Daily ratings over ≥2 cycles recommended for confirmation	ACOG (2023)
Differentiate from MDD/anxiety disorders	Symptoms must be temporally linked to menstrual cycle	DSM-5-TR (APA, 2022)
Assess functional impairment	Symptoms must significantly impact functioning	DSM-5-TR (APA, 2022)
Evaluate hormonal sensitivity	Symptoms related to hormonal fluctuations rather than baseline mood disorder	ACOG (2023)

C. Pharmacologic Options

Generic	Brand	Dose Range	Clinical Notes	Evidence Source
Sertraline	Zoloft	50–150 mg/day	Continuous or luteal-phase dosing	ACOG (2023)
Fluoxetine	Prozac	20–60 mg/day	Continuous or luteal-phase dosing	ACOG (2023)
Paroxetine CR	Paxil CR	12.5–25 mg/day	FDA-approved option for PMDD	FDA (2003); ACOG (2023)
Escitalopram	Lexapro	10–20 mg/day	Continuous or luteal-phase dosing; well tolerated	ACOG (2023)

Generic	Brand	Dose Range	Clinical Notes	Evidence Source
Venlafaxine XR	Effexor XR	75–150 mg/day	Useful when anxiety predominates; continuous or luteal-phase dosing	ACOG (2023)

Clinical note

SSRIs are the first-line pharmacologic treatment for PMDD. Symptom improvement may occur rapidly, allowing either continuous daily dosing or luteal-phase–only dosing. When SSRIs are ineffective or poorly tolerated, SNRIs such as venlafaxine are a reasonable alternative. Referral to gynecology should be considered for hormonal management in refractory cases.

9. PERIPARTUM DEPRESSION

A. OVERVIEW

Aspect	Detail	Evidence Source
Definition	Major depressive episode occurring during pregnancy or within 4 weeks postpartum (clinical window often extended)	DSM-5-TR (APA, 2022); ACOG (2023)
Core features	Depressed mood, anhedonia, fatigue, sleep disturbance, impaired bonding, guilt	DSM-5-TR (APA, 2022)
Clinical importance	Risk to mother and infant; requires careful medication risk–benefit evaluation	ACOG (2023)
Treatment approach	Psychotherapy ± SSRIs (e.g., sertraline preferred); consider zuranolone in severe cases	ACOG (2023); FDA (2023)

B. Diagnostic Considerations

Clinical Consideration	Clinical Notes	Evidence Source
Differentiate from postpartum blues	Symptoms persist >2 weeks and are more severe	DSM-5-TR (APA, 2022); ACOG (2023)
Assess maternal-infant bonding	Impairment may indicate severity	ACOG (2023)
Evaluate suicide risk	Includes passive thoughts and risk to infant	ACOG (2023); Clinical consensus
Review medication exposure	Consider risks/benefits of pharmacotherapy during pregnancy/lactation	ACOG (2023)
Screen for bipolar disorder	Important before initiating antidepressants	ACOG (2023); CANMAT (2023); Clinical consensus

C. Pharmacologic Options

Generic	Brand	Dose	Clinical Notes	Evidence Source
Sertraline	Zoloft	50–200 mg/day	Among the most commonly used SSRIs in pregnancy and lactation, with extensive clinical experience	ACOG (2023)
Escitalopram	Lexapro	10–20 mg/day	Often well tolerated; favorable side effect profile	ACOG (2023)
Fluoxetine	Prozac	20–60 mg/day	Effective option; long half-life may increase infant exposure during lactation — use with caution	ACOG (2023)
Nortriptyline	Pamelor	50–150 mg/day	Alternative if SSRIs not tolerated; monitor levels; limited use in current practice	ACOG (2023); Clinical consensus
Zuranolone	Zurzuvae	50 mg/day × 14 days	First oral medication specifically approved for postpartum depression; rapid onset; take in the evening with a fat-containing meal; carries a driving/CNS-impairment warning	FDA (2023)

Clinical note

SSRIs, particularly sertraline, are the first-line pharmacologic treatment for peripartum depression due to their favorable reproductive safety profile and extensive clinical experience. Zuranolone is the first oral agent specifically approved for postpartum depression in adults and may be considered in severe cases. It is not approved for major depressive disorder. All pharmacologic decisions require careful risk-benefit evaluation considering pregnancy and breastfeeding status. Psychotherapy remains a cornerstone of treatment

10. POSTPARTUM PSYCHOSIS (EMERGENCY)

A. OVERVIEW

Aspect	Detail	Evidence Source
Definition	Acute onset psychosis occurring in postpartum period, often within first 2 weeks	DSM-5-TR peripartum-onset specifier (APA, 2022)
Core features	Delusions, hallucinations, disorganized behavior, mood lability, confusion	DSM-5-TR (APA, 2022)
Clinical importance	Psychiatric emergency; high risk of suicide and infanticide	ACOG (2023)

Aspect	Detail	Evidence Source
Treatment approach	Immediate hospitalization; antipsychotics ± mood stabilizers; ECT if severe	ACOG (2023)

B. Diagnostic Considerations

Clinical Consideration	Clinical Notes	Evidence Source
Recognize rapid onset	Typically within first 2 weeks postpartum	DSM-5-TR (APA, 2022)
Assess for psychosis	Delusions, hallucinations, confusion	DSM-5-TR (APA, 2022)
Evaluate risk to infant	High risk of harm; requires immediate intervention	ACOG (2023)
Differentiate from severe depression	Presence of psychosis distinguishes condition	DSM-5-TR (APA, 2022)
Screen for bipolar disorder	Strong association with bipolar spectrum illness	Yatham et al. (2018); Keramatian et al. (2023)

C. Pharmacologic Options

Generic / Treatment	Brand	Dose Range	Clinical Notes	Evidence Source
Olanzapine	Zyprexa	5–20 mg/day	Commonly used for acute inpatient stabilization in postpartum psychosis	ACOG (2023)
Haloperidol	Haldol	2–20 mg/day	Commonly used for acute inpatient stabilization; monitor extrapyramidal symptoms (EPS)	ACOG (2023)
Quetiapine	Seroquel	100–800 mg/day	Useful when mood lability predominates; sedating	ACOG (2023); Clinical consensus
Risperidone	Risperdal	1–6 mg/day	Effective in acute psychosis; monitor EPS and prolactin	ACOG (2023); Clinical consensus
Lithium	Lithobid	Serum level 0.8–1.2 mEq/L	Effective mood stabilizer; requires careful monitoring due to maternal and neonatal risks; avoid during breastfeeding if possible	ACOG (2023)
Lorazepam	Ativan	Variable short-term dosing	Short-term adjunct for agitation and insomnia in postpartum psychosis	ACOG (2023)

Generic / Treatment	Brand	Dose Range	Clinical Notes	Evidence Source
ECT	—	—	Considered in severe, refractory, or life-threatening cases; highly effective in postpartum psychosis	ACOG (2023); Clinical consensus

Clinical note

Postpartum psychosis is a psychiatric emergency requiring immediate hospitalization. This table is intended as a reference for inpatient management and is outside the scope of routine outpatient psychiatric care. Risk to both mother and infant must be assessed immediately. All treatment decisions should be made in a supervised inpatient setting with close multidisciplinary collaboration.

Note: postpartum (puerperal) psychosis is not a distinct DSM-5-TR diagnosis; it is coded with the "with peripartum onset" specifier on a mood or psychotic disorder, most often bipolar I disorder.

REFERENCES

American College of Obstetricians and Gynecologists. (2023). Management of premenstrual disorders: ACOG Clinical Practice Guideline No. 7. *Obstetrics & Gynecology, 142*(6), 1516–1533.

American College of Obstetricians and Gynecologists. (2023). Treatment and management of mental health conditions during pregnancy and postpartum: ACOG Clinical Practice Guideline No. 5. *Obstetrics & Gynecology, 141*(6), 1262–1288. https://doi.org/10.1097/AOG.0000000000005202

American Psychiatric Association. (2022). *Diagnostic and statistical manual of mental disorders* (5th ed., text rev.; DSM-5-TR). American Psychiatric Publishing.

Keramatian, K., Chithra, N. K., & Yatham, L. N. (2023). The CANMAT and ISBD guidelines for the treatment of bipolar disorder: Summary and a 2023 update of evidence. *Focus, 21*(4), 344–353. https://doi.org/10.1176/appi.focus.20230009

Lam, R. W., Kennedy, S. H., Adams, C., et al. (2024). Canadian Network for Mood and Anxiety Treatments (CANMAT) 2023 clinical guidelines for the management of adults with major depressive disorder. *The Canadian Journal of Psychiatry*, 69(9), 641–687. https://doi.org/10.1177/07067437241245384

National Institute for Health and Care Excellence. (2022). *Depression in adults: Treatment and management (NICE Guideline NG222)*. NICE. https://www.nice.org.uk/guidance/ng222

Quitkin, F. M., Stewart, J. W., McGrath, P. J., et al. (1988). Phenelzine versus imipramine in the treatment of probable atypical depression: Defining syndrome boundaries of selective MAOI responders. *American Journal of Psychiatry, 145*(3), 306–311. https://doi.org/10.1176/ajp.145.3.306

Rush, A. J., Trivedi, M. H., Wisniewski, S. R., et al. (2006). Acute and longer-term outcomes in depressed outpatients requiring one or several treatment steps: A STAR*D report. *American Journal of Psychiatry, 163*(11), 1905–1917. https://doi.org/10.1176/ajp.2006.163.11.1905

The Joint Commission. (2023). *National Patient Safety Goals® effective January 2023 for the behavioral health care and human services program.* https://www.jointcommission.org/

U.S. Department of Veterans Affairs & U.S. Department of Defense. (2022). *VA/DoD clinical practice guideline for the management of major depressive disorder* (Version 4.0). https://www.healthquality.va.gov/guidelines/MH/mdd/

U.S. Food and Drug Administration. (2003). *Paxil CR (paroxetine hydrochloride) prescribing information.*

U.S. Food and Drug Administration. (2007). *Abilify (aripiprazole) prescribing information.*

U.S. Food and Drug Administration. (2009). *Seroquel XR (quetiapine fumarate) prescribing information.*

U.S. Food and Drug Administration. (2015). *Rexulti (brexpiprazole) prescribing information.*

U.S. Food and Drug Administration. (2017). *Prozac (fluoxetine hydrochloride) prescribing information.*

U.S. Food and Drug Administration. (2022). *Auvelity (dextromethorphan hydrobromide and bupropion hydrochloride) prescribing information.*

U.S. Food and Drug Administration. (2023). *Zurzuvae (zuranolone) prescribing information.*

U.S. Food and Drug Administration. (2023). *Exxua (gepirone hydrochloride extended-release tablets) prescribing information.*

U.S. Food and Drug Administration. (2019, updated 2025). Caplyta (lumateperone) prescribing information

Yatham, L. N., Kennedy, S. H., Parikh, S. V., et al. (2018). Canadian Network for Mood and Anxiety Treatments (CANMAT) and International Society for Bipolar Disorders (ISBD) 2018 guidelines for the management of patients with bipolar disorder. *Bipolar Disorders, 20*(2), 97–170. https://doi.org/10.1111/bdi.12609

IV. ANXIETY DISORDERS

SECTION INTRODUCTION

Anxiety disorders represent some of the most prevalent and clinically significant psychiatric conditions encountered in outpatient psychiatric practice. These disorders are associated with substantial functional impairment, reduced quality of life, increased healthcare utilization, occupational dysfunction, impaired interpersonal functioning, and significant psychosocial burden. Although anxiety disorders vary in presentation and severity, many share overlapping features including excessive fear, anticipatory anxiety, autonomic hyperarousal, avoidance behaviors, sleep disturbance, impaired concentration, emotional dysregulation, and chronic physiologic stress activation. Boxed warning (class): antidepressants carry an FDA boxed warning for an increased risk of suicidal thoughts and behaviors in patients aged 24 years and younger; monitor all patients for clinical worsening and emergent suicidality, especially early in treatment and after dose changes.

Anxiety disorders collectively affect a substantial proportion of the population across the lifespan, with lifetime prevalence estimates exceeding 25% in some epidemiologic studies. Generalized anxiety disorder (GAD), panic disorder, social anxiety disorder, agoraphobia, and specific phobias are among the most commonly encountered psychiatric conditions within primary care, emergency, and outpatient psychiatric settings. Many patients experience chronic or recurrent symptoms that significantly impair academic performance, occupational functioning, social interaction, medical stability, and overall quality of life.

The clinical presentation of anxiety disorders may vary considerably depending on symptom severity, psychosocial stressors, personality structure, developmental history, medical comorbidity, and coexisting psychiatric illness. Patients may present with excessive worry, panic attacks, somatic tension, autonomic symptoms, anticipatory fear, avoidance behaviors, irritability, insomnia, impaired concentration, fatigue, derealization, or progressive functional deterioration affecting work, relationships, and daily functioning. Because anxiety symptoms frequently overlap with medical, neurologic, endocrine, cardiac, respiratory, and substance-related conditions, careful diagnostic assessment remains essential prior to initiating treatment.

Comorbidity is extremely common across anxiety disorders. Major depressive disorder, bipolar disorder, obsessive-compulsive and related disorders, trauma-related disorders, ADHD, insomnia, chronic pain syndromes, personality pathology, and substance use disorders frequently coexist and may significantly complicate treatment response, prognosis, and medication selection. Inadequately treated anxiety disorders are associated with increased risk of depressive episodes, substance misuse, benzodiazepine dependence, chronic functional impairment, healthcare overutilization, and recurrent psychiatric instability.

Suicide risk should not be underestimated in patients with severe anxiety pathology, particularly when symptoms coexist with depression, hopelessness, panic symptoms, severe insomnia, impulsivity, chronic functional decline, or substance use disorders. Comprehensive psychiatric assessment should therefore include evaluation of suicide risk, substance use, psychosocial stressors, functional impairment, avoidance behaviors, sleep disturbance, and relevant medical contributors to psychiatric symptoms.

Although psychotherapy remains a foundational component of treatment, pharmacotherapy also plays a major role in the management of moderate-to-severe anxiety disorders. Selective serotonin reuptake inhibitors (SSRIs) and serotonin-norepinephrine reuptake inhibitors (SNRIs) remain first-line pharmacologic treatments across most anxiety disorders due to favorable efficacy and long-term safety profiles. Benzodiazepines, while potentially useful in selected short-term situations, require careful risk-benefit assessment because of tolerance, cognitive impairment, physiologic dependence, misuse potential, and withdrawal risk. Additional pharmacologic strategies may include buspirone, pregabalin, hydroxyzine, beta-blockers, and symptom-targeted adjunctive interventions depending on the specific anxiety presentation and comorbid clinical factors.

Treatment planning should remain individualized and longitudinal. Important clinical considerations include symptom severity, prior treatment response, comorbid psychiatric illness, substance use risk, sleep disturbance, occupational demands, medical comorbidity, psychosocial stressors, reproductive considerations, and patient preference. Clinicians should also monitor for medication-induced activation, adherence difficulties, avoidance reinforcement, functional decline, and the impact of chronic stress on long-term treatment outcomes.

The following sections provide a structured, evidence-informed framework for the evaluation and outpatient management of anxiety disorders commonly encountered in psychiatric practice. Recommendations are intended to support safe, consistent, and clinically individualized care while recognizing the importance of professional judgment, ongoing reassessment, collaborative treatment planning, and longitudinal therapeutic management.

1. GENERALIZED ANXIETY DISORDER (GAD)

A. OVERVIEW

Aspect	Detail	Evidence Source
Definition	Excessive anxiety and worry occurring more days than not for ≥6 months, difficult to control, associated with physical and cognitive symptoms	DSM-5-TR (APA, 2022)
Core features	Restlessness, fatigue, poor concentration, irritability, muscle tension, sleep disturbance	DSM-5-TR (APA, 2022)
Clinical importance	Chronic course with significant functional impairment; high comorbidity with MDD and other anxiety disorders	NICE (2011, updated 2020)
Treatment approach	First-line: SSRIs/SNRIs or CBT; combination recommended in moderate–severe or functionally impairing cases	NICE (2011, updated 2020)

B. Diagnostic Considerations

Clinical Consideration	Clinical Notes	Evidence Source
Rule out medical causes	Thyroid disease, arrhythmias, stimulant use, caffeine excess, and medication effects may mimic or worsen anxiety symptoms	DSM-5-TR (APA, 2022)
Screen for substance use	Alcohol, cannabis, stimulants, and sedative misuse may worsen anxiety or complicate treatment	NICE (2011, updated 2020)
Assess for comorbid depression	Major depressive disorder commonly co-occurs with GAD and may influence treatment planning	DSM-5-TR (APA, 2022)
Evaluate for panic disorder and social anxiety	Other anxiety disorders frequently co-occur and may alter pharmacologic and psychotherapeutic strategy	DSM-5-TR (APA, 2022)
DSM-5-TR diagnostic threshold	Excessive anxiety and worry more days than not for ≥6 months, difficult to control, with ≥3 of 6 associated symptoms (only 1 required in children) and clinically significant distress/impairment.	DSM-5-TR (APA, 2022)

C. First-Line Pharmacotherapy

Generic	Brand	Dose Range	Clinical Notes	Evidence Source
Sertraline	Zoloft	50–200 mg/day	First-choice SSRI per NICE due to cost-effectiveness	NICE (2011, updated 2020)
Escitalopram	Lexapro	10–20 mg/day	Well tolerated; minimal drug interactions	NICE (2011, updated 2020)
Paroxetine	Paxil	20–60 mg/day	More sedating; anticholinergic effects; discontinuation risk	NICE (2011, updated 2020)
Duloxetine	Cymbalta	30–120 mg/day	Also useful for neuropathic pain and fibromyalgia. In GAD, doses above 60 mg/day provide no clear added benefit; 60 mg/day is the usual target	NICE (2011, updated 2020)
Venlafaxine XR	Effexor XR	75–225 mg/day	May increase blood pressure at ≥150 mg/day; taper gradually to avoid discontinuation syndrome	NICE (2011, updated 2020)

Clinical note

First-line: sertraline preferred; alternative SSRIs or SNRIs if ineffective or not tolerated

D. Alternative / Off-Label Options

Generic	Brand	Dose Range	Clinical Notes	Evidence Source
Fluoxetine	Prozac	20–80 mg/day	Activating; long half-life	NICE (2011, updated 2020)
Mirtazapine	Remeron	15–45 mg/day	Sedating; useful with insomnia or poor appetite; risk of weight gain	Clinical consensus; limited supportive literature
Buspirone	Buspar	15–60 mg/day (given BID)	Non-sedating; no abuse potential; onset 2–4 weeks	Clinical consensus; limited evidence
Hydroxyzine	Vistaril	25–50 mg TID/PRN (up to 400 mg/day per FDA labeling)	Off-label; Non-habit forming; useful for acute anxiety; sedating — use with caution in older adults	FDA labeling; Clinical consensus
Pregabalin	Lyrica	150–600 mg/day	Consider if SSRIs/SNRIs are not tolerated or ineffective; not FDA-approved for GAD in U.S.; adjust for renal function	NICE (2011, updated 2020)

Generic	Brand	Dose Range	Clinical Notes	Evidence Source
Gabapentin	Neurontin	300–3600 mg/day	Off-label; limited evidence; selected treatment-resistant cases; monitor for sedation, dizziness, and misuse potential.	Limited evidence; Clinical consensus
Quetiapine XR	Seroquel XR	50–300 mg/day	Selected treatment-resistant cases; metabolic monitoring required	Limited evidence; Clinical consensus

Clinical note

Several medications used in GAD management may be considered off-label in the United States. Despite the absence of specific FDA approval, some agents are supported by guideline recommendations, clinical literature, or routine psychiatric practice when first-line treatments are ineffective or not tolerated.

E. Augmentation Strategies (After inadequate response to first-line SSRI/SNRI therapy)

Base Treatment	Add-On Agent	Dose Range	Clinical Notes	Evidence Source
SSRI/SNRI	Buspirone	15–60 mg/day	May be considered for persistent anxiety symptoms; modest efficacy	Clinical consensus; limited evidence
SSRI/SNRI	Pregabalin	150–600 mg/day	Evidence-supported option; adjust for renal function	NICE (2011, updated 2020)
SSRI/SNRI	Gabapentin	300–3600 mg/day	Off-label; limited evidence; monitor for sedation and dizziness; lower misuse risk than pregabalin	Limited evidence; Clinical consensus
SSRI/SNRI	Quetiapine XR	50–300 mg/day	Consider only in selected treatment-resistant cases after failure of first-line strategies; metabolic monitoring required.	Limited evidence; Clinical consensus

Clinical note

These agents are generally considered augmentation or second-/third-line options when first-line SSRI or SNRI therapy provides an inadequate response.

F. Short-Term Benzodiazepine Use (Adjunctive / Bridge Therapy)

Medication	Typical Dose Range	Clinical Notes	Evidence Source
Lorazepam	0.5–2 mg up to TID PRN	Intermediate half-life; commonly used for acute anxiety	Clinical consensus

Medication	Typical Dose Range	Clinical Notes	Evidence Source
Clonazepam	0.25–1 mg BID	Longer half-life; lower interdose rebound	Clinical consensus
Alprazolam	0.25–0.5 mg TID	Rapid onset and short half-life; associated with higher risk of rebound anxiety, physiologic dependence, and withdrawal symptoms.	Clinical consensus
All benzodiazepines (class)	Class-wide	Boxed warning (class): concomitant use with opioids may cause profound sedation, respiratory depression, coma, and death; benzodiazepines also carry risks of abuse, misuse, addiction, physical dependence, and withdrawal reactions. Use the lowest effective dose for the shortest duration and taper to discontinue.	FDA labeling (2020)

Clinical note

Benzodiazepines may be used transiently for symptomatic control while first-line treatments (SSRIs/SNRIs) begin to take effect. Guidelines recommend limiting use to short-term (generally ≤2–4 weeks) due to the risk of dependence, tolerance, and withdrawal syndrome.

G. Avoid or Use With Caution in GAD

Strategy	Clinical Notes	Evidence Source
Long-term benzodiazepine monotherapy	Dependence, cognitive impairment, falls; does not treat core disorder	NICE (2011, updated 2020); AGS Beers Criteria (2023)
Dual SSRI therapy	No added efficacy; increased adverse-effect burden	NICE (2011, updated 2020); Clinical consensus
Chronic antipsychotic use	Metabolic and neurologic adverse effects; reserve for refractory cases	Limited evidence; Clinical consensus

H. Practical Treatment Selection

Clinical Scenario	Preferred Treatment	Rationale	Avoid / Caution	Evidence Source
First-line uncomplicated GAD	SSRI (e.g., sertraline, escitalopram) or SNRI (duloxetine, venlafaxine XR)	Best evidence and tolerability across guidelines	—	NICE (2011, updated 2020)
Prominent somatic symptoms (pain, tension)	SNRI (duloxetine, venlafaxine XR)	Dual action on anxiety and pain	Monitor BP (venlafaxine)	NICE (2011, updated 2020)
Prominent insomnia	Consider mirtazapine or low-dose trazodone at bedtime in selected cases	Sedating properties may improve sleep	Weight gain (mirtazapine); next-day sedation	Clinical consensus

Clinical Scenario	Preferred Treatment	Rationale	Avoid / Caution	Evidence Source
Cognitive/rumination predominant	SSRI; consider buspirone in selected cases	Reduces excessive worry and rumination	Buspirone: delayed onset	Clinical consensus
Comorbid depression	SSRI or SNRI	Treats both conditions effectively	—	NICE (2011, updated 2020)
Substance use risk	SSRI preferred; consider buspirone	No abuse potential	Avoid benzodiazepines	NICE (2011, updated 2020); Clinical consensus
Partial response	Add buspirone, pregabalin, or switch SSRI ↔ SNRI	Augmentation or mechanism change	Monitor polypharmacy	NICE (2011, updated 2020); Clinical consensus
Severe acute anxiety (short-term)	Short-term benzodiazepine (≤2–4 weeks)	Rapid symptom relief	Dependence, withdrawal risk	NICE (2011, updated 2020); Clinical consensus
Treatment-resistant GAD	Pregabalin or quetiapine XR (selected cases)	Evidence-supported alternatives	Metabolic risk (SGA), misuse risk	NICE (2011, updated 2020); Limited evidence

2. PANIC DISORDER

A. OVERVIEW

Aspect	Detail	Evidence Source
Definition	Recurrent unexpected panic attacks with persistent concern about additional attacks or maladaptive behavioral changes	DSM-5-TR (APA, 2022)
Core features	Sudden episodes of intense fear with palpitations, dyspnea, chest pain, dizziness, fear of dying or losing control	DSM-5-TR (APA, 2022)
Clinical importance	High healthcare utilization; frequently misdiagnosed as cardiac or respiratory illness; often associated with agoraphobia	NICE (2011, updated 2020)
Treatment approach	First-line: SSRIs/SNRIs or CBT; combination often recommended in more severe cases; start low and titrate slowly to reduce activation	NICE (2011, updated 2020)

B. Diagnostic Considerations

Clinical Consideration	Clinical Notes	Evidence Source
Rule out cardiac causes	Palpitations, chest pain, and dyspnea may mimic cardiac disease (e.g., arrhythmias, ischemia)	DSM-5-TR (APA, 2022)

Clinical Consideration	Clinical Notes	Evidence Source
Assess for agoraphobia	Presence of agoraphobia influences severity, prognosis, and treatment planning	DSM-5-TR (APA, 2022)
Screen for substance use	Stimulants, caffeine, cannabis, and other substances may trigger or worsen panic symptoms	NICE (2011, updated 2020)
DSM 5 TR diagnostic threshold	Recurrent unexpected panic attacks plus ≥1 month of persistent concern about further attacks or maladaptive change in behavior related to them.	DSM-5-TR (APA, 2022)

C. First-Line Pharmacotherapy

Generic	Brand	Dose Range	Clinical Notes	Evidence Source
Sertraline	Zoloft	50–200 mg/day	Start low (12.5–25 mg) to reduce activation	NICE (2011, updated 2020)
Escitalopram	Lexapro	10–20 mg/day	Start low (5 mg) to reduce activation; well tolerated; minimal drug interactions	NICE (2011, updated 2020)
Fluoxetine	Prozac	20–80 mg/day	Long half-life; may be activating	NICE (2011, updated 2020)
Paroxetine	Paxil	20–60 mg/day	More sedating; higher discontinuation risk	NICE (2011, updated 2020)
Venlafaxine XR	Effexor XR	37.5–225 mg/day	Start low (37.5 mg/day XR); titrate gradually; monitor BP; taper to avoid discontinuation syndrome	NICE (2011, updated 2020)

Clinical note

Start low, go slow: initiate SSRIs at approximately half the usual starting dose (e.g., sertraline 12.5–25 mg/day, escitalopram 5 mg/day) to reduce early activation and improve tolerability. Patients with panic disorder are often highly sensitive to activating adverse effects during treatment initiation

D. Acute Symptom Relief (Short-Term Bridging)

Generic	Brand	Dose Range	Clinical Notes	Evidence Source
Clonazepam	Klonopin	0.25–1 mg BID	Longer half-life; lower rebound anxiety	Clinical consensus
Lorazepam	Ativan	0.5–2 mg up to TID PRN	Useful for acute panic episodes	Clinical consensus

Clinical note

Benzodiazepines should be limited to short-term bridging use (generally ≤2–4 weeks) because long-term treatment is associated with tolerance, physiologic dependence, withdrawal risk, cognitive impairment, and potential interference with exposure-based psychotherapeutic interventions.

E. Combination Strategies

Base Treatment	Add-On	Clinical Notes	Evidence Source
SSRI/SNRI	Short-term benzodiazepine	Bridge therapy during first 2–4 weeks	NICE (2011, updated 2020)
SSRI/SNRI	Cognitive Behavioral Therapy (CBT)	Combined therapy associated with best long-term outcomes	NICE (2011, updated 2020)
SSRI/SNRI	Short-term hypnotic	Consider if insomnia is prominent (e.g., trazodone, zolpidem short-term)	Clinical consensus; short-term symptomatic use only

F. Avoid or Use With Caution in Panic Disorder

Strategy	Clinical Notes	Evidence Source
Long-term benzodiazepine monotherapy	Dependence, tolerance, cognitive impairment; not recommended for chronic management	NICE (2011, updated 2020)
Dual serotonergic antidepressants	No added efficacy; increased adverse effects and risk of serotonin syndrome	NICE (2011, updated 2020); Clinical consensus
High-dose SSRI initiation	May worsen anxiety and panic early in treatment; start low and titrate gradually	NICE (2011, updated 2020)

G. Practical Treatment Selection

Clinical Scenario	Preferred Treatment	Rationale	Avoid / Caution	Evidence Source
First-line treatment	SSRI (sertraline, fluoxetine, paroxetine) or SNRI (venlafaxine XR)	Strong evidence base	Start low to avoid activation	NICE (2011, updated 2020)
Frequent panic attacks	SSRI/SNRI + short-term benzodiazepine	Provides short-term symptom stabilization while antidepressant response develops.	Limit BZD to ≤4 weeks	NICE (2011, updated 2020); Clinical consensus
High sensitivity to medications	Low-dose SSRI titration (start half-dose)	Improves tolerability	Avoid rapid titration	NICE (2011, updated 2020)
Prominent anticipatory anxiety	SSRI or SNRI	Reduces baseline anxiety	SNRIs may increase early anxiety	NICE (2011, updated 2020)
Comorbid depression	SSRI or SNRI	Treats both conditions	—	NICE (2011, updated 2020)
Partial response	Add CBT or switch SSRI ↔ SNRI	Combined therapy improves outcomes	—	NICE (2011, updated 2020)

Clinical Scenario	Preferred Treatment	Rationale	Avoid / Caution	Evidence Source
Treatment-resistant	Optimize CBT, switch class, or combination strategy	Addresses refractory symptoms	Avoid chronic benzodiazepine use	NICE (2011, updated 2020); Clinical consensus

3. SOCIAL ANXIETY DISORDER (SOCIAL PHOBIA)

A. OVERVIEW

Aspect	Detail	Evidence Source
Definition	Marked fear or anxiety about social situations involving possible scrutiny, leading to avoidance or intense distress ≥6 months	DSM-5-TR (APA, 2022)
Core features	Fear of embarrassment, avoidance of social/performance situations, anticipatory anxiety, physical symptoms (e.g., tremor, sweating)	DSM-5-TR (APA, 2022)
Clinical importance	Significant impact on occupational and academic functioning; often underdiagnosed; high comorbidity with depression	NICE (2013)
Treatment approach	First-line: SSRIs/SNRIs or CBT; combination recommended in severe cases; beta-blockers may be used for the performance-only subtype	NICE (2013); Clinical consensus

B. Diagnostic Considerations

Clinical Consideration	Clinical Notes	Evidence Source
Rule out medical causes	Hyperthyroidism, stimulant use, arrhythmias, or medication side effects may mimic anxiety symptoms	DSM-5-TR (APA, 2022)
Screen for substance use	Alcohol, cannabis, and sedative misuse are common due to self-medication	NICE (2013)
Assess for comorbid depression	Major depressive disorder commonly co-occurs with SAD	DSM-5-TR (APA, 2022)
Evaluate for other anxiety disorders	Panic disorder, GAD, and agoraphobia frequently co-occur	DSM-5-TR (APA, 2022)
Assess functional impairment	Evaluate impact on occupational, academic, and interpersonal functioning	DSM-5-TR (APA, 2022)
Distinguish from normal shyness	SAD involves persistent fear, avoidance, and clinically significant impairment ≥6 months	DSM-5-TR (APA, 2022)

Clinical Consideration	Clinical Notes	Evidence Source
Evaluate for performance-only subtype	Anxiety limited to performance situations; important for treatment selection	DSM-5-TR (APA, 2022)

C. First- and Second-Line Pharmacotherapy

Generic	Brand	Dose Range	Clinical Notes	Evidence Source
Sertraline	Zoloft	50–200 mg/day	Well tolerated; strong evidence	NICE (2013)
Escitalopram	Lexapro	10–20 mg/day	Well tolerated; minimal drug interactions	NICE (2013)
Venlafaxine XR	Effexor XR	75–225 mg/day	SNRI with strong evidence	NICE (2013)
Paroxetine	Paxil	20–60 mg/day	Effective but higher side-effect burden	NICE (2013)
Fluvoxamine	Luvox	100–300 mg/day	Alternative SSRI; off-label for SAD; consider when other SSRIs not tolerated or ineffective	NICE (2013)
Pregabalin	Lyrica	150–600 mg/day	Evidence in generalized SAD; consider after inadequate response to SSRIs/SNRIs; not FDA-approved for SAD; adjust for renal function	Clinical consensus

Clinical note

Sertraline and escitalopram are preferred first-line agents per NICE (2013). Venlafaxine XR is a second-line alternative when SSRIs are ineffective or not tolerated. Paroxetine is generally less preferred due to tolerability and discontinuation concerns. Fluvoxamine and pregabalin may be considered in selected cases after inadequate response to first-line agents.

D. Performance-Only / Social Anxiety

Generic	Brand	Dose Range	Clinical Notes	Evidence Source
Propranolol	Inderal	10–40 mg PRN	Use for performance-only situations; administer 30–60 minutes before performance; greater CNS penetration due to lipophilicity.	Clinical consensus
Atenolol	Tenormin	25–50 mg PRN	Use for performance-only situations; β1-selective with fewer CNS effects; alternative when propranolol is not tolerated.	Clinical consensus

Clinical note

Contraindications include uncontrolled asthma, bradycardia, heart block, and hypotension.

E. Combination Strategies

Base Treatment	Add-On	Dose Range	Clinical Notes	Evidence Source
SSRI/SNRI	CBT	—	Combined therapy associated with best outcomes	NICE (2013)
SSRI/SNRI	Propranolol	10–40 mg PRN	For residual performance anxiety only	Clinical consensus; NICE (2013)
SSRI/SNRI	Buspirone	15–60 mg/day	Very limited evidence; may help generalized anxiety component in selected cases	Limited evidence

F. Avoid or Use with Caution in Social Anxiety

Strategy	Clinical Notes	Evidence Source
Chronic benzodiazepine monotherapy	Dependence, cognitive impairment; may interfere with CBT	NICE (2013); AGS Beers Criteria (2023)
Beta-blockers in asthma or bradycardia	Risk of bronchospasm or bradycardia	Clinical consensus
High-dose SSRI initiation	May worsen anxiety initially; start low and titrate gradually	NICE (2013)

G. Practical Treatment Selection

Clinical Scenario	Preferred Treatment	Rationale	Avoid / Caution	Evidence Source
Generalized social anxiety	SSRI (sertraline) or SNRI (venlafaxine XR)	First-and second-line evidence-based options	Paroxetine: higher side-effect burden	NICE (2013)
Performance-only subtype	Propranolol PRN (10–40 mg)	Reduces autonomic symptoms during performance situations	Asthma, bradycardia, hypotension	Clinical consensus;
Comorbid depression	SSRI or SNRI (e.g., sertraline, venlafaxine XR)	May improve both anxiety and depressive symptoms	Monitor activation and tolerability	Clinical consensus; NICE (2013)
Severe avoidance / functional impairment	SSRI or SNRI + CBT	Combined treatment associated with best functional outcomes	—	NICE (2013)
Partial response	Add CBT or switch SSRI/SNRI	Augmentation or mechanism change may improve response	Avoid unnecessary polypharmacy	NICE (2013); Clinical consensus

Clinical Scenario	Preferred Treatment	Rationale	Avoid / Caution	Evidence Source
Treatment-resistant	Optimize CBT, switch SSRI ↔ SNRI, or consider selected off-label strategies	Alternative approach after inadequate first-line response	Limited evidence	NICE (2013); Clinical consensus

REFERENCES

American Geriatrics Society Beers Criteria® Update Expert Panel. (2023). American Geriatrics Society 2023 updated AGS Beers Criteria® for potentially inappropriate medication use in older adults. *Journal of the American Geriatrics Society*, *71*(7), 2052–2081. https://doi.org/10.1111/jgs.18372

American Psychiatric Association. (2022). *Diagnostic and statistical manual of mental disorders* (5th ed., text rev.; DSM-5-TR). American Psychiatric Publishing. https://doi.org/10.1176/appi.books.9780890425787

National Institute for Health and Care Excellence. (2011, updated 2020). *Generalized anxiety disorder and panic disorder in adults: Management (Clinical Guideline CG113).* https://www.nice.org.uk/guidance/cg113

National Institute for Health and Care Excellence. (2013). *Social anxiety disorder: Recognition, assessment and treatment (Clinical Guideline CG159).* https://www.nice.org.uk/guidance/cg159

V. TRAUMA- AND STRESSOR-RELATED DISORDERS

SECTION INTRODUCTION

Trauma-related disorders represent a major source of psychiatric morbidity across outpatient, emergency, primary care, and specialty mental health settings. Exposure to traumatic experiences—including interpersonal violence, childhood abuse, military combat, sexual assault, severe accidents, medical trauma, natural disasters, and sudden loss—may produce persistent alterations in emotional regulation, cognition, arousal, interpersonal functioning, stress reactivity, and neurobiological threat-processing systems. While many individuals demonstrate psychological recovery following trauma exposure, a substantial proportion develop clinically significant trauma-related symptoms associated with chronic distress, functional impairment, medical comorbidity, and elevated suicide risk. Boxed warning (class): antidepressants carry an FDA boxed warning for an increased risk of suicidal thoughts and behaviors in patients aged 24 years and younger; monitor all patients for clinical worsening and emergent suicidality, especially early in treatment and after dose changes.

Post-traumatic stress disorder (PTSD) is among the most extensively studied trauma-related conditions and is estimated to affect approximately 6–8% of individuals during their lifetime within the general U.S. population, with substantially higher prevalence observed among military veterans, survivors of interpersonal violence, first responders, refugees, and individuals exposed to repeated or prolonged trauma. Women are diagnosed with PTSD at significantly higher rates than men, partially related to differences in trauma exposure patterns, including higher rates of sexual violence and interpersonal trauma. Acute Stress Disorder (ASD), adjustment-related trauma reactions, and subthreshold post-traumatic syndromes are also commonly encountered in outpatient psychiatric practice and may significantly impair functioning even when full PTSD criteria are not met.

Trauma-related disorders rarely occur in isolation. Major depressive disorder, anxiety disorders, substance use disorders, chronic insomnia, dissociative symptoms, chronic pain syndromes, personality pathology, and medical illness frequently coexist and may complicate diagnostic formulation, treatment selection, and long-term prognosis. Patients with trauma-related disorders also demonstrate increased rates of suicidality, self-harm behaviors, emotional dysregulation, occupational impairment, relationship instability, and healthcare utilization compared to the general population. Sleep disturbance, hypervigilance, irritability, avoidance behaviors, emotional numbing, and physiologic hyperarousal commonly contribute to chronic functional decline and reduced quality of life.

The neurobiology of trauma-related disorders involves dysregulation across multiple interconnected systems, including fear conditioning pathways, stress hormone regulation, autonomic nervous system activation, emotional memory processing, and cortical-limbic circuitry. Functional neuroimaging and neurobiological research suggest abnormalities involving the amygdala, hippocampus, medial prefrontal cortex, hypothalamic-pituitary-adrenal (HPA) axis, and sympathetic nervous system activation. These alterations may contribute to persistent hyperarousal, exaggerated threat perception, intrusive recollections, impaired emotional regulation, dissociation, and maladaptive behavioral responses following trauma exposure.

Trauma-informed psychiatric care requires careful attention to safety, therapeutic alliance, emotional stabilization, and individualized pacing of treatment interventions. Pharmacotherapy may reduce symptom burden, improve sleep, decrease hyperarousal, and facilitate functional recovery; however, psychotherapy remains a central component of treatment for many trauma-related disorders. Evidence-based psychotherapeutic interventions—including trauma-focused cognitive behavioral therapy (TF-CBT), cognitive processing therapy (CPT), prolonged exposure therapy (PE), and eye movement desensitization and reprocessing (EMDR)—may substantially improve long-term outcomes when clinically appropriate and accessible.

Particular caution should be exercised regarding chronic benzodiazepine prescribing, polypharmacy, substance-related coping behaviors, dissociation, emotional dependency patterns, and coexisting personality pathology, as these factors may complicate treatment response and increase clinical risk. Clinicians should also remain attentive to medical contributors, ongoing trauma exposure, domestic violence, sleep disorders, chronic pain conditions, and social instability that may perpetuate symptom persistence or interfere with recovery.

The following sections provide a structured, evidence-informed framework for the evaluation and outpatient management of trauma-related disorders commonly encountered in psychiatric practice. Recommendations are intended to support safe, clinically individualized, trauma-informed care while recognizing that treatment decisions ultimately require ongoing reassessment, interdisciplinary collaboration, and individualized professional judgment.

1. POST-TRAUMATIC STRESS DISORDER (PTSD)

A. OVERVIEW

Aspect	Detail	Evidence Source
Definition	Disorder following exposure to trauma with symptoms in intrusion, avoidance, negative cognition/mood, and arousal domains lasting >1 month	DSM-5-TR (APA, 2022)
Core features	Flashbacks, nightmares, hypervigilance, avoidance, emotional numbing, negative cognitions	DSM-5-TR (APA, 2022)
Clinical importance	High risk of suicide, substance use disorders, and chronic disability; requires trauma-informed care	VA/DoD (2023); NICE (2018)
Treatment approach	First-line: trauma-focused psychotherapy; SSRIs (sertraline, paroxetine) as pharmacologic options. Only sertraline and paroxetine are FDA-approved for PTSD; venlafaxine and other agents are evidence-supported but used off-label.	VA/DoD (2023); NICE (2018)

B. Diagnostic Considerations

Clinical Consideration	Clinical Notes	Evidence Source
Assess trauma type and chronicity	Single vs. repeated trauma; recent vs. remote exposure	VA/DoD (2023)
Screen for dissociative symptoms	Depersonalization and derealization may indicate dissociative subtype	DSM-5-TR (APA, 2022)
Evaluate for comorbid MDD and SUD	Very common; influences treatment selection and prognosis	VA/DoD (2023)
Assess for nightmares and hypervigilance	Helps guide symptom-targeted interventions	VA/DoD (2023)
Assess suicide risk	PTSD is associated with increased suicide risk	VA/DoD (2023)

C. First-Line Pharmacotherapy

Generic	Brand	Dose Range	Clinical Notes	Evidence Source
Sertraline	Zoloft	50–200 mg/day	Most studied SSRI for PTSD	VA/DoD (2023); NICE (2018)
Paroxetine	Paxil	20–60 mg/day	Effective; higher side-effect burden	VA/DoD (2023); NICE (2018)

Generic	Brand	Dose Range	Clinical Notes	Evidence Source
Venlafaxine XR	Effexor XR	75–225 mg/day	SNRI with strong evidence for PTSD symptoms; monitor blood pressure (dose-related increases with venlafaxine) and for emergent suicidality; taper gradually to avoid discontinuation symptoms	VA/DoD (2023)

D. Evidence-Supported Off-Label Options

Generic	Brand	Dose Range	Clinical Notes	Evidence Source
Prazosin	Minipress	1–10 mg/day	May help trauma-related nightmares; start 1 mg HS and titrate; not recommended for routine overall PTSD treatment per VA/DoD (2023). Monitor blood pressure and orthostasis (first-dose hypotension); use caution with antihypertensives and avoid combination with PDE5 inhibitors because of additive hypotension	VA/DoD (2023)
Quetiapine	Seroquel	50–300 mg/day	Insufficient evidence per VA/DoD (2023); reserve only for selected refractory cases after failure of recommended agents; monitor metabolic effects	Limited evidence; Clinical consensus

Clinical note

VA/DoD (2023) recommends against prazosin for overall PTSD treatment but suggests it may be considered specifically for trauma-related nightmares.

E. Augmentation Strategies

Base Treatment	Add-On	Dose Range	Clinical Notes	Evidence Source
SSRI/SNRI	Prazosin	1–10 mg HS (individualized)	May help trauma-related nightmares; not recommended for routine overall PTSD treatment. Start 1 mg HS; titrate gradually based on nightmare response and tolerability. Typical outpatient range 1–10 mg HS; higher individualized total daily doses may be used with careful BP/orthostasis monitoring	VA/DoD (2023)
SSRI/SNRI	Quetiapine	50–300 mg/day	Limited evidence; reserve for selected refractory cases; monitor metabolic effects	VA/DoD (2023)
SSRI/SNRI	Risperidone	0.5–4 mg/day	Not recommended for routine augmentation due to negative trial evidence	VA/DoD (2023)

F. Avoid or Use With Caution in PTSD

Strategy	Clinical Notes	Evidence Source
Benzodiazepines	Discouraged; may interfere with fear extinction and trauma processing	VA/DoD (2023); NICE (2018)
Antipsychotic polypharmacy	No evidence of benefit; increased metabolic risk	VA/DoD (2023)
High-dose antipsychotics	Limited evidence; increased metabolic and neurologic adverse effects	VA/DoD (2023)
Risperidone	Not recommended for routine PTSD augmentation due to negative randomized trial evidence	VA/DoD (2023)

G. Practical Treatment Selection

Clinical Scenario	Preferred Treatment	Rationale	Avoid / Caution	Evidence Source
Core PTSD symptoms	SSRI (sertraline, paroxetine, venlafaxine) ± trauma-focused psychotherapy	Strongest evidence-based treatment approach	—	VA/DoD (2023); NICE (2018)
Persistent nightmares (refractory)	Consider prazosin in selected cases	May reduce trauma-related nightmares in some patients	Orthostatic hypotension	VA/DoD (2023)
Hyperarousal/insomnia	SSRI as core treatment; consider symptom-targeted sleep adjuncts	May address residual insomnia or hyperarousal	Metabolic risk with SGAs	VA/DoD (2023); Clinical consensus
Comorbid depression	SSRI or SNRI	May improve both PTSD and depressive symptoms	—	VA/DoD (2023)
Severe acute agitation / crisis symptoms	Symptom-specific stabilization	Prioritize safety, differential diagnosis, and level of care	Avoid routine benzodiazepine use	VA/DoD (2023); Clinical consensus
Partial response	Add prazosin or optimize psychotherapy	Symptom-targeted augmentation strategy	Limited evidence	VA/DoD (2023)

Clinical Scenario	Preferred Treatment	Rationale	Avoid / Caution	Evidence Source
Treatment-resistant	Switch SSRI ↔ SNRI or consider adjunct (SGA in select cases)	Alternative mechanism after inadequate response	Use cautiously	VA/DoD (2023); Limited evidence

2. ACUTE STRESS DISORDER

A. OVERVIEW

Aspect	Detail	Evidence Source
Definition	Trauma-related disorder occurring 3 days to 1 month after exposure, with ≥9 symptoms across defined domains	DSM-5-TR (APA, 2022)
Core features	Intrusion, dissociation, avoidance, negative mood, arousal following acute trauma	DSM-5-TR (APA, 2022)
Clinical importance	May resolve spontaneously or progress to PTSD; early identification improves outcomes	VA/DoD (2023); NICE (2018)
Treatment approach	First-line: trauma-focused psychotherapy; medications only for severe or persistent symptoms	VA/DoD (2023); NICE (2018)

B. Diagnostic Considerations

Clinical Consideration	Clinical Notes	Evidence Source
Confirm exposure to a traumatic event	Exposure to actual or threatened death, serious injury, or sexual violence (direct, witnessed, or indirect)	DSM-5-TR (APA, 2022)
Assess symptom timing	Symptoms must occur between 3 days and 1 month post-trauma; persistence beyond 1 month suggests PTSD	DSM-5-TR (APA, 2022)
Evaluate core symptom clusters	≥9 symptoms across intrusion, negative mood, dissociation, avoidance, and arousal domains	DSM-5-TR (APA, 2022)
Screen for dissociative symptoms	Depersonalization and derealization are common in acute trauma response	DSM-5-TR (APA, 2022)
Assess functional impairment	Symptoms must cause clinically significant distress or impairment	DSM-5-TR (APA, 2022)
Rule out substance or medical causes	Intoxication, withdrawal, TBI, or medical conditions may mimic ASD	DSM-5-TR (APA, 2022)

Clinical Consideration	Clinical Notes	Evidence Source
Evaluate suicide risk	Acute trauma exposure may increase suicidal ideation or impulsivity	VA/DoD (2023)
Monitor progression toward PTSD	A proportion of ASD cases progress to PTSD; close follow-up recommended	VA/DoD (2023); NICE (2018)

C. Treatment Approach

Aspect	Detail	Evidence Source
First-line treatment	Trauma-focused psychotherapy (CBT) is the primary intervention for acute stress disorder	VA/DoD (2023); NICE (2018)
Role of pharmacotherapy	Medications are not first-line; reserved for severe or persistent symptoms	VA/DoD (2023); NICE (2018)
Indications for medication	Consider short-term pharmacologic support for severe insomnia, hyperarousal, or marked impairment	VA/DoD (2023)
Treatment goal	Stabilize symptoms and reduce progression to PTSD	VA/DoD (2023); NICE (2018)
Duration of treatment	Use medications short-term with frequent reassessment	VA/DoD (2023)
Follow-up	Close monitoring is required due to risk of progression to PTSD	VA/DoD (2023); NICE (2018)

D. Symptom-Targeted Pharmacologic Support (Limited Evidence)

Generic	Brand	Dose Range	Clinical Notes	Evidence Source
Sertraline	Zoloft	50–150 mg/day	Not first-line; consider if symptoms persist or evolve toward PTSD	Limited evidence; VA/DoD (2023); Clinical consensus
Escitalopram	Lexapro	10–20 mg/day	May be considered in select cases with persistent distress	Limited evidence; VA/DoD (2023); Clinical consensus
Trazodone	Desyrel	25–100 mg HS	Symptom-targeted adjunct for insomnia; not disease-modifying	Clinical consensus; VA/DoD (2023)

E. Combination Strategies

Base Treatment	Add-On	Dose Range	Clinical Notes	Evidence Source
CBT	SSRI/SNRI	Per above	May be considered in persistent cases; evidence remains limited	Limited evidence; VA/DoD (2023)

Base Treatment	Add-On	Dose Range	Clinical Notes	Evidence Source
CBT	Short-term benzodiazepine	Clonazepam 0.25–1 mg BID; Lorazepam 0.5–2 mg PRN	Not routinely recommended; reserve only for exceptional short-term crisis situations.	Clinical consensus; VA/DoD (2023)

F. Avoid or Use with Caution in Acute Stress Disorder

Strategy	Clinical Notes	Evidence Source
Routine benzodiazepine use	Strongly discouraged; may worsen outcomes and does not prevent PTSD	VA/DoD (2023)
Escalation into chronic polypharmacy	No proven benefit; increased dependence and adverse-effect risk	Clinical consensus
Antipsychotic initiation	Avoid unless severe agitation or psychosis is present	Clinical consensus

G. Practical Treatment Selection

Clinical Scenario	Preferred Treatment	Rationale	Avoid / Caution	Evidence Source
Mild symptoms	Trauma-focused CBT alone	High spontaneous recovery rate	Avoid unnecessary medication	VA/DoD (2023); NICE (2018)
Severe insomnia	Short-term trazodone	May improve sleep	Avoid long-term use	Clinical consensus; VA/DoD (2023)
Severe anxiety/hyperarousal	Psychotherapy first; consider limited symptom-targeted medication support	Symptom stabilization when necessary	Avoid prolonged benzodiazepine use	Limited evidence; VA/DoD (2023); Clinical consensus
Functional impairment	Short-term symptom-targeted support + CBT	Supports stabilization and recovery	—	VA/DoD (2023); Clinical consensus
Persistent symptoms	Transition to PTSD treatment framework	Early intervention may reduce progression	—	VA/DoD (2023); NICE (2018)

REFERENCES

American Psychiatric Association. (2022). Diagnostic and statistical manual of mental disorders (5th ed., text rev.; DSM-5-TR). American Psychiatric Publishing. https://doi.org/10.1176/appi.books.9780890425787

National Institute for Health and Care Excellence. (2018). Post-traumatic stress disorder (NICE Guideline NG116). https://www.nice.org.uk/guidance/ng116

U.S. Department of Veterans Affairs & U.S. Department of Defense. (2023). VA/DoD clinical practice guideline for the management of posttraumatic stress disorder and acute stress disorder. https://www.healthquality.va.gov/guidelines/MH/ptsd/

VI. OBSESSIVE-COMPULSIVE AND RELATED DISORDERS

SECTION INTRODUCTION

Obsessive-compulsive and related disorders (OCRDs) comprise a group of psychiatric conditions characterized by intrusive thoughts, repetitive behaviors, compulsive rituals, preoccupations, or body-focused repetitive behaviors that cause clinically significant distress, functional impairment, or both. These disorders often involve maladaptive attempts to reduce anxiety, internal tension, distress, perceived incompleteness, or obsessive preoccupation through repetitive mental or behavioral acts that become difficult to control over time. Boxed warning (class): antidepressants carry an FDA boxed warning for an increased risk of suicidal thoughts and behaviors in patients aged 24 years and younger; monitor all patients for clinical worsening and emergent suicidality, especially early in treatment and after dose changes.

Obsessive-compulsive disorder (OCD) is among the most disabling psychiatric disorders and is associated with substantial occupational, academic, interpersonal, and psychosocial impairment when untreated. Lifetime prevalence estimates for OCD are approximately 2–3%, although subclinical obsessive-compulsive symptoms are considerably more common in the general population. Related disorders—including body dysmorphic disorder (BDD), hoarding disorder, trichotillomania, and excoriation (skin-picking) disorder—share overlapping features involving repetitive behaviors, compulsivity, impaired insight, and chronic functional impairment.

Patients with OCRDs frequently experience significant shame, secrecy, embarrassment, and delayed treatment-seeking behavior. As a result, symptoms may remain unrecognized for years before psychiatric evaluation occurs. Many individuals develop highly time-consuming rituals, avoidance behaviors, reassurance-seeking patterns, or repetitive behaviors that progressively interfere with work performance, academic functioning, relationships, self-care, and overall quality of life. Poor insight may further complicate diagnosis and treatment adherence in selected patients.

Obsessions commonly involve intrusive and unwanted thoughts, images, or urges related to contamination, harm, sexuality, religion, morality, symmetry, health concerns, or fear of losing control. Compulsions may include washing, checking, counting, ordering, reassurance seeking, mental rituals, or repetitive behaviors intended to reduce anxiety or prevent feared outcomes. In body-focused repetitive behavior disorders, repetitive hair pulling or skin picking may serve as tension-reducing or self-soothing behaviors despite resulting tissue damage, cosmetic consequences, or emotional distress.

Comorbidity is highly prevalent across obsessive-compulsive and related disorders. Major depressive disorder, anxiety disorders, tic disorders, ADHD, autism spectrum disorder, trauma-related disorders, eating disorders, and substance use disorders frequently coexist and may substantially influence prognosis and treatment selection. Suicide risk should also be carefully assessed, particularly in patients with severe OCD, body dysmorphic disorder, major depressive episodes, hopelessness, or marked psychosocial impairment. Body dysmorphic disorder, in particular, is associated with elevated rates of suicidal ideation, suicide attempts, and severe functional deterioration.

Evidence-based treatment typically involves a combination of psychotherapy and pharmacotherapy. Exposure and response prevention (ERP)-based cognitive behavioral therapy remains a foundational treatment for OCD and several related disorders. Selective serotonin reuptake inhibitors (SSRIs), often at higher therapeutic doses than those used for depressive disorders, remain first-line pharmacologic options for OCD. In treatment-resistant cases, augmentation strategies—including second-generation antipsychotics—may be considered when clinically appropriate. Treatment response is often gradual, requiring longer medication trials, longitudinal monitoring, and careful attention to adherence and tolerability.

Because obsessive-compulsive and related disorders are frequently chronic and fluctuating over time, clinicians should emphasize long-term treatment planning, psychoeducation, relapse prevention, and functional recovery. Careful assessment of insight, avoidance patterns, family accommodation behaviors, comorbid psychiatric illness, and medical or dermatologic complications remains essential during evaluation and ongoing treatment.

The following sections provide a structured, evidence-informed framework for the evaluation and treatment of obsessive-compulsive and related disorders within outpatient psychiatric practice. Recommendations are intended to support safe, individualized, and clinically consistent care while recognizing the importance of professional judgment, longitudinal reassessment, and patient-centered treatment planning.

1. OBSESSIVE-COMPULSIVE DISORDER (OCD)

A. OVERVIEW

Aspect	Detail	Evidence Source
Definition	Presence of obsessions, compulsions, or both causing distress or functional impairment	DSM-5-TR (APA, 2022)
Core features	Intrusive thoughts, urges, or images with repetitive behaviors or mental rituals aimed at reducing distress	DSM-5-TR (APA, 2022)
Clinical importance	Chronic and disabling condition with high comorbidity and elevated suicide risk	Fineberg et al. (2020)
Treatment approach	First-line: SSRI or ERP-based CBT; higher SSRI doses often required; combination is commonly used in moderate–severe cases	Fineberg et al. (2020)

B. Diagnostic Considerations

Clinical Consideration	Clinical Notes	Evidence Source
Assess insight	Insight level influences prognosis and need for augmentation strategies	DSM-5-TR (APA, 2022)
Rule out tic disorder	Comorbid tic disorders may predict better response to antipsychotic augmentation	Fineberg et al. (2020)
Screen for related disorders	Hoarding disorder and body dysmorphic disorder frequently co-occur	DSM-5-TR (APA, 2022)
Assess severity	Y-BOCS is the gold standard for severity assessment and monitoring	Goodman et al. (1989)
Assess functional impairment	Evaluate impact on social, occupational, and daily functioning	DSM-5-TR (APA, 2022)
Evaluate suicide risk	Increased suicide risk, especially with comorbid depression	Fineberg et al. (2020)
DSM-5-TR diagnostic threshold	Obsessions and/or compulsions that are time-consuming (>1 hr/day) or cause clinically significant distress/impairment; specify insight (good/fair, poor, or absent/delusional) and tic-related when applicable.	DSM-5-TR (APA, 2022)

C. First Line Pharmacotherapy

Generic	Brand	Dose Range	Clinical Notes	Evidence Source
Fluoxetine	Prozac	20–80 mg/day	Activating profile; higher doses often needed for OCD	Fineberg et al. (2020)
Fluvoxamine	Luvox	100–300 mg/day	Sedating profile; significant CYP interactions	Fineberg et al. (2020)
Paroxetine	Paxil	20–60 mg/day	Sedating; anticholinergic burden and discontinuation risk	Fineberg et al. (2020)
Sertraline	Zoloft	50–200 mg/day	Well tolerated; commonly used first-line SSRI	Fineberg et al. (2020)
Clomipramine	Anafranil	25–250 mg/day; consider plasma level monitoring	Highly effective; higher cardiac, anticholinergic, and seizure risk	Fineberg et al. (2020)

Clinical note

OCD requires higher SSRI doses and longer treatment trials (8–12 weeks) compared with major depressive disorder. Clomipramine is a TCA with significant anticholinergic effects, cardiac risk, and seizure risk >250 mg. Reserve for SSRI failures.

D. Alternative/Off-Label Pharmacologic Options

Generic	Brand	Dose Range	Clinical Notes	Evidence Source
Escitalopram	Lexapro	10–20 mg/day	Favorable tolerability; limited OCD evidence. Escitalopram (and citalopram) are off-label for OCD; FDA-approved agents for OCD are fluoxetine, fluvoxamine, sertraline, paroxetine, and clomipramine.	Limited evidence; Fineberg et al. (2020)
Venlafaxine XR	Effexor XR	75–225 mg/day	Limited evidence; may help refractory OCD; not routine treatment	Limited evidence; Denys et al. (2003)

Clinical note

These options may be considered when first-line SSRIs are not tolerated or ineffective; evidence remains less robust.

E. Augmentation Strategies (After Inadequate SSRI Response)

Base Treatment	Add-On Agent	Dose Range	Clinical Notes	Evidence Source
SSRI	Risperidone	0.5–4 mg/day	Strongest augmentation evidence; monitor prolactin and EPS	Fineberg et al. (2020)

Base Treatment	Add-On Agent	Dose Range	Clinical Notes	Evidence Source
SSRI	Aripiprazole	10–15 mg/day (RCT used fixed 15 mg dose)	Moderate augmentation evidence; lower metabolic burden	Moderate evidence; Muscatello et al. (2011)
SSRI	Quetiapine	50–300 mg/day	Mixed evidence; sedation common	Limited evidence; Fineberg et al. (2020)
SSRI or clomipramine	Olanzapine	2.5–20 mg/day (study range; clinical use often lower)	Very limited evidence; reserve for severe refractory OCD; high metabolic risk	Very limited evidence; Bystritsky et al. (2004)

Clinical note

Optimize SSRI dose and duration before augmentation. Antipsychotic augmentation improves symptoms in approximately 30% of SSRI-resistant OCD cases.

F. Avoid or Use with Caution in OCD

Strategy	Clinical Notes	Evidence Source
Dual SSRI therapy	No added benefit; increased adverse effects and serotonin syndrome risk	Fineberg et al. (2020)
SSRI + MAOI	Risk of life-threatening serotonin syndrome	FDA labeling; Clinical consensus
High-dose clomipramine without monitoring	Risk of arrhythmia, QT prolongation, and seizures	Fineberg et al. (2020); FDA labeling
Benzodiazepine monotherapy	No anti-obsessional benefit; risk of sedation, dependence, and cognitive impairment	Fineberg et al. (2020); AGS Beers Criteria (2023)
Rapid dose escalation	Increased adverse effects and reduced adherence	Fineberg et al. (2020); Clinical consensus

G. Practical Treatment Selection

Clinical Scenario	Preferred Treatment	Rationale	Avoid / Caution	Evidence Source
First-line uncomplicated OCD	SSRI (titrated to higher doses as needed) + ERP-based CBT	Best guideline-supported core treatment approach	Avoid underdosing	Fineberg et al. (2020)
Partial response	Optimize SSRI dose and duration	OCD requires high-dose, longer trials	Early switching	Fineberg et al. (2020)

Clinical Scenario	Preferred Treatment	Rationale	Avoid / Caution	Evidence Source
Non-response	Switch to another SSRI	A second SSRI may still be effective before premature augmentation	Premature augmentation	Fineberg et al. (2020)
Multiple SSRI failures	Clomipramine	Strong serotonergic efficacy	Cardiac and seizure risk	Fineberg et al. (2020)
Persistent symptoms	SSRI + risperidone or aripiprazole	Evidence-based augmentation	Polypharmacy	Fineberg et al. (2020)
Severe refractory OCD	Consider TMS	Option for treatment-resistant cases	Early invasive treatment	Limited evidence; Carmi et al. (2019)

2. BODY DYSMORPHIC DISORDER (BDD)

A. OVERVIEW

Aspect	Detail	Evidence Source
Definition	Preoccupation with perceived defects in appearance that are not observable or appear slight to others	DSM-5-TR (APA, 2022)
Core features	Repetitive behaviors (e.g., mirror checking, grooming) or mental acts in response to appearance concerns	DSM-5-TR (APA, 2022)
Clinical importance	High functional impairment and elevated suicide risk	Phillips et al. (2005, J Clin Psychiatry); Phillips et al. (2008, Am J Psychiatry)
Treatment approach	First-line: SSRI or CBT specific for BDD; combination recommended in moderate-severe cases	Fineberg et al. (2020); Phillips et al. (2008, Am J Psychiatry

B. Diagnostic Considerations

Clinical Consideration	Clinical Notes	Evidence Source
Assess insight	Poor or delusional insight is common and affects treatment approach	DSM-5-TR (APA, 2022)
Screen for suicidality	Elevated risk of suicidal ideation and attempts	Phillips et al. (2005, J Clin Psychiatry); Phillips et al. (2008, Am J Psychiatry)
Evaluate cosmetic-seeking behavior	Cosmetic procedures do not treat the disorder and may worsen symptoms	NICE (2022)

Clinical Consideration	Clinical Notes	Evidence Source
Rule out eating disorder	Differentiate when concerns primarily involve weight or body fat	DSM-5-TR (APA, 2022)
Assess functional impairment	Evaluate impact on social and occupational functioning	DSM-5-TR (APA, 2022)
Screen for comorbidities	Depression and anxiety commonly co-occur	Fineberg et al. (2020); Clinical consensus

C. First-Line Pharmacotherapy

Generic	Brand	Dose Range	Clinical Notes	Evidence Source
Fluoxetine	Prozac	40–80 mg/day (often requires high-dose SSRI)	Most studied SSRI; higher doses often required	Phillips et al. (2002); FDA labeling
Sertraline	Zoloft	100–200 mg/day	Effective SSRI; higher doses often needed	Fineberg et al. (2020); Clinical consensus
Escitalopram	Lexapro	10–20 mg/day	Favorable tolerability; direct BDD evidence remains limited	Clinical consensus

Clinical note

BDD typically requires higher SSRI doses and longer treatment trials (12–16 weeks) compared with major depressive disorder.

D. Alternative / Off-Label Options

Generic	Brand	Dose Range	Clinical Notes	Evidence Source
Venlafaxine XR	Effexor XR	75–225 mg/day	Very limited evidence; consider only after SSRI non-response	Limited evidence; Clinical consensus
Clomipramine	Anafranil	25–250 mg/day	Consider in refractory cases; higher anticholinergic, cardiac, and seizure risk	Fineberg et al. (2020); FDA labeling

E. Augmentation Strategies

Base Treatment	Add-On Agent	Dose Range	Clinical Notes	Evidence Source
SSRI	CBT (BDD-specific)	—	Most evidence-supported combined approach	Fineberg et al. (2020); Phillips et al. (2008, Am J Psychiatry)

Base Treatment	Add-On Agent	Dose Range	Clinical Notes	Evidence Source
SSRI	Risperidone / Aripiprazole	Standard dosing	Consider only in refractory cases or poor insight; evidence remains limited	Limited evidence; Clinical consensus
SSRI	Quetiapine / Olanzapine	Standard dosing	Very limited evidence; significant metabolic risk	Very limited evidence; Clinical consensus

Clinical note

CBT combined with SSRI remains the most evidence-supported treatment strategy.

F. Avoid or Use With Caution in BDD

Strategy	Clinical Notes	Evidence Source
Cosmetic procedures	Reinforces distorted beliefs and may worsen long-term outcomes	Phillips et al. (2008, Am J Psychiatry); Clinical consensus
Antipsychotic monotherapy	No established efficacy as monotherapy	Fineberg et al. (2020); Clinical consensus
Rapid SSRI discontinuation	High risk of symptom relapse	Fineberg et al. (2020); Clinical consensus

G. Practical Treatment Selection

Clinical Scenario	Preferred Treatment	Rationale	Avoid / Caution	Evidence Source
Mild–moderate BDD	BDD-specific CBT or SSRI; combination for more severe cases	Best-supported core treatments	Cosmetic procedures	Fineberg et al. (2020); Phillips et al. (2008, Am J Psychiatry)
Poor insight	High-dose SSRI; consider adjunctive SGA only in refractory cases	Poor insight is associated with greater severity	Antipsychotic monotherapy	Fineberg et al. (2020); Clinical consensus
Severe suicidality	Intensive psychiatric care + SSRI	High-risk population requiring close monitoring	Outpatient-only care	Phillips et al. (2005, J Clin Psychiatry); Clinical consensus

3. HOARDING DISORDER

A. OVERVIEW

Aspect	Detail	Evidence Source
Definition	Persistent difficulty discarding possessions regardless of value	DSM-5-TR (APA, 2022)
Core features	Clutter, excessive acquisition, and distress related to discarding	DSM-5-TR (APA, 2022)
Clinical importance	May cause fire hazards, falls, and severe functional impairment	Tolin et al. (2010); Clinical consensus
Treatment approach	Hoarding-specific CBT is first-line; pharmacotherapy evidence remains limited	Tolin et al. (2010); Clinical consensus

B. Diagnostic Considerations

Clinical Consideration	Clinical Notes	Evidence Source
Assess safety risks	Evaluate fire hazards, falls, sanitation issues, and unsafe living conditions	Tolin et al. (2010); Clinical consensus
Assess excessive acquiring	Excessive acquisition commonly worsens clutter severity	Tolin et al. (2010)
Assess insight	Poor or absent insight is common and may affect adherence	Tolin et al. (2010); Clinical consensus
Rule out medical contributors	Consider dementia, stroke, brain injury, or other neurocognitive disorders	DSM-5-TR (APA, 2022)
Assess comorbidities	Depression, anxiety, ADHD, and OCD-spectrum symptoms commonly co-occur	Tolin et al. (2010); Clinical consensus
Assess functional impairment	Evaluate impact on functioning, safety, and housing stability	DSM-5-TR (APA, 2022)

C. First-Line Treatment

Clinical Scenario	Preferred Treatment	Rationale	Avoid / Caution	Evidence Source
Core hoarding symptoms	CBT (hoarding-specific)	Strongest evidence for symptom reduction	Medication-only approaches	Clinical consensus
Poor insight	Motivational enhancement strategies + CBT	May improve engagement and adherence	Confrontational approaches	Clinical consensus

D. Pharmacotherapy (Adjunctive)

Generic	Brand	Dose Range	Clinical Notes	Evidence Source
Venlafaxine XR	Effexor XR	75–225 mg/day	Limited evidence; may help comorbid anxiety or depression, not core hoarding symptoms	Limited evidence; Clinical consensus
Paroxetine	Paxil	20–60 mg/day	Limited evidence; based on small non-replicated study	Limited evidence; Saxena et al. (2007)
SSRIs (various)	Various	Per agent	Primarily used for comorbid depression, anxiety, or OCD symptoms	Limited evidence; Clinical consensus

Clinical note

No medications are FDA-approved specifically for hoarding disorder.

E. Augmentation Strategies

Base Treatment	Add-On Agent	Dose Range	Clinical Notes	Evidence Source
CBT	SSRI	Standard dosing	May help comorbid depression or anxiety; limited effect on core hoarding symptoms	Clinical consensus

F. Avoid or Use With Caution in Hoarding Disorder

Strategy	Clinical Notes	Evidence Source
Polypharmacy without CBT	Medication alone rarely improves core hoarding symptoms and may delay effective treatment	Tolin et al. (2010); Clinical consensus
Antipsychotic monotherapy	No established benefit for core hoarding symptoms	Clinical consensus
Benzodiazepines	May worsen sedation, confusion, and fall risk, especially in older adults	AGS Beers Criteria (2023); Clinical consensus
Forced clean-outs without treatment plan	May increase distress, damage alliance, and lead to relapse	Tolin et al. (2010); Clinical consensus

G. Practical Treatment Selection

Clinical Scenario	Preferred Treatment	Rationale	Avoid / Caution	Evidence Source
Core symptoms	Hoarding-specific CBT	Strongest evidence for symptom improvement	Medication-only approaches	Tolin et al. (2010); Clinical consensus

Clinical Scenario	Preferred Treatment	Rationale	Avoid / Caution	Evidence Source
Comorbid depression	CBT + SSRI when clinically indicated	Targets comorbid depressive or anxiety symptoms	Expecting pharmacotherapy alone to improve core hoarding symptoms	Tolin et al. (2010); Clinical consensus

4. TRICHOTILLOMANIA (HAIR-PULLING DISORDER)

A. OVERVIEW

Aspect	Detail	Evidence Source
Definition	Recurrent hair pulling with attempts to stop	DSM-5-TR (APA, 2022)
Core features	Recurrent urges, tension, and repetitive hair-pulling behavior	DSM-5-TR (APA, 2022)
Clinical importance	Significant functional impairment and high rates of psychiatric comorbidity	Grant & Chamberlain (2021); Stein et al. (2021)
Treatment approach	First-line: behavioral therapy, particularly habit reversal training (HRT)	Grant & Chamberlain (2021); Bloch et al. (2007)

B. Diagnostic Considerations

Clinical Consideration	Clinical Notes	Evidence Source
Confirm DSM-5-TR diagnostic framework	Verify recurrent hair pulling, failed attempts to stop, and clinically significant distress/impairment	DSM-5-TR (APA, 2022)
Distinguish from OCD	Trichotillomania differs from OCD in symptom pattern, neurobiology, and treatment response	DSM-5-TR (APA, 2022); Grant & Chamberlain (2021)
Assess automatic vs. focused pulling	Determine whether pulling occurs outside awareness or in response to urges/tension	Woods et al. (2006); Grant & Chamberlain (2021)
Screen for co-occurring body-focused repetitive behaviors	Excoriation disorder and related grooming behaviors commonly coexist	Grant & Chamberlain (2021)
Assess psychiatric comorbidities	Depression, anxiety, OCD-spectrum, and attention-related symptoms commonly co-occur	Grant & Chamberlain (2021)

C. Pharmacologic Options (Off-Label)

Generic	Brand	Dose Range	Clinical Notes	Evidence Source
N-Acetylcysteine (NAC)	OTC	1200–2400 mg/day	Glutamate modulator; best-studied medication option; mixed but comparatively strongest evidence	Grant et al. (2009); Grant & Chamberlain (2021)
Fluoxetine	Prozac	20–80 mg/day	Limited/inconsistent benefit for core symptoms; may help comorbid depression or anxiety	Limited evidence; Bloch et al. (2007); Grant & Chamberlain (2021)
Sertraline	Zoloft	50–200 mg/day	No consistent benefit for core symptoms; may help comorbid OCD, anxiety, or depression	Limited evidence; Bloch et al. (2007); Grant & Chamberlain (2021)

Clinical note

Pharmacotherapy alone rarely produces full remission. Behavioral interventions remain the primary treatment modality.

D. Augmentation Strategies

Base Treatment	Add-On Agent	Dose Range	Clinical Notes	Evidence Source
Behavioral Therapy (Habit Reversal Training, HRT)	N-Acetylcysteine (NAC)	1200–2400 mg/day	Best-supported pharmacologic adjunct; may reduce urge-driven behaviors	Limited evidence; Grant et al. (2009); Grant & Chamberlain (2021)
Behavioral Therapy (HRT)	Other pharmacologic augmentation	No standard dosing established	Antipsychotics and other agents have very limited evidence; reserve for exceptional refractory cases	Very limited evidence; Clinical consensus; Grant & Chamberlain (2021)

E. Avoid or Use With Caution in Trichotillomania

Strategy	Clinical Notes	Evidence Source
Chronic antipsychotic escalation	Limited efficacy evidence; increased metabolic and neurologic risk	Limited evidence; Grant & Chamberlain (2021)
Medication without behavioral therapy	Inconsistent benefit for core symptoms; behavioral therapy remains primary treatment	Limited evidence; Bloch et al. (2007); Grant & Chamberlain (2021)

Strategy	Clinical Notes	Evidence Source
Benzodiazepines	No proven benefit for hair pulling; risk of disinhibition, dependence, and withdrawal	Clinical consensus

F. Practical Treatment Selection

Clinical Scenario	Preferred Treatment	Rationale	Avoid / Caution	Evidence Source
First-line	Habit Reversal Therapy (HRT)	Strongest evidence	Medication-only approaches	Grant & Chamberlain (2021); Bloch et al. (2007)
Persistent symptoms	HRT + NAC	Potential adjunctive benefit with limited evidence	Early antipsychotics	Limited evidence; Grant et al. (2009); Grant & Chamberlain (2021)

5. EXCORIATION (SKIN-PICKING) DISORDER

A. OVERVIEW

Aspect	Detail	Evidence Source
Definition	Recurrent skin picking causing lesions	DSM-5-TR (APA, 2022)
Core features	Recurrent urges, repetitive skin picking, and tissue damage	DSM-5-TR (APA, 2022)
Clinical importance	Risk of infection, scarring, and significant functional impairment	Grant & Chamberlain (2020); Grant & Chamberlain (2021)
Treatment approach	First-line: behavioral therapy, particularly habit reversal training (HRT)	Grant & Chamberlain (2020); Grant & Chamberlain (2021)

B. Diagnostic Considerations

Clinical Consideration	Clinical Notes	Evidence Source
Assess severity of skin damage	Evaluate lesions, infection risk, scarring, and functional impairment; consider dermatologic care when needed	DSM-5-TR (APA, 2022); Grant & Chamberlain (2020)
Rule out primary dermatologic conditions	Exclude dermatologic disorders driving scratching or picking behaviors	DSM-5-TR (APA, 2022)
Screen for trichotillomania and other body-focused repetitive behaviors	Excoriation disorder commonly co-occurs with other body-focused repetitive behaviors	Grant & Chamberlain (2020); Grant & Chamberlain (2021)
Assess psychiatric comorbidity	Depression, anxiety, OCD-spectrum, and substance use disorders commonly co-occur	Grant & Chamberlain (2020); Grant & Chamberlain (2021)

C. Pharmacologic Options (Off-label)

Generic	Brand	Dose Range	Clinical Notes	Evidence Source
N-Acetylcysteine (NAC)	OTC	1200–2400 mg/day	Best-studied option; glutamate modulation may reduce urge-driven picking	Grant et al. (2016); Grant & Chamberlain (2021)
Fluoxetine	Prozac	20–80 mg/day	Inconsistent benefit for core symptoms; may help comorbid OCD or depression	Limited evidence; Grant & Chamberlain (2020)
Sertraline	Zoloft	50–200 mg/day	Limited benefit for core symptoms; consider with comorbid anxiety, OCD, or depression	Limited evidence; Grant & Chamberlain (2020); Grant & Chamberlain (2021)
Clomipramine	Anafranil	25–250 mg/day	Possible benefit in refractory cases; higher anticholinergic and cardiac risk	Limited evidence; Grant & Chamberlain (2020); Grant & Chamberlain (2021)

Clinical note

Behavioral interventions remain first-line treatment for excoriation disorder; pharmacotherapy is typically used as an adjunct.

D. Alternative / Off-Label Options

Generic	Brand	Dose Range	Clinical Notes	Evidence Source
Olanzapine	Zyprexa	2.5–20 mg/day (study range; clinical use often lower)	Very limited evidence; high metabolic risk; not routine treatment for skin-picking symptoms	Very limited evidence; Clinical consensus

E. Augmentation Strategies

Base Treatment	Add-On Agent	Dose Range	Clinical Notes	Evidence Source
Behavioral therapy (HRT)	N-Acetylcysteine (NAC)	1200–2400 mg/day	Best-supported pharmacologic adjunct; may reduce urge-driven picking behaviors	Limited evidence; Grant et al. (2016); Grant & Chamberlain (2021)

F. Avoid or Use with Caution in Excoriation (Skin-Picking) Disorder

Strategy	Clinical Notes	Evidence Source
Poly-antidepressant therapy	No proven added benefit; increased adverse-effect risk	Clinical consensus

Strategy	Clinical Notes	Evidence Source
Antipsychotic monotherapy	Limited efficacy for core symptoms; risk of metabolic and neurologic adverse effects	Limited evidence; Grant & Chamberlain (2020)

G. Practical Treatment Selection

Clinical Scenario	Preferred Treatment	Rationale	Avoid / Caution	Evidence Source
Mild–moderate	Behavioral therapy (HRT)	First-line treatment	Medication-only approaches	Grant & Chamberlain (2020); Grant & Chamberlain (2021)
Persistent symptoms	HRT + N-acetylcysteine (NAC)	Potential adjunctive benefit with limited evidence	Polypharmacy	Limited evidence; Grant et al. (2016); Grant & Chamberlain (2021)

REFERENCES

American Geriatrics Society. (2023). American Geriatrics Society 2023 updated AGS Beers Criteria® for potentially inappropriate medication use in older adults. *Journal of the American Geriatrics Society, 71*(7), 2052–2081. https://doi.org/10.1111/jgs.18372

American Psychiatric Association. (2022). *Diagnostic and statistical manual of mental disorders* (5th ed., text rev.). American Psychiatric Association Publishing.

Bloch, M. H., Landeros-Weisenberger, A., Dombrowski, P. A., Kelmendi, B., Wegner, R., Nudel, J., & Coric, V. (2007). Systematic review: Pharmacological and behavioral treatment for trichotillomania. *Biological Psychiatry, 62*(8), 839–846. https://doi.org/10.1016/j.biopsych.2007.05.019

Bystritsky, A., Ackerman, D. L., Rosen, R. M., Vapnik, T., Gorbis, E., Maidment, K., & Saxena, S. (2004). Augmentation of serotonin reuptake inhibitors in refractory obsessive-compulsive disorder using adjunctive olanzapine. *Journal of Clinical Psychiatry, 65*(4), 565–568. https://doi.org/10.4088/JCP.v65n0418

Carmi, L., Tendler, A., Bystritsky, A., Hollander, E., Blumberger, D. M., Daskalakis, Z. J., Ward, H., Lapidus, K., Goodman, W., Casuto, L., Feifel, D., Barnea-Ygael, N., Roth, Y., Zangen, A., & Zohar, J. (2019). Efficacy and safety of deep transcranial magnetic stimulation for obsessive-compulsive disorder: A prospective multicenter randomized double-blind placebo-controlled trial. *American Journal of Psychiatry, 176*(11), 931–938. https://doi.org/10.1176/appi.ajp.2019.18101180

Denys, D., van Megen, H., van der Wee, N., & Westenberg, H. (2003). A double-blind comparison of venlafaxine and paroxetine in obsessive-compulsive disorder. *Journal of Clinical Psychopharmacology, 23*(6), 568–575. https://doi.org/10.1097/01.jcp.0000095342.32154.54

Fineberg, N. A., Hollander, E., Pallanti, S., Walitza, S., Grünblatt, E., Dell'Osso, B., & Stein, D. J. (2020). Clinical advances in obsessive-compulsive disorder: A position statement by the International College of Obsessive-Compulsive Spectrum Disorders. *International Clinical Psychopharmacology, 35*(4), 173–193. https://doi.org/10.1097/YIC.0000000000000314

Goodman, W. K., Price, L. H., Rasmussen, S. A., Mazure, C., Fleischmann, R. L., Hill, C. L., Heninger, G. R., & Charney, D. S. (1989). The Yale-Brown Obsessive Compulsive Scale. *Archives of General Psychiatry, 46*(11), 1006–1011. https://doi.org/10.1001/archpsyc.1989.01810110048007

Grant, J. E., Odlaug, B. L., & Kim, S. W. (2009). N-acetylcysteine, a glutamate modulator, in the treatment of trichotillomania. *Archives of General Psychiatry, 66*(7), 756–763. https://doi.org/10.1001/archgenpsychiatry.2009.60

Grant, J. E., Chamberlain, S. R., Redden, S. A., Leppink, E. W., & Odlaug, B. L. (2016). N-acetylcysteine in the treatment of excoriation disorder: A randomized clinical trial. *JAMA Psychiatry, 73*(5), 490–496. https://doi.org/10.1001/jamapsychiatry.2016.0060

Grant, J. E., & Chamberlain, S. R. (2021). Trichotillomania and skin-picking disorder: An update. Focus, 19(4), 405–412. https://doi.org/10.1176/appi.focus.20210013

Grant, J. E., & Chamberlain, S. R. (2020). Trichotillomania and skin-picking disorder. *New England Journal of Medicine, 382*(24), 2331–2339. https://doi.org/10.1056/NEJMcp1908142

Muscatello, M. R. A., Bruno, A., Pandolfo, G., Micò, U., Scimeca, G., Romeo, V. M., & Zoccali, R. A. (2011). Effect of aripiprazole augmentation of serotonin reuptake inhibitors in treatment-resistant obsessive-compulsive disorder. *Journal of Clinical Psychopharmacology, 31*(2), 174–179. https://doi.org/10.1097/JCP.0b013e31820e3db6

Phillips, K. A., Coles, M. E., Menard, W., Yen, S., Fay, C., & Weisberg, R. (2005). Suicidality in body dysmorphic disorder. *Journal of Clinical Psychiatry, 66*(6), 717–725. https://doi.org/10.4088/JCP.v66n0607

Phillips, K. A., Menard, W., Fay, C., & Pagano, M. (2005). Psychosocial functioning and quality of life in body dysmorphic disorder. *Comprehensive Psychiatry, 46*(4), 254–260. https://doi.org/10.1016/j.comppsych.2004.10.004

Phillips, K. A., Didie, E. R., Feusner, J., & Wilhelm, S. (2008). Body dysmorphic disorder: Treating an underrecognized disorder. *American Journal of Psychiatry, 165*(9), 1111–1118. https://doi.org/10.1176/appi.ajp.2008.07091413

Saxena, S., Brody, A. L., Maidment, K. M., & Baxter, L. R. (2007). Paroxetine treatment of compulsive hoarding. *Journal of Psychiatric Research, 41*(6), 481–487. https://doi.org/10.1016/j.jpsychires.2006.05.001

Stein, D. J., Costa, D. L. C., Lochner, C., Miguel, E. C., Reddy, Y. C. J., Shavitt, R. G., van den Heuvel, O. A., & Simpson, H. B. (2021). Obsessive-compulsive disorder. *Nature Reviews Disease Primers*, *7*(1), 1–21. https://doi.org/10.1038/s41572-021-00247-3

Tolin, D. F., Frost, R. O., & Steketee, G. (2010). A brief interview for assessing compulsive hoarding. *Psychiatry Research*, *178*(1), 147–152. https://doi.org/10.1016/j.psychres.2009.05.001

Woods, D. W., Flessner, C. A., Franklin, M. E., Wetterneck, C. T., Walther, M. R., Anderson, E. R., & Cardona, D. (2006). The trichotillomania impact project. *Journal of Clinical Psychiatry*, *67*(12), 1877–1888. https://doi.org/10.4088/JCP.v67n1207

VII. NEURODEVELOPMENTAL DISORDERS

SECTION INTRODUCTION

Neurodevelopmental disorders comprise a group of conditions characterized by developmental deficits affecting cognition, attention, executive functioning, communication, social interaction, behavioral regulation, learning, adaptive functioning, or motor performance. These disorders typically emerge during childhood or adolescence, although many persist into adulthood and continue to significantly affect academic achievement, occupational functioning, interpersonal relationships, emotional regulation, and overall quality of life across the lifespan.

Attention-deficit/hyperactivity disorder (ADHD), autism spectrum disorder (ASD), tic disorders, intellectual developmental disorder, and specific learning disorders represent some of the most frequently encountered neurodevelopmental conditions within psychiatric and outpatient clinical practice. Although symptom onset generally occurs early in development, many individuals remain underdiagnosed or are not formally identified until adolescence or adulthood, particularly in cases involving predominantly inattentive symptoms, high intellectual functioning, masking behaviors, or psychiatric comorbidity.

Neurodevelopmental disorders are highly heterogeneous in both presentation and severity. Patients may present with inattention, impulsivity, hyperactivity, executive dysfunction, emotional dysregulation, social communication difficulties, repetitive behaviors, sensory sensitivities, motor tics, academic impairment, behavioral disturbances, or adaptive functioning deficits. Symptom expression may vary substantially depending on developmental stage, environmental demands, cognitive ability, psychosocial support systems, and coexisting psychiatric or medical conditions.

Comorbidity is extremely common across neurodevelopmental disorders and frequently complicates diagnosis, treatment planning, and long-term prognosis. Anxiety disorders, depressive disorders, trauma-related disorders, obsessive-compulsive and related disorders, sleep disorders, substance use disorders, learning disabilities, and behavioral dysregulation commonly coexist with ADHD and ASD. Emotional dysregulation, low self-esteem, chronic academic difficulties, interpersonal rejection, and occupational impairment may further contribute to secondary psychiatric morbidity over time.

Careful longitudinal assessment is essential because symptom overlap may lead to diagnostic confusion with mood disorders, anxiety disorders, personality pathology, trauma-related conditions, or substance-related disorders. Comprehensive evaluation should therefore incorporate developmental history, educational performance, behavioral observations, family psychiatric history, psychosocial functioning, prior interventions, and collateral information whenever available. Assessment should also consider cultural, linguistic, environmental, and socioeconomic factors that may influence symptom recognition and access to care.

Although psychotherapy, behavioral interventions, educational accommodations, and psychosocial support remain foundational aspects of treatment, pharmacotherapy often plays an important role in symptom management and functional improvement. Stimulant medications remain first-line pharmacologic treatment for ADHD in many cases, while non-stimulant agents, alpha-2 agonists, antidepressants, and selected adjunctive treatments may be appropriate depending on symptom profile, comorbidity, tolerability, and clinical context. In autism spectrum disorder, pharmacologic treatment is generally symptom-targeted and may address irritability, aggression, impulsivity, anxiety, sleep disturbance, or repetitive behaviors rather than core social communication deficits.

Clinicians should remain attentive to medication safety, misuse potential, cardiovascular considerations, appetite suppression, sleep disruption, tic exacerbation, metabolic effects, and the impact of neurodevelopmental symptoms on academic, occupational, and social functioning. Particular attention should also be given to transition-of-care issues as pediatric patients move into adolescent and adult psychiatric systems, where continuity of diagnosis and treatment is frequently disrupted.

The following sections provide a structured, evidence-informed framework for the evaluation and treatment of neurodevelopmental disorders within outpatient psychiatric practice. Recommendations are intended to support safe, individualized, developmentally informed, and clinically consistent care while recognizing the importance of longitudinal reassessment, multidisciplinary collaboration, family involvement, and professional clinical judgment throughout the course of illness.

1. ATTENTION-DEFICIT/HYPERACTIVITY DISORDER (ADHD)

Applies primarily to adolescent and adult populations. Pediatric dosing may vary.

A. OVERVIEW

Aspect	Detail	Evidence Source
Definition	Persistent pattern of inattention and/or hyperactivity-impulsivity causing functional impairment across settings	DSM-5-TR (APA, 2022)
Core features	Inattention, disorganization, hyperactivity, impulsivity with onset in childhood and persistence into adulthood	DSM-5-TR (APA, 2022)
Epidemiology	Prevalence ~2.5–5% in adults; frequently underdiagnosed	NICE (2018); DSM-5-TR (APA, 2022)
Course	Chronic course; symptoms may evolve from hyperactivity to inattention in adulthood	DSM-5-TR (APA, 2022)
Functional impact	Impairment in academic, occupational, and interpersonal functioning; increased accident and substance use risk	NICE (2018)
First-line treatment approach	Stimulant pharmacotherapy with behavioral interventions as adjunct	NICE (2018); Bolea-Alamañac et al. (2014)

B. Diagnostic Considerations

Clinical Consideration	Clinical Notes	Evidence Source
Confirm diagnosis with collateral information	Multi-setting impairment required; collateral improves diagnostic accuracy	DSM-5-TR (APA, 2022); NICE (2018)
Rule out substance-induced symptoms	Stimulants, cannabis, cocaine may mimic ADHD symptoms	DSM-5-TR (APA, 2022); NICE (2018)
Assess psychiatric comorbidity	Anxiety, depression, bipolar disorder, SUD influence treatment choice	DSM-5-TR (APA, 2022); NICE (2018)
Screen cardiovascular history	Assess BP, HR, and cardiac history prior to stimulant initiation	NICE (2018); Vetter et al. (2008)
Assess for tic disorders	Tics influence medication selection (alpha-2 agonists preferred adjuncts)	DSM-5-TR (APA, 2022); NICE (2018)
Evaluate functional impairment	Confirm clinically significant impairment in daily functioning	DSM-5-TR (APA, 2022)

Clinical Consideration	Clinical Notes	Evidence Source
DSM-5-TR diagnostic threshold	≥6 inattentive and/or hyperactive–impulsive symptoms (≥5 if age ≥17) persisting ≥6 months; several present before age 12, across ≥2 settings, with functional impairment.	DSM-5-TR (APA, 2022)

Clinical note

EKG is recommended only if personal or family history suggests cardiac disease, syncope, or abnormal cardiovascular examination. NICE NG87 (2018, updated 2019)

C. Pharmacotherapy: Stimulants (First-Line)

Methylphenidate-Based

Generic	Brand	Dose Range	Clinical Notes	Evidence Source
Methylphenidate IR	Ritalin	10–60 mg/day	Short-acting (~3–4 h); multiple daily doses; useful for titration	NICE (2018); DSM-5-TR (APA, 2022)
Methylphenidate ER	Concerta	18–72 mg/day	Long-acting (~10–12 h); once-daily dosing improves adherence	NICE (2018); Bolea-Alamañac et al. (2014)
Dexmethylphenidate	Focalin	5–40 mg/day	d-isomer; effective at lower doses; available IR/XR	NICE (2018); Bolea-Alamañac et al. (2014)

Amphetamine-Based

Generic	Brand	Dose Range	Clinical Notes	Evidence Source
Mixed amphetamine salts	Adderall	5–40 mg/day	IR/XR forms; longer duration than IR methylphenidate; higher misuse risk; doses above 40 mg/day used in selected cases. Boxed warning: high potential for abuse and dependence (Schedule II). Doses above the FDA-labeled maximum are off-label and should be documented with explicit rationale and cardiovascular reassessment	NICE (2018); Bolea-Alamañac et al. (2014)
Lisdexamfetamine	Vyvanse	30–70 mg/day	Prodrug converted to dextroamphetamine; lower abuse potential; once-daily dosing	NICE (2018); Coghill et al. (2014)

Generic	Brand	Dose Range	Clinical Notes	Evidence Source
Dextroamphetamine	Dexedrine	5–40 mg/day	IR/ER forms; potent stimulant; option after methylphenidate failure	NICE (2018); Bolea-Alamañac et al. (2014)

Clinical note

Comparable efficacy at the population level, although individual response varies (Cortese et al., 2018).

D. Pharmacotherapy Non-Stimulants (FDA-Approved for ADHD)

Generic	Brand	Dose Range	Clinical Notes	Evidence Source
Atomoxetine	Strattera	40–100 mg/day	Selective norepinephrine reuptake inhibitor; no abuse potential; slower onset than stimulants (2–4 weeks); preferred in substance use risk. Boxed warning: increased risk of suicidal ideation in children and adolescents — monitor closely, especially early in treatment and after dose changes	NICE (2018); Bolea-Alamañac et al. (2014)
Guanfacine XR	Intuniv	1–4 mg/day	Alpha-2A agonist; useful for impulsivity/tics; limited adult evidence; monitor BP/HR; taper gradually to avoid rebound hypertension.	NICE (2018); Pringsheim et al. (2019)
Clonidine XR	Kapvay	0.1–0.4 mg/day	Sedating alpha-2 agonist; monitor BP/HR; taper gradually	NICE (2018); Pringsheim et al. (2019)
Viloxazine XR	Qelbree	200–600 mg/day	First novel non-stimulant approved for adults in 20 years; once-daily; no abuse potential; monitor for suicidal ideation; avoid with MAOIs. Boxed warning: increased risk of suicidal thoughts and behaviors in pediatric patients treated for ADHD — monitor closely, especially early in treatment and after dose changes	FDA (2022); FDA labeling

Clinical note

Substance use history, stimulant intolerance, comorbid tics/anxiety, or patient preference.

E. Off-Label Pharmacological Options

Generic	Brand	Dose Range	Clinical Notes	Evidence Source
Bupropion	Wellbutrin XL	150–450 mg/day	NDRI; Modest ADHD benefit; useful with comorbid depression; avoid in seizure/eating disorders	NICE (2018); Stuhec et al. (2015)
Modafinil	Provigil	100–200 mg/day	Wakefulness-promoting agent; Limited evidence; not routinely recommended; rare severe rash risk	NICE (2018); Cortese et al. (2018)

F. Augmentation Strategies

Base Treatment	Add-On Agent	Dose Range	Clinical Notes	Evidence Source
Stimulant	SSRI	Per SSRI	Treat comorbid anxiety or depressive disorders when present; monitor insomnia or activation	NICE (2018); DSM-5-TR (APA, 2022)
Stimulant	Guanfacine XR	1–4 mg/day	Useful for impulsivity, tics, or insomnia; monitor BP/HR	NICE (2018); Pringsheim et al. (2019)
Stimulant	Clonidine XR	0.1–0.4 mg/day	Helpful for hyperactivity/sleep; more sedating than guanfacine; taper gradually	NICE (2018); Pringsheim et al. (2019)
Atomoxetine	SSRI	Per SSRI	Use cautiously; CYP2D6 interactions may raise atomoxetine levels; monitor cardiovascular and adverse effects.	Limited evidence; Bolea-Alamañac et al. (2014); Clinical consensus

G. Avoid or Use with Caution in ADHD

Strategy	Clinical Notes	Evidence Source
Stimulant monotherapy in uncontrolled bipolar disorder	Risk of mania or mood destabilization; stabilize mood first	DSM-5-TR (APA, 2022); Yatham et al. (2018)
Dual stimulant therapy at full therapeutic doses	No evidence supports routine combined stimulant use at full therapeutic doses; Increased cardiovascular risk, insomnia, anxiety, and misuse	Clinical consensus; Bolea-Alamañac et al. (2014)
High-dose stimulant combined with SNRI	Risk of hypertension, tachycardia, and serotonin toxicity	NICE (2018); Cortese et al. (2018)

Strategy	Clinical Notes	Evidence Source
Immediate-release stimulants in patients with substance use disorder	Higher misuse/diversion risk; prefer ER or non-stimulants	NICE (2018); Bolea-Alamañac et al. (2014)
Abrupt stimulant discontinuation	Rebound fatigue, irritability, depression, or ADHD symptoms	NICE (2018); Cortese et al. (2018)

H. Practical Treatment Selection

Clinical Scenario	Preferred Treatment	Rationale	Avoid / Caution	Evidence Source
First-line uncomplicated ADHD	Long-acting stimulant	Strongest efficacy and adherence	Underdosing	NICE (2018); Bolea-Alamañac et al. (2014)
ADHD + substance use disorder	Lisdexamfetamine or atomoxetine	Lower misuse/diversion risk	Immediate-release (IR) stimulants	NICE (2018); Bolea-Alamañac et al. (2014)
ADHD + anxiety	Atomoxetine or stimulant + SSRI	Atomoxetine may improve ADHD and anxiety symptoms; stimulants may transiently worsen anxiety during initiation.	Rapid stimulant titration	NICE (2018); DSM-5-TR (APA, 2022)
ADHD + tic disorder	Stimulant + guanfacine XR (or clonidine XR)	Alpha-2 agonists may reduce tics	Ignoring tic worsening	NICE (2018); Pringsheim et al. (2019)
ADHD + bipolar disorder	Mood stabilizer or antipsychotic first, then cautious ADHD treatment	Mood stabilization reduces risk of treatment-emergent mania	Stimulant monotherapy	NICE (2018); DSM-5-TR (APA, 2022); Yatham et al. (2018)
Poor adherence	Long-acting stimulant formulations	Simplifies regimen and improves adherence	Multiple daily IR dosing	NICE (2018)

2. AUTISM SPECTRUM DISORDER (ASD) IRRITABILITY/AGITATION

A. OVERVIEW

Aspect	Detail	Evidence Source
Definition	Neurodevelopmental disorder with deficits in social communication and restricted/repetitive behaviors; irritability includes aggression, self-injury, and severe dysregulation	DSM-5-TR (APA, 2022)
Core features	Behavioral outbursts, aggression, self-injury, irritability often triggered by unmet needs or sensory overload	DSM-5-TR (APA, 2022); NICE (2013, updated 2021)
Epidemiology	Prevalence ~1–2%; irritability occurs in a significant subset with ASD	DSM-5-TR (APA, 2022)
Course	Chronic; severity fluctuates with environment, development, and interventions	NICE (2013, updated 2021)
Functional impact	Impairment in family, school, and social functioning; safety risks (self-injury, aggression)	NICE (2013, updated 2021)
First-line treatment approach	Behavioral/environmental interventions first; medication reserved for severe symptoms	NICE (2013, updated 2021); DSM-5-TR (APA, 2022)
Evidence basis for pharmacotherapy	ASD-associated irritability pharmacotherapy is supported by autism-specific FDA approvals (risperidone, aripiprazole), autism RCTs, and NICE; guidelines for other disorders — including the VA/DoD PTSD guideline — are not sources for ASD pharmacotherapy.	FDA labeling; NICE (2013, updated 2021)

B. Diagnostic Considerations

Clinical Consideration	Clinical Notes	Evidence Source
Rule out medical causes	Assess for pain, GI issues, sleep disorders, or infection	DSM-5-TR (APA, 2022); NICE (2013, updated 2021)
Assess communication deficits	Dysregulation may reflect inability to express needs	DSM-5-TR (APA, 2022)
Identify environmental triggers	Sensory overload, stress, or routine changes may precipitate agitation	NICE (2013, updated 2021)
Assess comorbid psychiatric conditions	ADHD, anxiety, or OCD symptoms may worsen irritability	DSM-5-TR (APA, 2022); NICE (2013, updated 2021)

Clinical Consideration	Clinical Notes	Evidence Source
Evaluate severity and safety risk	Determine need for pharmacologic intervention	NICE (2013, updated 2021)
Prioritize behavioral interventions	Reserve pharmacotherapy for severe or unsafe behaviors	NICE (2013, updated 2021)

C. Pharmacotherapy

Generic	Brand	Dose Range	Clinical Notes	Evidence Source
Risperidone	Risperdal	0.5–3 mg/day	Strongest evidence for irritability/aggression; monitor metabolic effects, prolactin, EPS. FDA-approved for irritability associated with autistic disorder in pediatric patients (ages 5–16), not in adults.	FDA (2006); NICE (2013, updated 2021); McCracken et al. (2002)
Aripiprazole	Abilify	2–15 mg/day	Effective with lower metabolic burden; monitor akathisia/activation. FDA-approved for irritability associated with autistic disorder in pediatric patients (ages 6–17), not in adults.	FDA (2009); NICE (2013, updated 2021); Owen et al. (2009)
Guanfacine XR	Intuniv	1–4 mg/day	Useful for hyperactivity/impulsivity; may be sedating	NICE (2013, updated 2021); Scahill et al. (2015)
Clonidine XR	Kapvay	0.1–0.4 mg/day	Sedating; may help sleep and dysregulation	NICE (2013, updated 2021); Pringsheim et al. (2019)
Fluoxetine	Prozac	10–40 mg/day	Not for core ASD symptoms; consider only for comorbid anxiety/OCD symptoms	Limited evidence; Williams et al. (2013)

D. Combination Strategies

Base Treatment	Add-On Agent	Dose Range	Clinical Notes	Evidence Source
Risperidone or Aripiprazole	Guanfacine XR	1–4 mg/day	Targets residual hyperactivity; monitor hypotension/sedation	NICE (2013, updated 2021); Scahill et al. (2015)
Risperidone or Aripiprazole	SSRI	Per SSRI	Only if comorbid anxiety/OCD; monitor activation	NICE (2013, updated 2021), Williams et al. (2013)

Base Treatment	Add-On Agent	Dose Range	Clinical Notes	Evidence Source
Behavioral therapy	Antipsychotic	Per agent	Pharmacotherapy adjunct for severe behaviors only	NICE (2013, updated 2021), DSM-5-TR (APA, 2022)

E. Avoid or Use With Caution in ASD

Strategy	Clinical Notes	Evidence Source
Dual antipsychotic therapy	No proven added benefit; increased metabolic, EPS, and sedation risk	NICE (2013, updated 2021); Correll et al. (2009)
Polypharmacy without behavioral plan	May overlook medical/environmental triggers and increase adverse effects	NICE (2013, updated 2021); DSM-5-TR (APA, 2022)
Benzodiazepines	Risk of paradoxical disinhibition, sedation, and dependence	Limited evidence; Clinical consensus; Posey et al. (2007)
Rapid dose escalation	Higher risk of sedation, EPS, and metabolic adverse effects	NICE (2013, updated 2021)
Antipsychotic without metabolic monitoring	Risk of obesity, diabetes, and dyslipidemia	American Diabetes Association & American Psychiatric Association (2004); NICE (2013, updated 2021)

F. Practical Treatment Selection

Clinical Scenario	Preferred Treatment	Rationale	Avoid / Caution	Evidence Source
Mild irritability	Behavioral interventions	Addresses underlying triggers	Early medication use	NICE (2013, updated 2021); DSM-5-TR (APA, 2022)
Moderate symptoms	Behavioral + consider SGA	Stepwise escalation	Polypharmacy	NICE (2013, updated 2021)
Severe aggression/self-injury	Risperidone or aripiprazole	Strongest evidence for irritability/aggression treatment	Delayed treatment	NICE (2013, updated 2021); McCracken et al. (2002); Owen et al. (2009)
ASD + ADHD features	Add guanfacine XR	Improves impulsivity/hyperactivity	Stimulant overuse	NICE (2013, updated 2021); Scahill et al. (2015)
ASD + anxiety/OCD	Add SSRI cautiously	Targets comorbid symptoms	Using SSRI for core ASD	NICE (2013, updated 2021); Williams et al. (2013)

Clinical Scenario	Preferred Treatment	Rationale	Avoid / Caution	Evidence Source
Poor response	Reassess triggers and diagnosis	Many cases environmental/medical	Dose escalation without reassessment	NICE (2013, updated 2021); DSM-5-TR (APA, 2022)

3. TIC DISORDER/TOURETTE DISORDER

A. OVERVIEW

Aspect	Detail	Evidence Source
Definition	Neurodevelopmental disorder with motor and/or vocal tics present for ≥1 year	DSM-5-TR (APA, 2022)
Core features	Sudden, rapid, recurrent, non-rhythmic motor movements or vocalizations	DSM-5-TR (APA, 2022)
Epidemiology	Prevalence ~0.3–1%; more common in males	DSM-5-TR (APA, 2022)
Course	Waxing and waning; often improves in adulthood	DSM-5-TR (APA, 2022)
Functional impact	Social impairment, stigma, academic disruption; comorbidities often drive severity	Pringsheim et al. (2019)
First-line treatment approach	Behavioral therapy (CBIT); pharmacotherapy if moderate–severe impairment	Pringsheim et al. (2019); NICE (2013)

B. Diagnostic Considerations

Clinical Consideration	Clinical Notes	Evidence Source
Assess severity and impairment	Many tics are mild and may not require medication; assess functional impact first	Pringsheim et al. (2019); DSM-5-TR (APA, 2022)
Screen psychiatric comorbidity	ADHD, OCD, anxiety, and mood disorders commonly co-occur and may drive impairment	Pringsheim et al. (2019); DSM-5-TR (APA, 2022)
Identify triggers	Stress, fatigue, excitement, or caffeine may worsen tics	Pringsheim et al. (2019); McGuire et al. (2015)
Differentiate tic vs stereotypy	Tics fluctuate and are suppressible; stereotypies are rhythmic and fixed	DSM-5-TR (APA, 2022)
Prioritize behavioral therapy as first-line	CBIT is first-line for impairing tics; medication is adjunctive when needed	Pringsheim et al. (2019)

C. Pharmacotherapy

C.1 First-Line Pharmacologic Options

Generic	Brand	Dose Range	Clinical Notes	Evidence Source
Guanfacine XR	Intuniv	1–4 mg/day	Alpha-2A agonist; useful with comorbid ADHD; may reduce tics and impulsivity; monitor BP/HR	Pringsheim et al. (2019)
Clonidine XR	Kapvay	0.1–0.4 mg/day	Alpha-2 agonist; reduces tics/hyperactivity; more sedating; may improve sleep	Pringsheim et al. (2019)

C.2 Antipsychotics (Moderate-Severe Tics)

Generic	Brand	Dose Range	Clinical Notes	Evidence Source
Risperidone	Risperdal	0.5–4 mg/day	Effective for moderate–severe tics; monitor metabolic effects, prolactin, and EPS	Clinical consensus; Pringsheim et al. (2019)
Aripiprazole	Abilify	2–20 mg/day	Effective for tic reduction; monitor akathisia and activation	Clinical consensus; Pringsheim et al. (2019)
Haloperidol	Haldol	1–10 mg/day	First-generation antipsychotic with proven efficacy; high EPS/tardive dyskinesia risk; reserve for severe cases	Pringsheim et al. (2019)
Pimozide	Orap	1–10 mg/day	FDA-approved for Tourette; FGA; monitor QTc prolongation and EPS; baseline ECG recommended; reserve for moderate–severe cases	FDA labeling; Pringsheim et al. (2019)

C.3 VMAT2 Inhibitors (Severe, Refractory Cases)

Generic	Brand	Dose Range	Clinical Notes	Evidence Source
Tetrabenazine	Xenazine	12.5–50 mg/day	Older VMAT2 inhibitor for refractory tics; specialist use only; monitor depression, parkinsonism, sedation, and QT prolongation	Limited evidence; Jankovic (2016)

Clinical note

Deutetrabenazine (Austedo) and Valbenazine (Ingrezza) are VMAT2 inhibitors FDA-approved for tardive dyskinesia and Huntington's, not Tourette's (off-label use). With strong CYP2D6 inhibitors or in CYP2D6 poor metabolizers, limit deutetrabenazine to a maximum of 36 mg/day, with a single dose not exceeding 18 mg.

D. Combination Strategies

Base Treatment	Add-On Agent	Clinical Notes	Evidence Source
Alpha-2 agonist (Guanfacine / Clonidine)	Low-dose second-generation antipsychotic	Consider for persistent impairing tics; monitor sedation, hypotension, and metabolic effects	Pringsheim et al. (2019)
CBIT (Comprehensive Behavioral Intervention for Tics)	Pharmacologic treatment (alpha-2 agonist or antipsychotic)	Combined behavioral and medication treatment may improve outcomes in severe cases	Pringsheim et al. (2019); McGuire et al. (2015)

E. Avoid or Use With Caution in Tic Disorders

Strategy	Clinical Notes	Evidence Source
Poly-antipsychotic therapy	No proven added benefit; increased EPS, metabolic, and sedation risk	Pringsheim et al. (2019)
High-dose stimulant use without appropriate monitoring	May worsen tics in some patients; monitor tic severity, BP, and HR	Pringsheim et al. (2019); NICE (2018)
Abrupt antipsychotic discontinuation	Risk of rebound or worsening tics; gradual taper recommended	Pringsheim et al. (2019)

F. Practical Treatment Selection

Clinical Scenario	Preferred Treatment	Rationale	Avoid / Caution	Evidence Source
Mild, non-impairing tics	Psychoeducation / monitoring	Many cases self-limited	Early medication	Pringsheim et al. (2019); DSM-5-TR (APA, 2022)
Moderate tics	CBIT	First-line non-pharmacologic	Skipping behavioral therapy	Pringsheim et al. (2019); McGuire et al. (2015)
Tics + ADHD	Guanfacine XR or stimulant + guanfacine	Treats both conditions	Ignoring tic worsening	Pringsheim et al. (2019); NICE (2018)
Severe tics	Antipsychotic (aripiprazole/risperidone)	Strongest efficacy	Delayed treatment	Pringsheim et al. (2019)

Clinical Scenario	Preferred Treatment	Rationale	Avoid / Caution	Evidence Source
Refractory tics	Consider VMAT2 inhibitor	Option for severe refractory cases; specialist oversight	Premature use	Jankovic (2016)

REFERENCES

American Diabetes Association, American Psychiatric Association, American Association of Clinical Endocrinologists, & North American Association for the Study of Obesity. (2004). Consensus development conference on antipsychotic drugs and obesity and diabetes. *Diabetes Care, 27*(2), 596–601.

American Psychiatric Association. (2022). *Diagnostic and statistical manual of mental disorders* (5th ed., text rev.). American Psychiatric Association Publishing.

Bolea-Alamañac, B., Nutt, D. J., Adamou, M., Asherson, P., Bazire, S., Coghill, D., Heal, D., Müller, U., Nash, J., Santosh, P., Sayal, K., Sonuga-Barke, E., & Young, S. J. (2014). Evidence-based guidelines for the pharmacological management of attention deficit hyperactivity disorder. *Journal of Psychopharmacology, 28*(3), 179–203.

Coghill, D., Banaschewski, T., Lecendreux, M., Soutullo, C., Johnson, M., Zuddas, A., Anderson, C., Civil, R., & Higgins, N. (2014). Lisdexamfetamine dimesylate in children and adolescents with ADHD. *European Neuropsychopharmacology, 24*(8), 1208–1218.

Correll, C. U., Manu, P., Olshanskiy, V., Napolitano, B., Kane, J. M., & Malhotra, A. K. (2009). Cardiometabolic risk of second-generation antipsychotics. *JAMA, 302*(16), 1765–1773.

Cortese, S., Adamo, N., Del Giovane, C., Mohr-Jensen, C., Hayes, A. J., Carucci, S., Atkinson, L. Z., Tessari, L., Banaschewski, T., Coghill, D., Hollis, C., Simonoff, E., Zuddas, A., Barbui, C., Purgato, M., Steinhausen, H. C., Shokraneh, F., Xia, J., & Cipriani, A. (2018). Comparative efficacy and tolerability of ADHD medications. *The Lancet Psychiatry, 5*(9), 727–738.

Jankovic, J. (2016). Tetrabenazine in hyperkinetic movement disorders. *Expert Review of Neurotherapeutics, 16*(7), 757–764.

McCracken, J. T., McGough, J., Shah, B., Cronin, P., Hong, D., Aman, M. G., Arnold, L. E., Lindsay, R., Nash, P., Hollway, J., McDougle, C. J., Posey, D., Swiezy, N., Kohn, A., Scahill, L., Martin, A., Koenig, K., Volkmar, F., Carroll, D., ... McMahon, D. (2002). Risperidone in autism with behavioral problems. *New England Journal of Medicine, 347*(5), 314–321.

McGuire, J. F., Piacentini, J., Brennan, E. A., Lewin, A. B., Murphy, T. K., Small, B. J., & Storch, E. A. (2015). Behavior therapy for Tourette syndrome: Meta-analysis. *Journal of Psychiatric Research, 62*, 17–25.

National Institute for Health and Care Excellence (NICE). (2013). *Autism spectrum disorder in under 19s: Support and management (CG170).* https://www.nice.org.uk/guidance/cg170

National Institute for Health and Care Excellence (NICE). (2018). *Attention deficit hyperactivity disorder: Diagnosis and management (NG87).* https://www.nice.org.uk/guidance/ng87

National Institute for Health and Care Excellence (NICE). (2021). *Autism spectrum disorder in adults: Diagnosis and management (NG227).* https://www.nice.org.uk/guidance/ng227

National Institute for Health and Care Excellence (NICE). (2021). *Autism spectrum disorder in under 19s: Diagnosis and management (NG228).* https://www.nice.org.uk/guidance/ng228

Owen, R., Sikich, L., Marcus, R. N., Corey-Lisle, P., Manos, G., McQuade, R. D., Carson, W. H., & Findling, R. L. (2009). Aripiprazole in the treatment of irritability in children and adolescents with autistic disorder. *Pediatrics, 124*(6), 1533–1540. https://doi.org/10.1542/peds.2008-3782

Posey, D. J., Stigler, K. A., Erickson, C. A., & McDougle, C. J. (2007). Antipsychotics in the treatment of autism. *Journal of Clinical Psychiatry, 68*(Suppl. 4), 9–15.

Pringsheim, T., Okun, M. S., Müller-Vahl, K., Martino, D., Jankovic, J., Cavanna, A. E., Woods, D. W., Robinson, M., Jarvie, E., Roessner, V., Oskoui, M., Holler-Managan, Y., & Piacentini, J. (2019). Treatment of tic disorders. *Neurology, 92*(19), 896–906.

Scahill, L., McCracken, J. T., King, B. H., Rockhill, C., Shah, B., Politte, L., Sanders, R., Minjarez, M., Cowen, J., Mullett, J., Page, C., Ward, D., Deng, Y., Loo, S., Dziura, J., & McDougle, C. J. (2015). Extended-release guanfacine for hyperactivity in children with autism spectrum disorder. *American Journal of Psychiatry, 172*(12), 1197–1206. https://doi.org/10.1176/appi.ajp.2015.15010055

Stuhec, M., Munda, B., Svab, V., & Locatelli, I. (2015). Comparative efficacy and acceptability of atomoxetine, lisdexamfetamine, bupropion and methylphenidate in treatment of attention deficit hyperactivity disorder in children and adolescents: A meta-analysis with focus on bupropion. *Journal of Affective Disorders, 178*, 149–154. https://doi.org/10.1016/j.jad.2015.02.052

U.S. Food and Drug Administration. (2006). *Risperdal (risperidone) prescribing information.*

U.S. Food and Drug Administration. (2009). *Abilify (aripiprazole) prescribing information.*

Vetter, V. L., Elia, J., Erickson, C., Berger, S., Blum, N., Uzark, K., & Webb, C. L. (2008). Cardiovascular monitoring in ADHD. *Circulation, 117*(18), 2407–2423.

Williams, K., Brignell, A., Randall, M., Silove, N., & Hazell, P. (2013). Selective serotonin reuptake inhibitors (SSRIs) for autism spectrum disorders (ASD). *Cochrane Database of Systematic Reviews*, (8), CD004677. https://doi.org/10.1002/14651858.CD004677.pub3

VIII. PSYCHOTIC DISORDERS

SECTION INTRODUCTION

Psychotic disorders comprise a group of severe psychiatric conditions characterized by abnormalities in perception, thought processes, reality testing, cognition, behavior, and emotional regulation. Core features may include delusions, hallucinations, disorganized thinking, disorganized or catatonic behavior, negative symptoms, impaired insight, and varying degrees of functional deterioration. These disorders are frequently associated with substantial psychosocial impairment, occupational dysfunction, recurrent hospitalization, medical comorbidity, and elevated suicide risk.

Schizophrenia spectrum and other psychotic disorders typically emerge during late adolescence or early adulthood, although onset may occur across a broader age range depending on the underlying condition. Schizophrenia affects approximately 1% of the population worldwide and remains among the most disabling psychiatric illnesses due to its chronic course, cognitive impairment, social dysfunction, and long-term functional consequences. Early identification and sustained treatment are strongly associated with improved clinical outcomes, reduced relapse risk, and better preservation of social and occupational functioning.

Psychotic symptoms may occur in the context of primary psychotic disorders, mood disorders with psychotic features, substance-induced conditions, neurologic illness, medical disorders, medication effects, autoimmune syndromes, or severe trauma-related pathology. Accurate differential diagnosis is therefore essential, particularly during first-episode psychosis. Comprehensive psychiatric and medical evaluation should assess symptom chronology, substance use, mood symptoms, cognitive changes, neurologic findings, developmental history, and potential medical contributors to psychosis.

The clinical presentation of psychotic disorders is highly heterogeneous. Positive symptoms may include hallucinations, delusions, paranoia, disorganized speech, or bizarre behavior, while negative symptoms may involve affective flattening, avolition, anhedonia, social withdrawal, reduced speech output, and impaired motivation. Cognitive dysfunction—including impaired executive functioning, attention deficits, working memory impairment, and slowed processing speed—is also common and may substantially contribute to long-term disability and poor functional recovery.

Comorbidity is extremely common among patients with psychotic disorders. Mood disorders, anxiety disorders, substance use disorders, trauma-related disorders, metabolic disease, nicotine dependence, sleep disorders, and cognitive impairment frequently coexist and may complicate diagnosis, treatment adherence, and prognosis. Substance use—particularly cannabis, stimulants, hallucinogens, and alcohol—may precipitate, worsen, or mimic psychotic symptoms in vulnerable individuals. Medical comorbidity also contributes substantially to reduced life expectancy in patients with chronic psychotic illness.

Suicide risk remains a major clinical concern across psychotic disorders, particularly during first-episode psychosis, depressive episodes, periods of insight recovery, medication nonadherence, substance misuse, and recent hospitalization. Patients may also demonstrate impaired judgment, behavioral dysregulation, paranoia, or reduced ability to recognize medical or psychiatric deterioration. Comprehensive risk assessment, safety planning, and continuity of care are therefore critical components of longitudinal management.

Antipsychotic medications remain the cornerstone of pharmacologic treatment for schizophrenia spectrum disorders and other primary psychotic illnesses. Treatment selection should consider efficacy, prior response, metabolic risk, extrapyramidal symptoms, prolactin elevation, sedation, cardiovascular effects, adherence history, and patient preference. Clozapine remains the gold-standard treatment for treatment-resistant schizophrenia and recurrent suicidality but requires specialized monitoring because of risks including agranulocytosis, myocarditis, seizures, constipation, and metabolic complications. Long-acting injectable antipsychotics may significantly improve adherence and reduce relapse risk in selected patients. Boxed warning (class): both first- and second-generation antipsychotics are associated with increased mortality in elderly patients with dementia-related psychosis and are not approved for that indication.

Effective management of psychotic disorders extends beyond symptom reduction and should include psychoeducation, psychosocial rehabilitation, cognitive and functional support, substance use treatment, family involvement, supported employment or educational interventions, and coordination of medical care. Longitudinal monitoring should emphasize relapse prevention, medication adherence, metabolic surveillance, suicide risk assessment, and preservation of functional capacity whenever possible.

The following sections provide a structured, evidence-informed framework for the evaluation and treatment of psychotic disorders within outpatient psychiatric practice. Recommendations are intended to support safe, consistent, and clinically individualized care while recognizing the importance of multidisciplinary management, longitudinal reassessment, and professional clinical judgment throughout the course of illness.

1. SCHIZOPHRENIA

A. OVERVIEW

Clinical Principle	Clinical Notes	Evidence Source
Antipsychotic treatment is the foundation of care	Antipsychotics remain the core treatment for acute and maintenance schizophrenia; selection should consider response history, adverse effects, comorbidities, and patient preference	APA (2020); NICE (2014, updated 2019)
Antipsychotic monotherapy is preferred as the standard initial approach	Monotherapy reduces cumulative adverse effects and allows clearer assessment of efficacy and tolerability	APA (2020); NICE (2014, updated 2019)
Clozapine is the treatment of choice for treatment-resistant schizophrenia	Consider after failure of ≥2 adequate antipsychotic trials; strongest evidence for persistent psychosis	APA (2020); NICE (2014, updated 2019); Kane et al. (1988)
Long-acting injectable antipsychotics should be considered when adherence risk is high	Appropriate for recurrent relapse, poor adherence, limited insight, or patient preference	APA (2020); NICE (2014, updated 2019)
Metabolic and neurologic monitoring are essential	Monitor weight, glucose/A1c, lipids, EPS, tardive dyskinesia, prolactin, and QTc as indicated	APA (2020); American Diabetes Association & American Psychiatric Association (2004)
Treatment planning should include psychosocial recovery goals	Combine medication with psychoeducation, relapse prevention, and functional rehabilitation	APA (2020); NICE (2014, updated 2019)

B. Diagnostic Considerations

Diagnostic Consideration	Clinical Notes	Evidence Source
Confirm core psychotic symptoms	Assess for delusions, hallucinations, disorganized speech/behavior, catatonia, and negative symptoms per DSM-5-TR criteria	DSM-5-TR (APA, 2022)
Assess longitudinal functional decline	Evaluate deterioration in social, academic, occupational, or self-care functioning	DSM-5-TR (APA, 2022)
Exclude substance-induced psychosis	Assess cannabis, stimulants, hallucinogens, alcohol withdrawal, and medication-related causes	DSM-5-TR (APA, 2022); APA (2020)
Exclude medical and neurologic causes	Consider seizures, autoimmune encephalitis, CNS lesions, infections, delirium, or metabolic disorders	DSM-5-TR (APA, 2022); APA (2020)

Diagnostic Consideration	Clinical Notes	Evidence Source
Distinguish from mood disorders with psychotic features	Determine whether psychosis occurs outside mood episodes	DSM-5-TR (APA, 2022)
Assess suicidality, aggression risk, and inability to care for self	Safety assessment guides level of care and hospitalization need	APA (2020); NICE (2014, updated 2019)
Identify catatonia or severe agitation early	May require urgent stabilization or higher level of care	APA (2020); DSM-5-TR (APA, 2022)
DSM-5-TR diagnostic threshold	≥2 Criterion A symptoms for a significant portion of ≥1 month (at least one being delusions, hallucinations, or disorganized speech), with continuous signs of disturbance for ≥6 months.	DSM-5-TR (APA, 2022)

C. First-Generation Antipsychotics (FGAs)

Drug	Brand	Dose	Clinical Notes	Evidence Source
Haloperidol	Haldol	2–20 mg/day	High-potency FGA; effective for positive symptoms/agitation; high EPS and QTc risk	APA (2020); NICE (2014, updated 2019)
Perphenazine	Trilafon	8–64 mg/day	Mid-potency FGA; lower metabolic burden; clinically relevant EPS risk	APA (2020); NICE (2014, updated 2019)
Chlorpromazine	Thorazine	200–800 mg/day	Low-potency FGA; more sedation, orthostasis, and anticholinergic effects	APA (2020); NICE (2014, updated 2019)
Thiothixene	Navane	5–60 mg/day	High-potency FGA with significant EPS risk	APA (2020); NICE (2014, updated 2019)
Trifluoperazine	Stelazine	5–40 mg/day	High-potency FGA; less sedating but higher EPS/tardive dyskinesia risk	APA (2020); NICE (2014, updated 2019)
Fluphenazine	Prolixin	2.5–20 mg/day	High-potency FGA available oral/LAI; notable EPS and tardive dyskinesia risk	APA (2020); NICE (2014, updated 2019)

D. Second-Generation Antipsychotics (SGAs)

Drug	Brand	Dose	Clinical Notes	Evidence Source
Risperidone	Risperdal	1–6 mg/day	Effective and commonly used; prolactin elevation and dose-related EPS may occur	APA (2020); NICE (2014, updated 2019)

Drug	Brand	Dose	Clinical Notes	Evidence Source
Paliperidone	Invega	3–12 mg/day	Active risperidone metabolite; fewer CYP interactions; prolactin/EPS risk persists	APA (2020); NICE (2014, updated 2019)
Olanzapine	Zyprexa	5–20 mg/day	Highly effective; among the highest metabolic and weight gain risks	APA (2020); NICE (2014, updated 2019)
Quetiapine	Seroquel	300–800 mg/day	Lower EPS burden; sedating; monitor orthostasis and metabolic effects	APA (2020); NICE (2014, updated 2019)
Ziprasidone	Geodon	40–160 mg/day	Lower metabolic burden; take with food; monitor QTc	APA (2020); NICE (2014, updated 2019)
Aripiprazole	Abilify	10–30 mg/day	Lower metabolic burden; akathisia and activation may limit tolerability	APA (2020); NICE (2014, updated 2019)
Lurasidone	Latuda	40–160 mg/day	Lower metabolic burden; requires food; akathisia/EPS may occur	APA (2020); NICE (2014, updated 2019)
Cariprazine	Vraylar	1.5–6 mg/day	Partial dopamine agonist; may help negative symptoms; akathisia common	APA (2020); NICE (2014, updated 2019)
Asenapine	Saphris	10–20 mg/day	Sublingual; avoid eating/drinking after dosing; oral numbness common	APA (2020); NICE (2014, updated 2019)
Iloperidone	Fanapt	6–24 mg/day	Slow titration required due to orthostasis; QTc caution	APA (2020); NICE (2014, updated 2019)
Milsaperidone	Bysanti	12–24 mg/day (6–12 mg BID)	Active metabolite of iloperidone; 7-day titration due to orthostasis; QTc caution; reduce dose in CYP2D6 poor metabolizers or with strong CYP2D6/3A4 inhibitors	FDA labeling (2026)
Clozapine	Clozaril	200–900 mg/day	Gold standard for treatment-resistant schizophrenia; requires ANC monitoring	APA (2020); NICE (2014, updated 2019); Kane et al. (1988)

Drug	Brand	Dose	Clinical Notes	Evidence Source
Lumateperone	Caplyta	42 mg/day	Favorable metabolic profile; long-term comparative data remain limited. 42 mg/day is the standard adult dose. Reduce to 21 mg/day with moderate CYP3A4 inhibitors or moderate-to-severe (Child-Pugh B/C) hepatic impairment, and to 10.5 mg/day with strong CYP3A4 inhibitors; avoid CYP3A4 inducers	FDA labeling ; Correll et al. (2020)

E. Novel Mechanism Agents

Drug	Brand	Dose	Clinical Notes	Evidence Source
Xanomeline / Trospium	Cobenf y	50/20 mg to 125/30 mg BID	Muscarinic agonist combined with a peripheral anticholinergic; non-D2-based mechanism; low EPS and prolactin burden; GI adverse effects common	FDA (2024); Kaul et al. (2024

F. Long-Acting Injectables (LAIs)

Drug	Brand	Dose	Clinical Notes	Evidence Source
Risperidone IM	Risperdal Consta	12.5–50 mg every 2 weeks	Requires oral overlap during initiation	APA (2020)
Risperidone SQ	Uzedy	50–250 mg monthly or every 2 months	SQ formulation; establish oral tolerability first	APA (2020)
Paliperidone palmitate monthly	Invega Sustenna	39–234 mg monthly	No prolonged oral overlap after loading strategy	APA (2020)
Paliperidone palmitate every 3 months	Invega Trinza	273–819 mg every 3 months	Use after stabilization on monthly paliperidone	APA (2020)
Paliperidone palmitate every 6 months	Invega Hafyera	1092–1560 mg every 6 months	For carefully stabilized patients; extended dosing interval	APA (2020)
Paliperidone palmitate monthly	Erzofri	Product-specific strengths monthly	Follow product-specific labeling/interchangeability guidance	FDA (2024); Janssen Pharmaceuticals (2024)
Aripiprazole monohydrate	Abilify Maintena	300–400 mg monthly	Requires oral overlap during initiation	APA (2020)

Drug	Brand	Dose	Clinical Notes	Evidence Source
Aripiprazole lauroxil	Aristada	441–1064 mg every 4–8 weeks	Requires product-specific overlap or loading strategy	APA (2020)
Olanzapine pamoate	Zyprexa Relprevv	150–405 mg every 2–4 weeks	Requires post-injection monitoring for delirium/sedation syndrome (PDSS): administer only in a registered/restricted healthcare facility, with continuous observation by a healthcare professional for at least 3 hours after each injection	APA (2020); FDA (2017)
Fluphenazine decanoate	Prolixin Decanoate	Product-specific individualized dosing every 2–4 weeks	High-potency FGA LAI with significant EPS risk	APA (2020); NICE (2014, updated 2019)
Haloperidol decanoate	Haldol Decanoate	Product-specific individualized dosing every 4 weeks	Common FGA LAI; akathisia and EPS remain limiting	APA (2020); NICE (2014, updated 2019)

G. Augmentation

Clinical Scenario	Preferred Treatment	Rationale	Clinical Notes	Avoid / Caution	Evidence Source
Partial response to first antipsychotic	Switch to another antipsychotic monotherapy	Better supported than early polypharmacy	Reassess adherence, substance use, dose adequacy, and diagnosis first	Avoid reflexive dose escalation	APA (2020); NICE (2014, updated 2019)
Persistent symptoms with adherence concerns	Transition to an LAI	Addresses covert nonadherence and relapse risk	Useful with inconsistent oral adherence	Establish oral tolerability first when required	APA (2020); NICE (2014, updated 2019)
Severe agitation or insomnia during acute stabilization	Short-term adjunctive benzodiazepine	May reduce agitation while antipsychotic benefit emerges	Use short-term with frequent reassessment	Avoid chronic benzodiazepine continuation	APA (2020); NICE (2014, updated 2019)

H. Treatment-Resistant / Refractory Schizophrenia

Step	Preferred Treatment	Rationale	Clinical Notes	Avoid / Caution	Evidence Source
Failure of two adequate antipsychotic trials	Clozapine monotherapy	Most evidence-based treatment for resistant schizophrenia	Document dose, duration, and adherence; monitor ANC and major adverse effects	Avoid delaying clozapine with repeated ineffective trials	APA (2020); NICE (2014, updated 2019); Kane et al. (1988)
Incomplete response to optimized clozapine	Reassess dose, adherence, serum level, substance use, and diagnosis	Apparent nonresponse may reflect underexposure or comorbidity	Evaluate constipation, sedation, seizures, myocarditis risk, and smoking effects	Avoid labeling failure before optimization	APA (2020); NICE (2014, updated 2019)
Persistent severe symptoms despite optimized clozapine	Clozapine augmentation in selected specialist-managed cases	Augmentation evidence is mixed and generally modest	Use only with clear rationale and risk-benefit review	Routine augmentation is not strongly supported	APA (2020); Correll et al. (2017)

I. Risks / Monitoring

Monitoring Domain	Clinical Notes	Evidence Source
Weight and metabolic risk	Monitor weight/BMI, glucose or A1c, and lipids at baseline and periodically; risk highest with clozapine and olanzapine	American Diabetes Association & American Psychiatric Association (2004); APA (2020)
EPS and tardive dyskinesia	Assess regularly for parkinsonism, dystonia, akathisia, and tardive dyskinesia	APA (2020)
Prolactin-related effects	Monitor for amenorrhea, galactorrhea, sexual dysfunction, gynecomastia, and bone-related effects	APA (2020)
QTc risk	Use caution with ziprasidone, haloperidol, iloperidone, chlorpromazine, and QT-prolonging combinations	APA (2020); NICE (2014, updated 2019)

Monitoring Domain	Clinical Notes	Evidence Source
Clozapine hematologic and systemic adverse effects	Monitor ANC and watch for myocarditis, seizures, ileus/constipation, sedation, and metabolic syndrome. Start a proactive bowel regimen from initiation (clozapine-induced GI hypomotility can progress to ileus, bowel obstruction, and death); assess bowel function at each visit and treat constipation promptly	FDA labeling (2025); APA (2020)
Anticholinergic burden	Excess anticholinergic exposure may worsen cognition, constipation, urinary retention, blurred vision, and fall risk	Beers Criteria (2023); APA (2020)

J. Practical Treatment Selection

Clinical Scenario	Preferred Treatment	Rationale	Clinical Notes	Avoid / Caution	Evidence Source
First episode or uncomplicated schizophrenia	Antipsychotic monotherapy	Standard first-line treatment across guidelines	Select agent based on response history, comorbidities, adverse effects, and adherence factors	Avoid premature polypharmacy	APA (2020); NICE (2014, updated 2019)
Need to minimize extrapyramidal symptoms	Lower-EPS SGA (e.g., quetiapine)	Lower EPS liability than high-potency FGAs	Balance EPS benefit against sedation, orthostasis, and metabolic burden	Aripiprazole may cause akathisia; quetiapine may cause sedation and orthostasis	APA (2020); NICE (2014, updated 2019)
Prominent metabolic vulnerability	Lower-metabolic-risk agent (e.g., aripiprazole, ziprasidone, lurasidone, lumateperone)	May reduce cardiometabolic burden	Continue metabolic monitoring	Ziprasidone/ lurasidone require food; ziprasidone has QTc risk	APA (2020); Correll et al. (2020)
Prominent nonadherence or repeated relapse	Long-acting injectable antipsychotic	Improves treatment continuity and may reduce relapse	Discuss early in treatment course	Confirm oral tolerability when required	APA (2020); NICE (2014, updated 2019)

Clinical Scenario	Preferred Treatment	Rationale	Clinical Notes	Avoid / Caution	Evidence Source
Persistent symptoms after two adequate trials	Clozapine	Most evidence-supported treatment for resistant schizophrenia	Requires ANC monitoring and gradual titration	Avoid delaying clozapine with repeated ineffective trials	APA (2020); NICE (2014, updated 2019); Kane et al. (1988)
D2-intolerant patient or EPS/prolactin burden with prior SGAs	Xanomeline/ trospium (Cobenfy)	Non-D2 mechanism; no EPS or prolactin elevation	GI adverse effects common (nausea, vomiting, dyspepsia); titrate slowly; not yet established as first-line	Avoid in patients with active GI conditions or significant anticholinergic sensitivity	FDA (2024); Kaul et al. (2024)

2. SCHIZOAFFECTIVE DISORDER

A. OVERVIEW

Clinical Principle	Clinical Notes	Evidence Source
Antipsychotic treatment remains foundational	Management centers on antipsychotic therapy, with adjunctive treatment guided by mood pathology	APA (2020); NICE (2014, updated 2019)
Mood symptoms must be treated directly when clinically significant	Bipolar-type illness may require mood stabilizers; depressive-type illness may require antidepressant augmentation	APA (2020); NICE (2014, updated 2019)
Diagnostic clarification is essential	Differentiate schizoaffective disorder from schizophrenia or mood disorders with psychotic features by assessing the longitudinal relationship between mood and psychosis	DSM-5-TR (APA, 2022)

B. Diagnostic Considerations

Diagnostic Consideration	Clinical Notes	Evidence Source
Confirm uninterrupted illness with psychosis and mood syndrome	DSM-5-TR requires psychosis plus a major mood episode, with ≥2 weeks of psychosis without mood symptoms during the illness course	DSM-5-TR (APA, 2022)
Define bipolar type versus depressive type	Subtyping guides mood stabilizer- versus antidepressant-based treatment strategies	DSM-5-TR (APA, 2022)

Diagnostic Consideration	Clinical Notes	Evidence Source
Rule out substance-induced and medical causes	Substance use and medical illness may mimic psychotic/mood syndromes	DSM-5-TR (APA, 2022); APA (2020)
DSM-5-TR diagnostic threshold	Major mood episode concurrent with Criterion A, plus ≥2 weeks of psychosis without a major mood episode; mood symptoms present for the majority of total illness duration.	DSM-5-TR (APA, 2022)

C. First-Line Treatment

Clinical Scenario	Preferred Treatment	Rationale	Clinical Notes	Avoid / Caution	Evidence Source
Psychotic symptoms across subtypes	Antipsychotic	Foundational treatment for psychosis	Maintain antipsychotic coverage unless diagnosis changes	Avoid mood-only treatment when psychosis is persistent	APA (2020); NICE (2014, updated 2019)
Bipolar-type schizoaffective disorder	Antipsychotic plus mood stabilizer when indicated	Addresses mania, cycling, and mood instability	Lithium or valproate commonly used; lamotrigine more useful for bipolar depression	Monitor organ-specific risks and drug interactions	APA (2020); NICE (2014, updated 2019)
Depressive-type schizoaffective disorder	Antipsychotic plus antidepressant when indicated	Treats depressive symptoms while maintaining psychosis coverage	Monitor for activation, mixed symptoms, or diagnostic reconsideration	Avoid antidepressant monotherapy	APA (2020); NICE (2014, updated 2019)

D. Pharmacotherapy

Drug	Brand	Dose	Clinical Notes	Evidence Source
Paliperidone	Invega	3–12 mg/day	FDA-approved for schizoaffective disorder; oral and LAI forms available	FDA labeling
Risperidone	Risperdal	1–6 mg/day	Effective for psychosis; prolactin elevation and EPS increase at higher doses	APA (2020); Clinical consensus

Drug	Brand	Dose	Clinical Notes	Evidence Source
Quetiapine	Seroquel	300–800 mg/day	May help when depressive burden or EPS sensitivity is prominent; sedating and metabolically relevant	APA (2020); Clinical consensus
Olanzapine	Zyprexa	5–20 mg/day	Effective but associated with high metabolic burden	APA (2020); Clinical consensus
Aripiprazole	Abilify	10–30 mg/day	Lower metabolic burden; may help bipolar-spectrum symptoms; akathisia/activation may occur	APA (2020); Clinical consensus
Cariprazine	Vraylar	1.5–6 mg/day	Evidence extrapolated from schizophrenia RCTs; may help negative symptoms and bipolar-type presentations; akathisia common	APA (2020); Clinical consensus
Clozapine	Clozaril	200–900 mg/day	Reserve for treatment-resistant schizoaffective disorder; requires ongoing ANC monitoring (REMS enrollment discontinued June 13, 2025; ANC monitoring remains recommended per FDA prescribing information)	APA (2020); Kane et al. (1988)

Clinical note

With the exception of paliperidone, pharmacological recommendations for schizoaffective disorder are largely extrapolated from schizophrenia and bipolar disorder evidence. Treatment should be individualized based on predominant symptom polarity, prior response, and tolerability.

E. Second-Line / Augmentation

Clinical Scenario	Preferred Treatment	Rationale	Clinical Notes	Avoid / Caution	Evidence Source
Bipolar-type with inadequate mood control	Add mood stabilizer	Targets mania or persistent mood instability	Lithium may reduce suicide risk; valproate useful in mania; lamotrigine more useful for bipolar depression/maintenance	Monitor renal, thyroid, hepatic, hematologic, and teratogenic risks	APA (2020); NICE (2014, updated 2019)
Depressive-type with persistent depression	Add antidepressant to antipsychotic	Treats depression while maintaining psychosis coverage	Reassess if activation, mood switching, or worsening psychosis occurs	Avoid antidepressant monotherapy	APA (2020); NICE (2014, updated 2019)

F. Risks / Monitoring

Monitoring Domain	Clinical Notes	Evidence Source
Mood switching or activation	Particularly relevant when antidepressants are used in bipolar-type or diagnostically uncertain presentations	APA (2020); Clinical consensus
Antipsychotic metabolic and neurologic burden	Monitoring principles parallel schizophrenia treatment	APA (2020); American Diabetes Association & American Psychiatric Association (2004)
Mood stabilizer-specific toxicity	Lithium requires renal, thyroid, and serum monitoring; valproate requires LFTs/platelets; lamotrigine requires slow titration and rash monitoring	APA (2020); Clinical consensus

G. Practical Treatment Selection

Clinical Scenario	Preferred Treatment	Rationale	Clinical Notes	Avoid / Caution	Evidence Source
Bipolar-type schizoaffective disorder with recurrent mania	Antipsychotic plus mood stabilizer	Addresses psychosis and recurrent mood instability	Lithium or valproate commonly used based on comorbidity and tolerability	Avoid antidepressant-led strategy	APA (2020); Clinical consensus
Depressive-type schizoaffective disorder with persistent depressive syndrome	Antipsychotic plus antidepressant	Treats depression while preserving psychosis control	Monitor for activation or emerging manic features	Avoid antidepressant monotherapy	APA (2020); Clinical consensus
Recurrent nonadherence	LAI antipsychotic-based regimen	Supports continuity of treatment	Particularly useful with unreliable oral adherence	Ensure mood treatment remains subtype-concordant	APA (2020); Clinical consensus

3. DELUSIONAL DISORDER

A. OVERVIEW

Clinical Principle	Clinical Notes	Evidence Source
Lower antipsychotic doses may be sufficient	Patients may respond to and better tolerate lower doses than those used in schizophrenia	APA (2020); NICE CG178 (2014, updated 2019); Clinical consensus
Therapeutic alliance is central	Early direct confrontation of fixed beliefs is often counterproductive; focus on distress, safety, and functioning	APA (2020); NICE CG178 (2014, updated 2019); Clinical consensus
Rule out medical and substance causes carefully	Delusional syndromes may be secondary to neurologic, endocrine, substance-related, or neurocognitive disorders	DSM-5-TR (APA, 2022); APA (2020)

B. Diagnostic Considerations

Diagnostic Consideration	Clinical Notes	Evidence Source
Confirm delusional disorder phenomenology	Functioning may remain relatively preserved outside the delusional system	DSM-5-TR (APA, 2022)
Exclude schizophrenia-spectrum features suggestive of another diagnosis	Marked disorganization, persistent non-thematic hallucinations, or prominent negative symptoms may indicate schizophrenia	DSM-5-TR (APA, 2022)
Assess comorbid depression and anxiety	Mood and anxiety symptoms commonly contribute to distress and help-seeking	APA (2020); Clinical consensus

C. First-Line Treatment

Clinical Scenario	Preferred Treatment	Rationale	Clinical Notes	Avoid / Caution	Evidence Source
Delusional disorder with distress or functional impairment	Low-dose antipsychotic + supportive alliance-based care	May reduce conviction, preoccupation, or behavioral consequences	Titrate gradually and focus on distress/functioning rather than directly challenging beliefs	Avoid early confrontational approaches	APA (2020); NICE CG178 (2014, updated 2019); Clinical consensus
Prominent comorbid depression/anxiety	Treat comorbidity when clearly present	Reduces overall distress and functional burden	Antidepressants may be appropriate for true depressive or anxiety disorders	Monitor for activation or worsening suspiciousness	APA (2020); DSM-5-TR (APA, 2022)

D. Pharmacotherapy

Drug	Brand	Dose	Clinical Notes	Evidence Source
Risperidone	Risperdal	0.5–4 mg/day	Commonly used; often effective at lower doses than those used in schizophrenia	Limited evidence; Clinical consensus
Aripiprazole	Abilify	5–20 mg/day	Lower metabolic burden; akathisia or activation may occur	Limited evidence; Clinical consensus
Olanzapine	Zyprexa	5–15 mg/day	Effective but limited by weight gain and metabolic burden	Limited evidence; Clinical consensus
Haloperidol	Haldol	2–10 mg/day	Effective but EPS and tardive dyskinesia risk may limit tolerability	Limited evidence; Clinical consensus

Clinical note

No randomized controlled trials exist specifically for delusional disorder. Pharmacological recommendations are based on case reports, case series, and clinical consensus. Antipsychotic response rates are inconsistent and adherence is often a significant challenge.

E. Practical Treatment Selection

Clinical Scenario	Preferred Treatment	Rationale	Clinical Notes	Avoid / Caution	Evidence Source
Older or medically fragile patient	Lowest effective dose with slow titration	Reduces adverse-effect burden	Orthostasis, EPS, sedation, and anticholinergic effects are more clinically relevant	Avoid aggressive titration	Limited evidence; Clinical consensus; Beers Criteria (2023)
Strong suspiciousness and poor alliance	Lower-dose, better-tolerated option with supportive framing	Improves treatment acceptability and adherence	Emphasize distress reduction, sleep, and functioning	Avoid directly challenging delusional beliefs early	Limited evidence; Clinical consensus

4. BRIEF PSYCHOTIC DISORDER/ACUTE PSYCHOSIS

A. OVERVIEW

Clinical Principle	Clinical Notes	Evidence Source
Safety and level-of-care assessment come first	Assess suicidality, homicidality, severe disorganization, inability to care for self, agitation, medical instability, and support reliability	APA (2020); DSM-5-TR (APA, 2022)
Hospitalize when outpatient care is unsafe	Inpatient treatment is indicated when risk, impairment, or diagnostic uncertainty exceeds outpatient capacity	APA (2020); NICE (2014, updated 2019)
Antipsychotic treatment is generally short term with frequent reassessment	Duration depends on diagnosis evolution, remission, recurrence risk, and tolerability	APA (2020); NICE (2014, updated 2019)

B. Diagnostic Considerations

Diagnostic Consideration	Clinical Notes	Evidence Source
Clarify diagnostic subtype	Differentiate brief psychotic disorder from substance-induced psychosis, mania with psychosis, delirium, or first-episode schizophrenia-spectrum illness	DSM-5-TR (APA, 2022); APA (2020)
Assess for medical precipitants	Rule out fever, intoxication, withdrawal, autoimmune, neurologic, and endocrine causes when indicated	DSM-5-TR (APA, 2022)
Review supports and supervision	Outpatient care requires reliable monitoring, medication access, and rapid follow-up	APA (2020); NICE (2014, updated 2019)
DSM-5-TR diagnostic threshold	At least one positive psychotic symptom lasting ≥1 day but <1 month, with eventual full return to premorbid level of functioning.	DSM-5-TR (APA, 2022)

C. First-Line Treatment

Clinical Scenario	Preferred Treatment	Rationale	Clinical Notes	Avoid / Caution	Evidence Source
Acute psychosis manageable outpatient	Antipsychotic + very close follow-up	Reduces psychotic symptoms while diagnosis evolves	Follow-up should be prompt and repeated; involve supports when possible	Avoid outpatient management if reliability is poor	APA (2020); NICE (2014, updated 2019)
Severe agitation	Antipsychotic + short-term benzodiazepine when necessary	Reduces acute behavioral dysregulation and immediate risk	Use in a documented, time-limited manner	Avoid chronic benzodiazepine continuation	APA (2020); NICE (2014, updated 2019)
Any meaningful safety compromise	Hospitalization	Provides stabilization and diagnostic clarification	Includes dangerousness, severe agitation, inability to care for self, or absent support	Do not force outpatient treatment when unsafe	APA (2020); NICE (2014, updated 2019)

D. Pharmacotherapy

Drug	Brand	Dose	Clinical Notes	Evidence Source
Risperidone	Risperdal	1–4 mg/day	Practical first-line option for acute psychosis; monitor prolactin and EPS at higher doses	APA (2020); NICE (2014, updated 2019)
Olanzapine	Zyprexa	5–15 mg/day	May help when sedation is clinically useful; metabolic burden remains relevant	APA (2020); NICE (2014, updated 2019)
Aripiprazole	Abilify	10–20 mg/day	Lower metabolic burden; less sedating; akathisia or activation may limit tolerability	APA (2020); NICE (2014, updated 2019)
Haloperidol	Haldol	2–10 mg/day	Effective for acute agitation and psychosis; EPS and QTc caution apply	APA (2020); NICE (2014, updated 2019)
Quetiapine	Seroquel	150–400 mg/day	Lower EPS burden; useful when anxiety or insomnia prominent; sedating; monitor orthostasis	Clinical consensus
Ziprasidone	Geodon	40–160 mg/day	Lower metabolic burden; take with food; monitor QTc; IM formulation available for acute agitation	Clinical consensus

Clinical note

No randomized controlled trials exist specifically for brief psychotic disorder. Pharmacological recommendations are extrapolated from acute psychosis and schizophrenia treatment frameworks. Treatment duration should be reassessed frequently given the expected short course of illness.

E. Practical Treatment Selection

Clinical Scenario	Preferred Treatment	Rationale	Clinical Notes	Avoid / Caution	Evidence Source
Need sedation and strong acute calming effect	Olanzapine or haloperidol depending on presentation	Often useful for agitation and acute psychosis	Balance EPS risk against sedation/metabolic burden	Avoid long-term continuation without reassessment	APA (2020); NICE (2014, updated 2019)

Clinical Scenario	Preferred Treatment	Rationale	Clinical Notes	Avoid / Caution	Evidence Source
Concern about longer-term metabolic risk during evolving diagnosis	Aripiprazole or risperidone depending on presentation	More practical when ongoing treatment may be needed	Monitor for akathisia with aripiprazole	Frequent reassessment remains essential	APA (2020); NICE (2014, updated 2019)

5. CLOZAPINE PROTOCOL SUMMARY

A. OVERVIEW

Clinical Principle	Clinical Notes	Evidence Source
Clozapine is the gold-standard treatment for treatment-resistant schizophrenia	Use after failure of ≥2 adequate antipsychotic trials with documented adherence	APA (2020); NICE (2014, updated 2019); Kane et al. (1988)
Clozapine requires structured monitoring infrastructure	Hematologic, cardiovascular, neurologic, gastrointestinal, and metabolic risks require close follow-up	APA (2020); FDA REMS
Slow titration improves tolerability and safety	Gradual titration reduces risk of orthostasis, oversedation, and early adverse effects	APA (2020); FDA REMS

B. First-Line Use Case

Clinical Scenario	Preferred Treatment	Rationale	Clinical Notes	Avoid / Caution	Evidence Source
Treatment-resistant schizophrenia	Clozapine	Most evidence-supported treatment after failure of two adequate antipsychotic trials	Document prior trials, dose, duration, adherence, and outcome carefully	Avoid delaying clozapine through repeated ineffective alternatives	APA (2020); NICE (2014, updated 2019); Kane et al. (1988)

C. Operational Requirements

Requirement	Clinical Notes	Evidence Source
REMS enrollment	REMS enrollment no longer required (eliminated June 13, 2025); ANC monitoring strongly recommended per FDA prescribing information	FDA labeling (2025); APA (2020)
ANC monitoring	Weekly for first 6 months, every 2 weeks for next 6 months, then monthly if eligible	FDA labeling (2025); APA (2020)
Documentation of treatment resistance	Record prior antipsychotic trials, doses, duration, adherence, and reasons for failure	APA (2020); NICE (2014, updated 2019)
Metabolic monitoring	Obtain baseline and periodic weight/BMI, glucose or A1c, and lipid profile	American Diabetes Association & American Psychiatric Association (2004); APA (2020)
Constipation surveillance	Severe constipation and ileus may be life-threatening; proactive bowel management is essential	FDA REMS; APA (2020)
Myocarditis and seizure vigilance. Obtain baseline and weekly CRP and troponin during the first ~4 weeks of clozapine treatment; evaluate promptly if cardiac symptoms occur	Monitor clinically during titration; seizure risk increases with higher doses and rapid titration	Ronaldson et al. (2011); Leung et al. (2023); Clinical consensus

D. Practical Treatment Selection

Clinical Scenario	Preferred Treatment	Rationale	Clinical Notes	Avoid / Caution	Evidence Source
Persistent psychosis after two adequate trials	Clozapine initiation	Best chance of meaningful response in treatment resistance	Educate patient and family regarding monitoring, constipation, fever, chest pain, sedation, and smoking-related level changes	Avoid clozapine without monitoring capacity	APA (2020); NICE (2014, updated 2019); Kane et al. (1988)

Clinical Scenario	Preferred Treatment	Rationale	Clinical Notes	Avoid / Caution	Evidence Source
Partial response after clozapine initiation	Optimize clozapine before augmentation	Many apparent nonresponses reflect underdosing, nonadherence, or inadequate time	Plasma levels may help when available	Avoid premature augmentation	APA (2020); NICE (2014, updated 2019)

E. Dosing Protocol

Phase	Dose	Clinical Notes	Evidence Source
Initiation	12.5–25 mg/day	Start low to minimize orthostasis, oversedation, and early adverse effects	APA (2020); FDA labeling
Titration	Increase by 25–50 mg/day every 1–2 days as tolerated	Slower titration recommended in elderly, medically compromised, or highly sensitive patients	APA (2020); FDA labeling
Therapeutic range	200–450 mg/day	Most patients respond within this range; divide doses BID or TID	APA (2020); FDA labeling
Maximum dose	Up to 900 mg/day in refractory cases	Use only with clear clinical justification and specialist oversight	FDA labeling
Plasma level target	≥250 ng/mL; optimal response often at ≥350 ng/mL	Plasma level monitoring recommended when response is suboptimal or toxicity is suspected	APA (2020); Clinical consensus

REFERENCES

American Diabetes Association, & American Psychiatric Association. (2004). Consensus development conference on antipsychotic drugs and obesity and diabetes. *Diabetes Care*, *27*(2), 596–601. https://doi.org/10.2337/diacare.27.2.596

American Geriatrics Society Beers Criteria® Update Expert Panel. (2023). American Geriatrics Society 2023 updated AGS Beers Criteria® for potentially inappropriate medication use in older adults. *Journal of the American Geriatrics Society*, *71*(7), 2052–2081. https://doi.org/10.1111/jgs.18372

American Psychiatric Association. (2020). *The American Psychiatric Association practice guideline for the treatment of patients with schizophrenia* (3rd ed.). American Psychiatric Publishing.

American Psychiatric Association. (2022). *Diagnostic and statistical manual of mental disorders* (5th ed., text rev.; DSM-5-TR). American Psychiatric Publishing.

Correll, C. U., Rubio, J. M., Inczedy-Farkas, G., Birnbaum, M. L., Kane, J. M., & Leucht, S. (2017). Efficacy and safety of antipsychotic combinations for schizophrenia: A meta-analysis of randomized controlled trials. *JAMA Psychiatry, 74*(7), 675–684. https://doi.org/10.1001/jamapsychiatry.2017.0624

Correll, C. U., Davis, R. E., Weingart, M., Saillard, J., O'Gorman, C., Kane, J. M., & Vanover, K. E. (2020). Efficacy and safety of lumateperone for treatment of schizophrenia: A randomized clinical trial. *JAMA Psychiatry, 77*(4), 349–358. https://doi.org/10.1001/jamapsychiatry.2019.4379

Janssen Pharmaceuticals. (2024). *Erzofri (paliperidone palmitate) prescribing information*.

Kaul, I., Sawchak, S., Walling, D. P., Tamminga, C. A., Breier, A., Zhu, H., Miller, A. C., Paul, S. M., & Brannan, S. K. (2024). Efficacy and safety of xanomeline-trospium chloride in schizophrenia: A randomized clinical trial. *JAMA Psychiatry, 81*(8), 749–756. https://doi.org/10.1001/jamapsychiatry.2024.0785

Kane, J., Honigfeld, G., Singer, J., & Meltzer, H. (1988). Clozapine for the treatment-resistant schizophrenic: A double-blind comparison with chlorpromazine. *Archives of General Psychiatry, 45*(9), 789–796. https://doi.org/10.1001/archpsyc.1988.01800330013001

National Institute for Health and Care Excellence. (2014). *Psychosis and schizophrenia in adults: Prevention and management (CG178)*. Updated 2019. https://www.nice.org.uk/guidance/cg178

U.S. Food and Drug Administration. (2017). *Zyprexa Relprevv (olanzapine pamoate) prescribing information*. https://www.accessdata.fda.gov

U.S. Food and Drug Administration. (2024). *Cobenfy (xanomeline and trospium chloride) prescribing information*. https://www.accessdata.fda.gov

U.S. Food and Drug Administration. (2024). *Erzofri (paliperidone palmitate) prescribing information*. https://www.accessdata.fda.gov

U.S. Food and Drug Administration. (2025). *Discontinuation of the Clozapine REMS program (effective June 13, 2025)*. Absolute neutrophil count monitoring remains recommended per FDA prescribing information.

U.S. Food and Drug Administration. (n.d.). *Clozapine prescribing information (package insert)*. https://www.accessdata.fda.gov

IX. NEUROCOGNITIVE DISORDERS

SECTION INTRODUCTION

Neurocognitive disorders comprise a group of conditions characterized by acquired decline in cognitive functioning affecting memory, attention, executive functioning, language, visuospatial ability, learning, processing speed, social cognition, or overall adaptive functioning. These disorders are associated with progressive or clinically significant impairment in independence, occupational functioning, medication management, financial decision-making, interpersonal functioning, and overall quality of life. Neurocognitive disorders frequently require multidisciplinary management because of their complex interaction with medical illness, psychiatric symptoms, neurologic deterioration, caregiver burden, and functional decline.

Major and mild neurocognitive disorders become increasingly prevalent with advancing age and represent a growing public health concern due to population aging and increasing life expectancy. Alzheimer's disease remains the most common cause of neurocognitive decline, although vascular disease, Lewy body disease, Parkinson's disease, traumatic brain injury, frontotemporal degeneration, substance-related conditions, HIV-associated neurocognitive disorder, and other medical or neurologic illnesses may also contribute to cognitive impairment. Early recognition and diagnostic clarification are essential because selected causes of cognitive decline may be partially reversible or modifiable when appropriately identified.

The clinical presentation of neurocognitive disorders is highly heterogeneous and depends on the underlying etiology, severity of impairment, premorbid functioning, medical comorbidity, and psychosocial support system. Patients may present with progressive memory loss, executive dysfunction, language impairment, impaired judgment, behavioral changes, personality changes, visuospatial deficits, disorientation, apathy, hallucinations, agitation, or reduced ability to perform activities of daily living. In many cases, family members or caregivers initially recognize functional decline before the patient demonstrates insight into symptoms.

Differential diagnosis remains critically important because psychiatric conditions may mimic or worsen cognitive impairment. Depression, bipolar disorder, psychosis, substance use disorders, delirium, sleep disorders, medication adverse effects, sensory impairment, thyroid disease, vitamin deficiencies, neurologic illness, and chronic medical conditions may contribute to reversible or partially reversible cognitive symptoms. Comprehensive evaluation should therefore include psychiatric assessment, neurologic review, medication reconciliation, laboratory testing, collateral information, and consideration of neuroimaging or formal neuropsychological testing when clinically indicated.

Behavioral and psychiatric symptoms frequently coexist with neurocognitive disorders and may substantially increase caregiver burden, institutionalization risk, hospitalization, and safety concerns. Agitation, psychosis, wandering, impulsivity, sleep disturbance, depression, anxiety, disinhibition, and aggression are common across multiple dementia syndromes and often require careful behavioral and pharmacologic management. Clinicians should remain particularly cautious regarding antipsychotic use in elderly populations because of increased risks of cerebrovascular events, sedation, falls, metabolic complications, and mortality in dementia-related psychosis.

Assessment of safety and functional capacity represents a core component of neurocognitive evaluation. Important clinical considerations include driving safety, medication adherence, financial vulnerability, fall risk, firearms access, wandering behavior, caregiver support, elder abuse risk, and ability to perform activities of daily living. Advance care planning, caregiver education, and long-term support planning should be incorporated early in the course of illness whenever possible.

Although current pharmacologic treatments provide limited disease-modifying benefit for most neurodegenerative conditions, medications such as cholinesterase inhibitors and memantine may provide symptomatic benefit in selected patients. Equally important are nonpharmacologic interventions including cognitive support strategies, sleep regulation, environmental modification, caregiver education, structured routines, sensory optimization, and management of medical comorbidities. Treatment planning should remain individualized and should balance symptom management, quality of life, safety, tolerability, and preservation of functional independence.

The following sections provide a structured, evidence-informed framework for the evaluation and treatment of neurocognitive disorders within outpatient psychiatric practice. Recommendations are intended to support safe, compassionate, and clinically individualized care while recognizing the importance of longitudinal reassessment, interdisciplinary collaboration, caregiver involvement, and professional clinical judgment throughout the course of illness.

1. MAJOR NEUROCOGNITIVE DISORDER DUE TO ALZHEIMER'S DISEASE (ALZHEIMER DEMENTIA)

A. OVERVIEW

Aspect	Clinical Notes	Evidence Source
Definition	Progressive neurocognitive disorder with decline in memory and other cognitive domains sufficient to impair independence; Alzheimer's disease is the most common cause of major neurocognitive disorder	DSM-5-TR (APA, 2022); NICE (2018)
Core features	Gradual progressive decline in memory, language, executive function, visuospatial ability, and daily functioning; behavioral symptoms may emerge over time	DSM-5-TR (APA, 2022); NICE (2018)
Clinical importance	Major contributor to disability, caregiver burden, institutionalization, and mortality; early recognition supports safety planning and caregiver support	APA Dementia Guideline (2016); NICE (2018)
Treatment approach	Management includes diagnostic clarification, non-pharmacologic support, caregiver education, and selected cognitive enhancers; medication benefits are generally modest	APA Dementia Guideline (2016); NICE (2018); NICE (2022)

B. Diagnostic Considerations

Consideration	Clinical Notes	Evidence Source
Confirm diagnosis with standardized cognitive testing	Use validated tools (e.g., MMSE, MoCA, SLUMS) to establish baseline and monitor progression	APA Dementia Guideline (2016); DSM-5-TR (APA, 2022); NICE (2018)
Rule out reversible or contributing causes	Evaluate B12 deficiency, thyroid dysfunction, syphilis, medication effects, and consider neuroimaging when indicated	APA Dementia Guideline (2016); NICE (2018)
Assess for behavioral and psychological symptoms	Screen for agitation, psychosis, depression, and sleep disturbance, which often drive morbidity and treatment decisions	APA Dementia Guideline (2016); NICE (2018)
Evaluate caregiver stress and support systems	Caregiver burden strongly affects outcomes, safety, and level-of-care needs	APA Dementia Guideline (2016); NICE (2018)
Assess for delirium	Acute or fluctuating cognitive changes suggest delirium; evaluate for infection, medications, metabolic disturbances, or acute illness	DSM-5-TR (APA, 2022); NICE (2018)

C. Pharmacotherapy for Cognitive Symptoms

C.1. Cholinesterase Inhibitors

Generic	Brand	Dose Range	Clinical Notes	Evidence Source
Donepezil	Aricept	5–23 mg/day	Once-daily dosing; start 5 mg/day for 4–6 weeks, then increase to 10 mg/day; monitor bradycardia, syncope, and GI effects. The 23 mg/day dose is reserved for moderate-to-severe Alzheimer's disease and only after at least 3 months of stability on 10 mg/day	NICE NG97 (2018)
Rivastigmine (transdermal)	Exelon Patch	4.6–13.3 mg/24h	Patch formulation may reduce GI side effects; useful with poor oral tolerance; monitor weight loss and bradycardia	APA Dementia Guideline (2016); NICE (2018)
Galantamine ER	Razadyne ER	8–24 mg/day	Extended-release once daily; titrate gradually; monitor GI effects, hydration, and bradycardia. Reduce the dose in moderate renal or hepatic impairment (maximum 16 mg/day) and avoid in severe impairment (CrCl <9 mL/min or Child-Pugh C)	APA Dementia Guideline (2016); NICE (2018)

Clinical note

All cholinesterase inhibitors are equally efficacious. Choice depends on tolerability, dosing convenience, and caregiver preference

C.2. NMDA Receptor Antagonist (Moderate – Severe)

Generic	Brand	Dose Range	Clinical Notes	Evidence Source
Memantine	Namenda	5–20 mg/day	NMDA receptor antagonist; titrate gradually to target dose; may provide modest cognitive, functional, and behavioral benefit; can be combined with cholinesterase inhibitors	APA Dementia Guideline (2016); NICE (2018)

D. Combination Strategies

Base Treatment	Add-On	Clinical Notes	Evidence Source
Cholinesterase inhibitor (e.g., donepezil, rivastigmine, galantamine)	Memantine	Consider in moderate–severe Alzheimer's disease; combination may provide modest additional cognitive and functional benefit	APA Dementia Guideline (2016); NICE (2018)
Donepezil	Memantine ER (fixed-dose combination)	Fixed-dose combination may simplify regimen and improve adherence	APA Dementia Guideline (2016); NICE (2018); Tariot et al. (2004)

Clinical note

Combination therapy shows modest benefit in cognition and function compared to monotherapy.

E. Avoid or Use with Caution in Alzheimer's Dementia

Strategy	Clinical Notes	Evidence Source
Routine dual cholinesterase inhibitor use	No added benefit; increased cholinergic adverse effects (bradycardia, syncope, nausea, diarrhea)	APA Dementia Guideline (2016); NICE (2018)
Escalating cognitive enhancers without reassessment	May overlook nonadherence, adverse effects, delirium, or disease progression	APA Dementia Guideline (2016); NICE (2018)
Anticholinergic medications	May worsen cognition and increase delirium, constipation, urinary retention, and fall risk	APA Dementia Guideline (2016); NICE (2018); Beers Criteria (2023)
Benzodiazepine use	Increased risk of falls, sedation, cognitive impairment, and delirium	APA Dementia Guideline (2016); NICE (2018); Beers Criteria (2023)
Cholinesterase inhibitors in cardiac conduction disease, active or prior peptic ulcer or GI bleeding, COPD/asthma, or seizure history	Use with caution: may cause symptomatic bradycardia, syncope, or AV block; increased gastric acid secretion and GI bleeding risk; bronchoconstriction; and lowered seizure threshold. Assess cardiac and GI risk before initiation.	FDA labeling; APA Dementia Guideline (2016)

2. MILD NEUROCOGNITIVE DISORDER (MCI)

A. OVERVIEW

Aspect	Clinical Notes	Evidence Source
Definition	Mild neurocognitive disorder involves modest decline in one or more cognitive domains without loss of independence, though compensatory strategies may be needed	DSM-5-TR (APA, 2022)
Core features	Subjective and objective cognitive decline with preserved basic functioning and absence of major neurocognitive disorder	DSM-5-TR (APA, 2022); NICE (2018)
Clinical importance	MCI may remain stable, improve if reversible causes are treated, or progress to major neurocognitive disorder	APA Dementia Guideline (2016); NICE (2018)
Treatment approach	Focus on diagnostic clarification, treatment of reversible causes, vascular/lifestyle optimization, and longitudinal monitoring; pharmacotherapy is not routinely recommended	APA Dementia Guideline (2016); NICE (2018)

B. Core Principles

Principle	Clinical Notes	Evidence Source
Focus on diagnostic clarity and reversible causes	Evaluate B12 deficiency, thyroid dysfunction, medication effects, depression, and sleep disorders; distinguish MCI from normal aging or early dementia	APA Dementia Guideline (2016); DSM-5-TR (APA, 2022); NICE (2018)
Address vascular risk factors	Optimize hypertension, diabetes, dyslipidemia, and smoking cessation to reduce dementia progression risk	APA Dementia Guideline (2016); NICE (2018)
Optimize sleep, hearing, and vision	Treat sleep disorders, correct sensory deficits, and review cognition-impairing medications	APA Dementia Guideline (2016); NICE (2018)
Encourage cognitive, physical, and social activity	Cognitive stimulation, exercise, and social engagement may help support cognition and delay decline	APA Dementia Guideline (2016); NICE (2018)

Clinical note

Pharmacotherapy is not routinely recommended for mild neurocognitive disorder. Management focuses on diagnostic clarification, treatment of reversible contributors, vascular/lifestyle optimization, cognitive and physical activity, and longitudinal monitoring. Cognitive enhancers should generally be reserved for selected specialist-guided cases.

Emerging Therapies Note:

Anti-amyloid monoclonal antibodies (lecanemab [Leqembi], FDA 2023; donanemab [Kisunla], FDA 2024) are approved for early symptomatic Alzheimer's disease with confirmed amyloid pathology. Use is currently limited to specialized settings because of infusion requirements,

ARIA monitoring, and restricted trial generalizability. These agents are outside the scope of this manual's routine pharmacotherapy framework. — *FDA (2023, 2024); van Dyck et al. (2023); Sims et al. (2023)*

3. VASCULAR NEUROCOGNITIVE DISORDER (VASCULAR DEMENTIA)

A. OVERVIEW

Aspect	Clinical Notes	Evidence Source
Definition	Neurocognitive disorder caused by cerebrovascular disease, often with stepwise or mixed progression linked to vascular injury	DSM-5-TR (APA, 2022)
Core features	Executive dysfunction, slowed processing, attention deficits, gait impairment, and focal neurologic findings may predominate; memory loss may be less prominent early	DSM-5-TR (APA, 2022); NICE (2018)
Clinical importance	Frequently coexists with Alzheimer pathology; management emphasizes vascular risk reduction and stroke prevention	APA Dementia Guideline (2016); NICE (2018)
Treatment approach	Focus on vascular risk-factor control, secondary stroke prevention, rehabilitation, and supportive care; cognitive enhancers may help selected mixed-pathology cases	APA Dementia Guideline (2016); NICE (2018)

B. Core Principles

Principle	Clinical Notes	Evidence Source
Primary management is vascular risk control	Optimize hypertension, diabetes, dyslipidemia, and smoking cessation; emphasize secondary stroke prevention	APA Dementia Guideline (2016); NICE (2022)
Use guideline-directed vascular therapies	Use antiplatelets, antihypertensives, statins, and glycemic control when indicated	APA Dementia Guideline (2016); NICE (2018)
Consider Alzheimer's cognitive agents in mixed pathology	Cholinesterase inhibitors or memantine may help selected mixed Alzheimer's/vascular cases, though benefits are modest	APA Dementia Guideline (2016); NICE (2018)

4. LEWY BODY DEMENTIA (LBD) / PARKINSON'S DISEASE DEMENTIA (PDD)

A. OVERVIEW

Aspect	Clinical Notes	Evidence Source
Definition	Progressive neurocognitive disorders associated with Lewy body pathology; timing of cognitive versus motor symptoms helps distinguish LBD from PDD	DSM-5-TR (APA, 2022); McKeith et al. (2017)

Aspect	Clinical Notes	Evidence Source
Core features	Fluctuating cognition, visual hallucinations, REM sleep behavior disorder, parkinsonism, and attentional/executive dysfunction	McKeith et al. (2017); NICE (2018)
Clinical importance	Marked antipsychotic sensitivity may cause severe EPS worsening, sedation, autonomic decline, or neuroleptic malignant syndrome	McKeith et al. (2017); APA Dementia Guideline (2016); NICE (2018)
Treatment approach	Emphasize cholinesterase inhibitors, minimization of offending medications, and highly cautious antipsychotic use only for severe dangerous symptoms	McKeith et al. (2017); APA Dementia Guideline (2016); NICE (2018)

B. Core Principles

Principle	Clinical Notes	Evidence Source
High sensitivity to dopamine blockade	Antipsychotics may cause severe EPS, sedation, or neuroleptic malignant syndrome; avoid typical antipsychotics	APA Dementia Guideline (2016); NICE (2018); McKeith et al. (2017)
If antipsychotics are required, use extreme caution	Reserve for severe dangerous psychosis/agitation; start low, titrate slowly, and prefer lower-EPS agents such as quetiapine	APA Dementia Guideline (2016); NICE (2018); McKeith et al. (2017)
Cholinesterase inhibitors are first-line cognitive therapy	Rivastigmine and related agents may improve cognition, attention, and hallucinations	APA Dementia Guideline (2016); NICE (2018); McKeith et al. (2017)

Clinical note

Antipsychotics in LBD/PDD can cause severe, irreversible Parkinsonism and increased mortality.

5. AGITATION ASSOCIATED WITH DEMENTIA DUE TO ALZHEIMER'S DISEASE

A. OVERVIEW

Aspect	Clinical Notes	Evidence Source
Definition	Agitation in dementia involves excessive motor activity, aggression, or emotional distress not better explained by delirium, pain, or another untreated cause	APA Dementia Guideline (2016); DSM-5-TR (APA, 2022)
Core features	Restlessness, verbal/physical aggression, resistance to care, disinhibition, or distress impairing safety or care	APA Dementia Guideline (2016); NICE (2018)
Clinical importance	Major contributor to caregiver burden, institutionalization, emergency visits, and unsafe antipsychotic use	APA Dementia Guideline (2016); NICE (2018)

Aspect	Clinical Notes	Evidence Source
Treatment approach	Rule out delirium, pain, medical triggers, and environmental precipitants first; prioritize non-pharmacologic strategies and reserve medication for severe or dangerous symptoms	APA Dementia Guideline (2016); NICE (2018)

B. Core Principles

Principle	Clinical Notes	Evidence Source
Always rule out delirium and medical causes first	Evaluate infection, pain, constipation, dehydration, medication effects, and metabolic disturbances; acute changes should be presumed delirium until excluded	APA Dementia Guideline (2016); DSM-5-TR (APA, 2022); NICE (2018)
Prioritize non-pharmacologic interventions	Use behavioral/environmental strategies, caregiver education, structured routines, and trigger reduction before medication	APA Dementia Guideline (2016); NICE (2018)
Reserve pharmacologic treatment for severe or dangerous symptoms	Use medication only for severe, persistent agitation/aggression causing major distress or safety risk; use the lowest effective dose for the shortest duration	APA Dementia Guideline (2016); NICE (2018)

C. FDA-Approved Option (First Approval for This Indication)

Generic	Brand	Dose Range	Clinical Notes	Evidence Source
Brexpiprazole	Rexulti	0.5–3 mg/day	FDA-approved for agitation associated with Alzheimer's dementia; scheduled (not PRN) dosing; titrate gradually to target 2 mg/day; monitor akathisia, sedation, and metabolic effects; boxed warning for increased mortality in elderly patients with dementia-related psychosis	FDA Labeling (2023); APA Dementia Guideline (2016)

Clinical note

Increased mortality in elderly patients with dementia-related psychosis. Not approved for dementia-related psychosis without agitation.

D. Other Antipsychotics (Off-Label)

Generic	Brand	Geriatric Dose Range	Clinical Notes	Evidence Source
Risperidone	Risperdal	0.25–2 mg/day	Most evidence among off-label agents for BPSD; reserve for severe agitation or psychosis; monitor EPS, prolactin, stroke, and mortality risk	APA Dementia Guideline (2016); NICE (2018)
Olanzapine	Zyprexa	2.5–10 mg/day	May reduce agitation and psychosis; high risk of sedation, weight gain, and metabolic effects; increased stroke/mortality risk in dementia	APA Dementia Guideline (2016); NICE (2018)
Quetiapine	Seroquel	12.5–200 mg/day	Lower EPS risk; often preferred with parkinsonism or Lewy body dementia; monitor orthostasis and sedation	APA Dementia Guideline (2016); NICE (2018)
Haloperidol	Haldol	0.5–5 mg/day	High EPS and QTc risk; reserve for severe acute agitation and short-term use only	APA Dementia Guideline (2016); NICE (2018)

Clinical note

All antipsychotics carry the same black box warning for increased mortality in elderly dementia patients. FDA labeling; APA Dementia Guideline (2016)

E. Combination Strategies

Base Treatment	Add-On	Clinical Notes	Evidence Source
Non-pharmacologic interventions + medical trigger management	Brexpiprazole (Rexulti)	Consider only for persistent severe agitation after failure of non-pharmacologic measures and correction of underlying causes; document rationale carefully	FDA Labeling (2023); NICE (2018)
Brexpiprazole (Rexulti)	Cholinesterase inhibitor or memantine	May address both cognitive and behavioral symptoms in moderate–severe disease; reassess regularly for cumulative adverse effects	APA Dementia Guideline (2016); NICE (2018)
Off-label antipsychotic	Cholinesterase inhibitor or memantine	Consider for persistent severe agitation or psychosis despite cognitive therapy; use lowest effective dose and reassess frequently	APA Dementia Guideline (2016); NICE (2018)

F. Avoid or Use with Caution in Agitation in Alzheimer's

Strategy	Clinical Notes	Evidence Source
Concurrent use of two antipsychotics	No clear added benefit; increased mortality, stroke, EPS, sedation, and metabolic risk	APA Dementia Guideline (2016); NICE (2018)
PRN-only antipsychotic strategy without reassessment	May lead to inappropriate chronic use without monitoring or defined goals	APA Dementia Guideline (2016); NICE (2018)
Dose escalation without addressing delirium or medical triggers	May overlook reversible causes such as infection, pain, constipation, dehydration, or medication effects	APA Dementia Guideline (2016); DSM-5-TR (APA, 2022); NICE (2018)
Benzodiazepine use	Increased risk of falls, paradoxical disinhibition, sedation, cognitive worsening, and delirium	APA Dementia Guideline (2016); NICE (2018); Beers Criteria (2023)
Antipsychotic use for mild or non-distressing agitation	Mortality and stroke risks may outweigh benefit in mild cases	APA Dementia Guideline (2016); NICE (2018)
Valproate / Divalproex for agitation	No evidence of benefit for agitation in dementia based on multiple RCTs and Cochrane review; not recommended by NICE; associated with sedation, cognitive worsening, and falls in elderly patients	Baillon et al. (2018) — Cochrane Review; NICE NG97 (2018)
Continuing antipsychotics without a reassessment and deprescribing plan	After agitation or psychosis stabilizes, reassess at regular intervals and attempt gradual dose reduction or withdrawal; many patients can taper without symptom recurrence. Define indication, goals, and review dates, and use the lowest effective dose for the shortest duration.	APA Dementia Guideline (2016); NICE (2018)

6. PARKINSON'S DISEASE PSYCHOSIS (PDP)

A. OVERVIEW

Aspect	Clinical Notes	Evidence Source
Definition	Psychosis occurring in Parkinson's disease, usually involving hallucinations or delusions related to disease progression and dopaminergic therapy	DSM-5-TR (APA, 2022); Seppi et al. (2019)
Core features	Visual hallucinations are most common; illusions, passage phenomena, delusions, sleep disturbance, and cognitive impairment may occur	Seppi et al. (2019); NICE (2018)

Aspect	Clinical Notes	Evidence Source
Clinical importance	Associated with caregiver burden, falls, institutionalization, worse quality of life, and increased morbidity	Seppi et al. (2019); NICE (2018)
Treatment approach	Rule out delirium, infection, metabolic causes, and medication toxicity first; optimize Parkinson's regimen before adding antipsychotics	APA Dementia Guideline (2016); NICE (2018); Seppi et al. (2019)

B. Core Principles

Principle	Clinical Notes	Evidence Source
Rule out medical and reversible causes first	Evaluate infection, metabolic disturbances, delirium, and medication toxicity; acute changes should be presumed delirium until excluded	APA Dementia Guideline (2016); DSM-5-TR (APA, 2022); NICE (2018)
Optimize Parkinson's regimen before antipsychotics	Gradually reduce psychosis-provoking agents when possible while balancing motor versus psychiatric symptoms	APA Dementia Guideline (2016); NICE (2022); Seppi et al. (2019)
Initiate treatment only if psychosis is distressing or dangerous	Mild non-distressing hallucinations may not require medication	APA Dementia Guideline (2016); NICE (2018)

C. FDA-Approved Agent for PDP

Generic	Brand	Dose Range	Clinical Notes	Evidence Source
Pimavanserin	Nuplazid	34 mg/day	Selective 5-HT2A inverse agonist; does not worsen motor symptoms; once-daily dosing without titration; monitor QTc and CYP3A4 interactions; boxed warning for increased mortality in elderly patients with dementia-related psychosis	FDA Labeling (2016); APA Dementia Guideline (2016); NICE (2018)

Clinical note

Selective serotonin 5-HT2A inverse agonist; no dopamine blockade → no worsening of motor symptoms.

D. Combination Strategies

Base Treatment	Add-On	Clinical Notes	Evidence Source
Optimization of Parkinson's regimen	Pimavanserin	Consider for persistent distressing hallucinations or delusions despite dopaminergic optimization; document prior medication adjustments and functional impact	APA Dementia Guideline (2016); NICE (2018)
Pimavanserin	Levodopa-containing regimen	Dopaminergic therapy may continue for motor symptoms; pimavanserin generally does not worsen motor function; monitor QTc and CYP3A4 interactions	APA Dementia Guideline (2016); FDA Labeling (2016); NICE (2018)

E. Avoid or Use with Caution in PDP

Strategy	Clinical Notes	Evidence Source
Routine use of high-potency D2 antagonists (e.g., haloperidol)	May severely worsen parkinsonism; high risk of EPS and neuroleptic malignant syndrome	APA Dementia Guideline (2016); NICE (2018); Seppi et al. (2019)
Poly-antipsychotic combinations	No clear added benefit; increased sedation, orthostasis, QTc prolongation, and mortality risk	APA Dementia Guideline (2016); NICE (2018)
Starting antipsychotics before optimizing Parkinson's regimen	May overlook psychosis improvement achievable through dopaminergic adjustment	APA Dementia Guideline (2016); NICE (2018); Seppi et al. (2019)

7. AMANTADINE: CLINICAL POSITIONING

A. OVERVIEW

Aspect	Clinical Notes	Evidence Source
Definition	Amantadine is an NMDA receptor antagonist used in Parkinson's disease mainly for dyskinesia and motor fluctuation management, not psychosis treatment	Seppi et al. (2019); NICE (2018)
Core uses	May reduce levodopa-induced dyskinesia and improve "off" symptoms; available in IR and ER formulations	Seppi et al. (2019); NICE (2018); FDA Labeling (2017); FDA Labeling (2018)
Clinical importance	May worsen hallucinations, confusion, and psychosis, especially in older adults, cognitively impaired patients, or renal impairment	Seppi et al. (2019); NICE (2018)

Aspect	Clinical Notes	Evidence Source
Treatment approach	Use only when clinically indicated for motor symptoms; avoid or reduce in active psychosis, cognitive vulnerability, or poor renal clearance	NICE (2018); Seppi et al. (2019)

B. Indication Anchor

Indication	Context	Clinical Notes	Evidence Source
Parkinson's disease	Dyskinesia, "off" episodes	NMDA receptor antagonist; may reduce levodopa-induced dyskinesia and improve motor fluctuations; typically used adjunctively with dopaminergic therapy	APA Dementia Guideline (2016); NICE (2022); Seppi et al. (2019)
Not indicated for psychosis treatment	May worsen psychosis	Can exacerbate hallucinations, confusion, and agitation, especially in older adults or neurocognitive disorders	APA Dementia Guideline (2016); NICE (2018)

C. Formulations and Dosing

Generic	Brand	Dose Range	Clinical Notes	Evidence Source
Amantadine IR	Symmetrel	100–400 mg/day	Immediate-release; usually BID–TID dosing; requires renal adjustment; may cause confusion, hallucinations, and insomnia, especially in older adults	APA Dementia Guideline (2016); NICE (2018)
Amantadine ER	Osmolex ER	129–322 mg/day	Once-daily morning ER formulation for Parkinson's disease and drug-induced EPS; requires renal adjustment	FDA Labeling (2018); NICE (2018)
Amantadine ER	Gocovri	137–274 mg/day	Bedtime ER formulation approved for levodopa-induced dyskinesia and "off" episodes; may increase hallucinations and confusion	FDA Labeling (2017); NICE (2018)

D. Key Neuropsychiatric Safety Warning

Warning	Clinical Notes	Evidence Source
Amantadine treatment or abrupt withdrawal may cause confusion, hallucinations, or psychosis	Monitor during initiation, titration, and discontinuation; taper gradually when possible	APA Dementia Guideline (2016); NICE (2018); Seppi et al. (2019)
Increased neuropsychiatric adverse-effect risk	Risk is higher with renal impairment, dementia, advanced age, or concomitant anticholinergic use; consider dose reduction and close monitoring	APA Dementia Guideline (2016); NICE (2018)

REFERENCES

Acadia Pharmaceuticals Inc. (2016). *Nuplazid (pimavanserin) prescribing information*. https://www.nuplazid.com

American Geriatrics Society Beers Criteria® Update Expert Panel. (2023). American Geriatrics Society 2023 updated AGS Beers Criteria® for potentially inappropriate medication use in older adults. *Journal of the American Geriatrics Society, 71*(7), 2052–2081. https://doi.org/10.1111/jgs.18372

American Psychiatric Association. (2016). *The American Psychiatric Association practice guideline on the use of antipsychotics to treat agitation or psychosis in patients with dementia*. American Psychiatric Publishing.

American Psychiatric Association. (2022). *Diagnostic and statistical manual of mental disorders* (5th ed., text rev.; DSM-5-TR). American Psychiatric Publishing.

Baillon, S. F., Narayana, U., Luxenberg, J. S., & Clifton, A. V. (2018). Valproate preparations for agitation in dementia. *Cochrane Database of Systematic Reviews*, (10), CD003945. https://doi.org/10.1002/14651858.CD003945.pub4

McKeith, I. G., Boeve, B. F., Dickson, D. W., Halliday, G., Taylor, J.-P., Weintraub, D., Aarsland, D., Galvin, J., Attems, J., Ballard, C. G., Bayston, A., Beach, T. G., Blanc, F., Bohnen, N., Bonanni, L., Bras, J., Brundin, P., Burn, D., Chen-Plotkin, A., ... Kosaka, K. (2017). Diagnosis and management of dementia with Lewy bodies: Fourth consensus report of the DLB Consortium. *Neurology, 89*(1), 88–100. https://doi.org/10.1212/WNL.0000000000004058

National Institute for Health and Care Excellence. (2018). *Dementia: Assessment, management and support for people living with dementia and their carers (NG97)*. https://www.nice.org.uk/guidance/ng97

Otsuka Pharmaceutical Co., Ltd. (2023). *Rexulti (brexpiprazole) prescribing information*. https://www.rexulti.com

Seppi, K., Ray Chaudhuri, K., Coelho, M., Fox, S. H., Katzenschlager, R., Perez Lloret, S., Weintraub, D., Sampaio, C., & the collaborators of the Parkinson's Disease Update on Non-Motor Symptoms Study Group on behalf of the Movement Disorders Society Evidence-Based Medicine Committee. (2019). Update on treatments for nonmotor symptoms of Parkinson's disease—An evidence-based medicine review. *Movement Disorders, 34*(2), 180–198. https://doi.org/10.1002/mds.27602

Sims, J. R., Zimmer, J. A., Evans, C. D., Lu, M., Ardayfio, P. A., Sparks, J., Wessels, A. M., Shcherbinin, S., Wang, H., Monkul Nery, E. S., Collins, E. C., Solomon, P., Salloway, S., Apostolova, L. G., Hansson, O., Ritchie, C., Brooks, D. A., Mintun, M. A., & Skovronsky, D. M. (2023). Donanemab in early symptomatic Alzheimer's disease: The TRAILBLAZER-ALZ 2 randomized clinical trial. *JAMA, 330*(6), 512–527. https://doi.org/10.1001/jama.2023.13239

Tariot, P. N., Farlow, M. R., Grossberg, G. T., Graham, S. M., McDonald, S., & Gergel, I. (2004). Memantine treatment in patients with moderate to severe Alzheimer disease already receiving donepezil: A randomized controlled trial. *JAMA, 291*(3), 317–324. https://doi.org/10.1001/jama.291.3.317

van Dyck, C. H., Swanson, C. J., Aisen, P., Bateman, R. J., Chen, C., Gee, M., Kanekiyo, M., Li, D., Reyderman, L., Cohen, S., Froelich, L., Katayama, S., Sabbagh, M., Vellas, B., Watson, D., Dhadda, S., Irizarry, M., Kramer, L. D., & Iwatsubo, T. (2023). Lecanemab in early Alzheimer's disease. *New England Journal of Medicine, 388*(1), 9–21. https://doi.org/10.1056/NEJMoa2212948

U.S. Food and Drug Administration. (2017). *Gocovri (amantadine) prescribing information*. https://www.accessdata.fda.gov

U.S. Food and Drug Administration. (2017). *Razadyne ER (galantamine hydrobromide) prescribing information*. Janssen Pharmaceuticals. https://www.accessdata.fda.gov

U.S. Food and Drug Administration. (2023). FDA approves first drug to treat agitation symptoms associated with dementia due to Alzheimer's disease [FDA news release]. https://www.fda.gov/drugs/news-events-human-drugs/fda-approves-first-drug-treat-agitation-symptoms-associated-dementia-due-alzheimers-disease

X. SUBSTANCE USE DISORDERS

SECTION INTRODUCTION

Substance use disorders (SUDs) comprise a group of chronic and frequently relapsing conditions characterized by impaired control over substance use, compulsive use despite harmful consequences, physiologic dependence, craving, tolerance, withdrawal symptoms, and progressive functional impairment. These disorders are associated with substantial psychiatric, medical, occupational, legal, interpersonal, and socioeconomic consequences and represent a major source of morbidity and mortality across outpatient, emergency, inpatient, and community healthcare settings. Under DSM-5-TR, a substance use disorder is diagnosed when at least 2 of 11 criteria occur within a 12-month period, with severity graded by the number of criteria met: mild (2–3), moderate (4–5), and severe (6 or more).

Substance use disorders commonly involve alcohol, opioids, stimulants, cannabis, sedative-hypnotics, nicotine, hallucinogens, and other psychoactive substances. Alcohol use disorder remains among the most prevalent substance-related conditions worldwide, while opioid-related overdose deaths and stimulant-related psychiatric complications continue to represent major public health concerns. Many patients experience recurrent cycles of intoxication, withdrawal, relapse, and psychosocial deterioration that require longitudinal, multidisciplinary treatment approaches rather than short-term crisis management alone.

The clinical presentation of substance use disorders is highly variable and may include intoxication syndromes, withdrawal states, craving, compulsive use patterns, cognitive impairment, mood instability, psychosis, anxiety symptoms, sleep disturbance, impulsivity, behavioral dysregulation, and severe functional decline. Substance use may directly precipitate psychiatric symptoms, worsen preexisting mental illness, impair treatment adherence, or complicate diagnostic clarification. Careful longitudinal assessment is therefore essential to distinguish primary psychiatric disorders from substance-induced conditions whenever possible.

Comorbidity is extremely common among patients with substance use disorders. Major depressive disorder, bipolar disorder, anxiety disorders, trauma-related disorders, ADHD, psychotic disorders, personality pathology, chronic pain syndromes, insomnia, and medical illnesses frequently coexist and may substantially influence prognosis, relapse risk, and treatment planning. Trauma exposure, adverse childhood experiences, chronic stress, and social instability are also strongly associated with increased vulnerability to substance misuse and recurrent relapse.

Substance use disorders are associated with elevated suicide risk, accidental overdose, impulsive behavior, violence exposure, medical complications, and premature mortality. Suicide risk assessment should therefore be integrated into all psychiatric evaluations involving substance use, particularly in the presence of intoxication, withdrawal, hopelessness, severe psychiatric comorbidity, chronic pain, or polysubstance misuse. Patients with opioid use disorder, alcohol use disorder, stimulant use disorder, and sedative-hypnotic dependence may also experience life-threatening withdrawal syndromes or overdose complications requiring urgent medical intervention.

Withdrawal management and medical stabilization represent critical aspects of psychiatric and addiction-related care. Alcohol and benzodiazepine withdrawal may lead to seizures, delirium tremens, autonomic instability, and death if inadequately treated. Opioid withdrawal, while generally not fatal, may produce severe distress, relapse risk, dehydration, and medical instability. Stimulant withdrawal frequently contributes to depression, suicidality, fatigue, and relapse vulnerability. Clinicians should therefore remain familiar with evidence-based detoxification strategies, medications for opioid use disorder (MOUD), overdose management, and emergency stabilization procedures.

Evidence-based treatment of substance use disorders generally involves a combination of pharmacotherapy, psychotherapy, relapse-prevention strategies, psychosocial support, and longitudinal recovery-oriented care. Medications such as buprenorphine, methadone, naltrexone, acamprosate, disulfiram, nicotine replacement therapies, varenicline, and selected adjunctive agents may significantly improve outcomes in appropriately selected patients. Motivational interviewing, cognitive behavioral therapy, contingency management, peer recovery programs, trauma-informed treatment, and family involvement also play important roles in long-term recovery and functional stabilization.

Treatment planning should remain individualized and longitudinal, recognizing that relapse may occur as part of the chronic course of illness rather than as evidence of treatment failure. Important clinical considerations include overdose risk, withdrawal severity, co-occurring psychiatric illness, housing instability, legal involvement, social support, chronic pain, medical comorbidity, pregnancy, and readiness for change. Harm-reduction strategies, naloxone education, infectious disease screening, and coordination of medical and psychiatric care should also be incorporated whenever clinically appropriate.

The following sections provide a structured, evidence-informed framework for the evaluation and treatment of substance use disorders within outpatient psychiatric practice. Recommendations are intended to support safe, compassionate, and clinically individualized care while recognizing the importance of longitudinal recovery planning, multidisciplinary collaboration, relapse prevention, and professional clinical judgment throughout the course of illness. Note on sources: the ASAM (2020) clinical practice guideline cited in this chapter addresses alcohol withdrawal management specifically; recommendations for alcohol use disorder maintenance pharmacotherapy and for non-alcohol substances rely on the other cited sources (e.g., VA/DoD 2021, SAMHSA TIP 63, NICE).

1. ALCOHOL USE DISORDER (AUD)

A. OVERVIEW

Withdrawal management alone is insufficient	Detoxification treats physiologic dependence but not the underlying AUD; relapse-prevention planning remains essential	VA/DoD (2021)
Relapse-prevention treatment should begin once stable	Early pharmacotherapy and psychosocial intervention improve engagement and outcomes	VA/DoD (2021)
Pharmacotherapy is recommended for moderate–severe AUD	Medications reduce heavy drinking and support abstinence but remain underutilized	VA/DoD (2021); NICE (2022); Kranzler & Soyka (2018)
Behavioral interventions should accompany medication treatment	CBT, motivational approaches, relapse-prevention counseling, and mutual-help participation improve recovery outcomes	VA/DoD (2021)

B. First-Line Pharmacotherapy

Drug	Brand	Dose	Clinical Notes	Evidence Source
Naltrexone (oral)	Revia	50 mg/day	Reduces heavy drinking and binge risk; avoid with current opioid use; monitor liver-related considerations when indicated	VA/DoD (2021); Kranzler & Soyka (2018)
Naltrexone XR (IM)	Vivitrol	380 mg IM every 4 weeks	Monthly formulation may improve adherence; requires opioid-free interval before initiation	VA/DoD (2021); Kranzler & Soyka (2018)
Acamprosate	Campral	666 mg TID	Best for maintaining abstinence after cessation; renally cleared; diarrhea common	VA/DoD (2021); Kranzler & Soyka (2018)

C. Selected / Situational Pharmacotherapy

Drug	Brand	Dose	Clinical Notes	Evidence Source
Disulfiram	Antabuse	125–500 mg/day	Best for highly motivated patients with reliable supervision; monitor hepatotoxicity risk	VA/DoD (2021); Kranzler & Soyka (2018)

Drug	Brand	Dose	Clinical Notes	Evidence Source
Topiramate	Topamax	25–300 mg/day	Not FDA-approved for AUD; strong recommendation in VA/DoD (2021) based on RCT evidence; titrate slowly; cognitive slowing, paresthesias, and weight loss may occur	VA/DoD (2021); Johnson et al. (2007); Kranzler & Soyka (2018)
Gabapentin	Neuronti n	900–1800 mg/day	May help insomnia, anxiety, and protracted withdrawal symptoms; monitor sedation and misuse potential	VA/DoD (2021); Mason et al. (2014); Kranzler & Soyka (2018)

D. Combination Strategies

Clinical Scenario	Preferred Treatment	Rationale	Clinical Notes	Avoid / Caution	Evidence Source
Moderate–severe AUD after stabilization	Behavioral treatment + naltrexone or acamprosate	Best-supported relapse-prevention approach	Naltrexone for reducing heavy drinking; acamprosate for abstinence maintenance	Do not rely on detox alone	VA/DoD (2021); Kranzler & Soyka (2018)
Inadequate response to first-line treatment	Switch to or consider another evidence-based agent	Different mechanisms may improve response	Reassess adherence, alcohol use, medical factors, and treatment goals first	Avoid escalation without reassessment	VA/DoD (2021); Kranzler & Soyka (2018)
Early recovery with insomnia or anxiety	Behavioral treatment + targeted adjunct (e.g., gabapentin)	May improve tolerability and engagement in recovery	Use with clear targets, defined duration, and misuse monitoring	Do not present adjuncts as equivalent to core AUD treatment	VA/DoD (2021)

E. Risks / Monitoring

Monitoring Domain	Clinical Notes	Evidence Source
Liver-related considerations	Monitor hepatic status when indicated, especially with naltrexone or disulfiram	VA/DoD (2021)
Renal considerations	Acamprosate requires renal dose adjustment and may be preferred when hepatic burden is a concern	VA/DoD (2021)
Misuse risk with adjunctive agents	Gabapentin may carry misuse risk in selected populations	Kranzler & Soyka (2018); VA/DoD (2021)

Monitoring Domain	Clinical Notes	Evidence Source
Supervision requirements	Disulfiram is best reserved for highly motivated patients with reliable supervision	Kranzler & Soyka (2018)

F. Practical Treatment Selection

Clinical Scenario	Preferred Treatment	Rationale	Clinical Notes	Avoid / Caution	Evidence Source
Strong cravings or recurrent heavy drinking	Naltrexone	Useful when reducing heavy drinking or craving is the primary goal	Confirm no active opioid use	Avoid with opioid use or anticipated opioid analgesics	VA/DoD (2021); Kranzler & Soyka (2018)
Abstinent patient focused on maintaining sobriety	Acamprosate	Supports abstinence maintenance	Useful when hepatic burden is a concern	Renal limitations apply	VA/DoD (2021)
Highly motivated patient with reliable supervision	Disulfiram	Most effective when adherence is supervised	Patient should understand and accept the aversive model	Avoid unsupervised use	Kranzler & Soyka (2018)

G. Alcohol Withdrawal Management (Brief Outpatient Anchor)

Practical Risk Stratification

Criteria	Outpatient Appropriate	To higher Level of Care	Clinical Notes	Evidence Source
Withdrawal severity	Mild symptoms only	Moderate–severe symptoms	Severe withdrawal requires closer monitoring or inpatient care	ASAM (2020); VA/DoD (2021)
History of seizures or delirium tremens	No	Yes	Prior severe withdrawal predicts higher complication risk	ASAM (2020)
Medical comorbidity	Stable	Unstable	Liver disease, cardiac illness, pregnancy, or electrolyte abnormalities increase risk	ASAM (2020); VA/DoD (2021)
Psychiatric comorbidity	Mild and stable	Severe or unstable	Suicidality, psychosis, or severe mood instability complicate outpatient management	ASAM (2020); VA/DoD (2021)

Criteria	Outpatient Appropriate	To higher Level of Care	Clinical Notes	Evidence Source
Social support	Reliable sober support	Unsafe or unreliable setting	Outpatient detox requires supervision and access to urgent care	ASAM (2020)

2. OPIOID USE DISORDER (OUD)

A. OVERVIEW

Clinical Principle	Clinical Notes	Evidence Source
Medications for OUD are first-line	MOUD improves retention and reduces opioid use, overdose risk, and mortality	SAMHSA TIP 63 (2021)
Buprenorphine and methadone have the strongest mortality data	XR-naltrexone is effective for selected patients, but mortality evidence is strongest for buprenorphine and methadone	SAMHSA TIP 63 (2021)
MOUD should not be withheld if counseling is unavailable	Behavioral support helps, but medication treatment should not be delayed	SAMHSA TIP 63 (2021)
Naloxone should be co-prescribed	Overdose education and naloxone access should be routine safety measures	SAMHSA TIP 63 (2021); CDC (2022)

B. FDA-Approved MOUD

Drug	Brand / Setting	Dose	Clinical Notes	Evidence Source
Buprenorphine/ Naloxone SL	Suboxone	Induction usually 2–4 mg; maintenance commonly 8–24 mg/day	Start when objective withdrawal is present to reduce precipitated withdrawal risk; low-dose induction may be considered in selected patients	SAMHSA TIP 63 (2021)
Buprenorphine ER	Sublocade	300 mg monthly × 2, then commonly 100 mg monthly	Requires prior stabilization on transmucosal buprenorphine; may improve adherence	SAMHSA TIP 63 (2021); FDA labeling

Drug	Brand / Setting	Dose	Clinical Notes	Evidence Source
Methadone	OTP	Individualized dosing	Dispensed through regulated opioid treatment programs; monitor sedation, interactions, and QT-related risk when indicated. Boxed warnings: QT prolongation/torsades de pointes, life-threatening respiratory depression, and addiction, abuse, and misuse. For OUD, initiation/induction should occur through authorized opioid treatment programs	SAMHSA TIP 63 (2021)
Naltrexone XR	Vivitrol	380 mg IM every 4 weeks	Requires complete opioid-free interval before initiation	SAMHSA TIP 63 (2021)

C. Overdose Prevention

Drug	Brand	Dose	Clinical Notes	Evidence Source
Naloxone nasal spray	Narcan	4 mg intranasal per spray	Administer promptly in suspected overdose; may repeat every 2–3 minutes while activating EMS	SAMHSA TIP 63 (2021); CDC (2022)

D. Combination Strategies

Clinical Scenario	Preferred Treatment	Rationale	Clinical Notes	Avoid / Caution	Evidence Source
Any patient receiving MOUD	Naloxone kit + harm-reduction counseling	Standard overdose-prevention approach	Include fentanyl exposure and relapse-risk education when appropriate	Avoid MOUD without overdose planning	SAMHSA TIP 63 (2021); CDC (2022)
MOUD with comorbid mood or anxiety disorder	Treat comorbidity while continuing MOUD	Improves functioning and retention	SSRIs/SNRIs may be used when indicated; monitor interactions and sedation	Do not discontinue MOUD because psychiatric symptoms persist	SAMHSA TIP 63 (2021); Clinical consensus

Clinical Scenario	Preferred Treatment	Rationale	Clinical Notes	Avoid / Caution	Evidence Source
Methadone treatment	Coordinated care with OTP and other prescribers	Improves safety and continuity of care	Communication is critical for sedatives, QT-prolonging agents, and pain treatment	Avoid fragmented prescribing	SAMHSA TIP 63 (2021)

E. Risks / Monitoring

Monitoring Domain	Clinical Notes	Evidence Source
Precipitated withdrawal risk	Buprenorphine and naltrexone require careful opioid timing; naltrexone requires a full opioid-free interval	SAMHSA TIP 63 (2021)
Sedative co-use	Benzodiazepines, alcohol, and other sedatives increase overdose risk and require close monitoring	SAMHSA TIP 63 (2021)
Retention in treatment	Continued MOUD is protective; discontinuation increases relapse and overdose risk	SAMHSA TIP 63 (2021)

F. Practical Treatment Selection

Clinical Scenario	Preferred Treatment	Rationale	Clinical Notes	Avoid / Caution	Evidence Source
Most outpatient patients with OUD	Buprenorphine	Accessible and effective for office-based treatment	Start when objective withdrawal is present	Avoid initiating too soon after opioid use	SAMHSA TIP 63 (2021)
Patient benefits from structured daily dispensing	Methadone	Highly effective in regulated treatment settings	Useful in high-tolerance patients or when buprenorphine is insufficient	Requires close coordination and monitoring	SAMHSA TIP 63 (2021)
Fully detoxified patient preferring antagonist treatment	Naltrexone XR	Evidence-based option after opioid-free interval	Best for selected, motivated patients with reliable follow-up	Avoid before complete detoxification	SAMHSA TIP 63 (2021)

3. STIMULANT USE DISORDER (COCAINE/METHAMPHETAMINE)

A. OVERVIEW

Clinical Principle	Clinical Notes	Evidence Source
No FDA-approved medications exist for stimulant use disorder	No medication is FDA-approved for cocaine or methamphetamine use disorder	VA/DoD (2021); NICE (2022)
Behavioral treatment is first-line	Contingency management, CBT, and structured treatment programs have the strongest evidence	VA/DoD (2021); NICE (2022)
Adjunctive pharmacotherapy may be considered selectively	Off-label options may help selected patients, particularly in methamphetamine use disorder	VA/DoD (2021); Trivedi et al. (2021)

B. Evidence-Based Adjuncts for Methamphetamine Use Disorder

Drug	Brand	Dose	Clinical Notes	Evidence Source
Naltrexone XR	Vivitrol	380 mg IM every 4 weeks	Studied with bupropion for methamphetamine use disorder; requires opioid-free status	Trivedi et al. (2021); VA/DoD (2021)
Bupropion ER	Wellbutrin XL	Up to 450 mg/day	Combined with naltrexone showed modest benefit in selected patients; monitor insomnia, anxiety, BP, and seizure risk	Trivedi et al. (2021); VA/DoD (2021)

C. Combination Strategies

Clinical Scenario	Preferred Treatment	Rationale	Clinical Notes	Avoid / Caution	Evidence Source
Stimulant use disorder without contraindication to behavioral care	Contingency management + CBT	Strongest overall evidence base	Behavioral treatment remains first-line	Avoid presenting medications as equivalent substitutes	VA/DoD (2021); NICE (2022)
Methamphetamine use disorder with inadequate response to behavioral care	Behavioral treatment + naltrexone XR/bupropion ER in selected patients	Large trial showed modest benefit	Requires adherence monitoring and careful patient selection	Benefit is modest and not universal	Trivedi et al. (2021)
Comorbid depression or anxiety	Treat comorbid disorder directly	Improves overall functioning	Do not overstate indirect effects on stimulant abstinence	Avoid unnecessary polypharmacy	VA/DoD (2021)

D. Avoid / Caution

Strategy	Clinical Notes	Evidence Source
Escalating antipsychotics without reassessing stimulant exposure	May mask ongoing stimulant use and increase metabolic and neurologic burden	VA/DoD (2021)
Repeated benzodiazepine prescribing for crash symptoms	Increases misuse, dependence, and sedative-use-disorder risk	VA/DoD (2021)
Routine stimulant replacement therapy	Not routinely recommended; evidence remains limited and inconsistent	VA/DoD (2021); NICE (2022)

4. SEDATIVE/HYPNOTIC/ANXIOLYTIC USE DISORDER (BENZODIAZEPINES)

A. OVERVIEW

Clinical Principle	Clinical Notes	Evidence Source
Structured taper is the primary treatment	Abrupt discontinuation may cause severe withdrawal, seizures, or delirium; taper gradually and individually	NICE (2022)
Withdrawal risk must be assessed carefully	High-dose, long-term, polysedative, or medically complex use may require higher-level monitoring	NICE (2022)
Outpatient taper is appropriate only for selected patients	Patients should be medically stable and able to engage in close follow-up	Brunner et al. (2025)
Long-acting benzodiazepines may facilitate taper	Conversion to diazepam or chlordiazepoxide may improve tolerability, especially with short-acting agents	NICE (2022)

B. Symptom-Targeted Adjuncts

Drug	Brand	Dose	Clinical Notes	Evidence Source
Hydroxyzine	Vistaril	25–100 mg/day PRN	May reduce short-term anxiety or agitation; sedation and anticholinergic effects may limit use	NICE (2022)
Gabapentin	Neuronti n	300–1800 mg/day	May help insomnia or anxiety during taper; monitor sedation and misuse risk	VA/DoD (2021)
Propranolol	Inderal	10–40 mg BID–TID	May reduce autonomic symptoms such as tremor or tachycardia; monitor BP and pulse	Brunner et al. (2025); Clinical consensus

Drug	Brand	Dose	Clinical Notes	Evidence Source
Chlordiazepoxide	Librium	25–100 mg QID initial; individualized taper	Long-acting agent commonly used for withdrawal taper; gradual dose reduction improves tolerability	Brunner et al. (2025); NICE (2022)
Diazepam	Valium	5–20 mg QID initial; individualized taper	Useful for conversion taper from short-acting benzodiazepines; monitor accumulation in older adults and hepatic impairment	Brunner et al. (2025); NICE (2022)
Clonazepam	Klonopin	0.5–2 mg BID–TID initial; individualized taper	Intermediate-to-long-acting option sometimes used in patients with comorbid anxiety or seizure history	Brunner et al. (2025); NICE (2022)

C. Combination Strategies

Clinical Scenario	Preferred Treatment	Rationale	Clinical Notes	Avoid / Caution	Evidence Source
Benzodiazepine use disorder with comorbid anxiety or depression	Structured taper + treatment of underlying disorder	Addresses physiologic dependence and psychiatric vulnerability	SSRIs/SNRIs may reduce long-term relapse risk in selected patients	Do not confuse psychiatric treatment with withdrawal management	NICE (2022)
Significant insomnia or anxiety during taper	Short-term targeted adjunct	May improve taper tolerability	Use with clear targets, short duration, and stop plan	Avoid indefinite sedating polypharmacy	Brunner et al. (2025); Clinical consensus

D. Avoid or Use with Caution in patients with Sedative Use Disorder

Strategy	Clinical Notes	Evidence Source
Replacing one benzodiazepine with another without a taper plan	May perpetuate dependence; substitution should occur only within a structured taper strategy	NICE (2022)
Concurrent benzodiazepines with opioids or alcohol	Significantly increases respiratory depression and overdose risk	CDC (2022)
Combining multiple sedatives	Increases risk of CNS depression, falls, cognitive impairment, and delirium, especially in older adults	Beers Criteria (2023)

5. CANNABIS USE DISORDER

A. OVERVIEW

Clinical Principle	Clinical Notes	Evidence Source
No FDA-approved medications exist for cannabis use disorder	Treatment remains primarily behavioral	VA/DoD (2021); NICE (2022)
Behavioral treatment is first-line	CBT, motivational enhancement therapy, and contingency management have the strongest evidence	VA/DoD (2021); NICE (2022)
Medications should be limited to short-term symptom targets	Adjuncts may help insomnia, anxiety, or irritability but do not replace behavioral treatment	VA/DoD (2021)

B. Off-Label / Adjunct Options

Drug	Brand	Dose	Clinical Notes	Evidence Source
N-acetylcysteine	OTC	1200–2400 mg/day	Evidence remains mixed; may be considered only as a selective adjunct with realistic expectations	Gray et al. (2012); VA/DoD (2021)
Gabapentin	Neurontin	300–1800 mg/day	May help sleep or anxiety symptoms in early recovery; evidence remains limited	VA/DoD (2021)

C. Combination Strategies

Clinical Scenario	Preferred Treatment	Rationale	Clinical Notes	Avoid / Caution	Evidence Source
Cannabis use disorder with early withdrawal-related insomnia or anxiety	Behavioral treatment + short-term symptom-targeted medication if needed	May improve comfort and treatment engagement	Define target symptoms, duration, and stop plan	Avoid long-term sedative prescribing	VA/DoD (2021); NICE (2022)
Patient interested in adjunctive OTC treatment	Behavioral treatment + selective NAC trial	May help some patients, though evidence is inconsistent	Continue only if measurable benefit is observed	Avoid overstating evidence	Gray et al. (2012); VA/DoD (2021)

D. Avoid or Use with Caution in Patients with Cannabis Use Disorder

Strategy	Clinical Notes	Evidence Source
Escalating sedatives for withdrawal insomnia	May lead to secondary dependence and obscure recovery assessment	VA/DoD (2021); NICE (2022)
Polypharmacy without measurable targets	Increases adverse-effect burden without clear evidence of benefit	VA/DoD (2021)
Antipsychotic use without a psychotic disorder	Not indicated for cannabis use disorder itself; reserve for true psychotic syndromes	VA/DoD (2021); DSM-5-TR (APA, 2022)

REFERENCES

American Geriatrics Society Beers Criteria® Update Expert Panel. (2023). American Geriatrics Society 2023 updated AGS Beers Criteria® for potentially inappropriate medication use in older adults. *Journal of the American Geriatrics Society, 71*(7), 2052–2081. https://doi.org/10.1111/jgs.18372

American Psychiatric Association. (2022). *Diagnostic and statistical manual of mental disorders* (5th ed., text rev.; DSM-5-TR). American Psychiatric Publishing.

American Society of Addiction Medicine. (2020). The ASAM clinical practice guideline on alcohol withdrawal management. *Journal of Addiction Medicine, 14*(3S Suppl. 1), 1–72. https://doi.org/10.1097/ADM.0000000000000668

Brunner, E., Chen, C.-Y. A., Klein, T., et al. (2025). Joint clinical practice guideline on benzodiazepine tapering: Considerations when risks outweigh benefits. *Journal of General Internal Medicine, 40*(12), 2814–2859. https://doi.org/10.1007/s11606-025-09499-2

Centers for Disease Control and Prevention. (2022). *CDC clinical practice guideline for prescribing opioids for pain — United States, 2022. MMWR Recommendations and Reports, 71*(3), 1–95. https://doi.org/10.15585/mmwr.rr7103a1

Gray, K. M., Carpenter, M. J., Baker, N. L., DeSantis, S. M., Kryway, E., Hartwell, K. J., McRae-Clark, A. L., & Brady, K. T. (2012). A double-blind randomized controlled trial of N-acetylcysteine in cannabis-dependent adolescents. *American Journal of Psychiatry, 169*(8), 805–812. https://doi.org/10.1176/appi.ajp.2012.12010055

Johnson, B. A., Rosenthal, N., Capece, J. A., Wiegand, F., Mao, L., Beyers, K., McKay, A., Ait-Daoud, N., Anton, R. F., Ciraulo, D. A., Kranzler, H. R., Mann, K., O'Malley, S. S., Swift, R. M., & Topiramate for Alcoholism Advisory Board and the Topiramate for Alcoholism Study Group. (2007). Topiramate for treating alcohol dependence: A randomized controlled trial. *JAMA, 298*(14), 1641–1651. https://doi.org/10.1001/jama.298.14.1641

Kranzler, H. R., & Soyka, M. (2018). Diagnosis and pharmacotherapy of alcohol use disorder: A review. *JAMA, 320*(8), 815–824. https://doi.org/10.1001/jama.2018.11406

Mason, B. J., Quello, S., Goodell, V., Shadan, F., Kyle, M., & Begovic, A. (2014). Gabapentin treatment for alcohol dependence: A randomized clinical trial. *JAMA Internal Medicine, 174*(1), 70–77. https://doi.org/10.1001/jamainternmed.2013.11950

National Institute for Health and Care Excellence. (2011). *Alcohol-use disorders: Diagnosis, assessment and management of harmful drinking and alcohol dependence (CG115)*. Updated 2022. https://www.nice.org.uk/guidance/cg115

National Institute for Health and Care Excellence. (2022). *Medicines associated with dependence or withdrawal symptoms (NG215)*. https://www.nice.org.uk/guidance/ng215

Substance Abuse and Mental Health Services Administration. (2021). *TIP 63: Medications for opioid use disorder*. U.S. Department of Health and Human Services. https://store.samhsa.gov

Trivedi, M. H., Walker, R., Ling, W., Dela Cruz, A., Sharma, G., Carmody, T., Ghitza, U. E., Wahle, A., Kim, M., Shores-Wilson, K., Sparenborg, S., Coffin, P., Schmitz, J., Wiest, K., Bart, G., Sonne, S. C., Wakhlu, S., Rush, A. J., Nunes, E. V., & Shoptaw, S. (2021). Bupropion and naltrexone in methamphetamine use disorder. *New England Journal of Medicine, 384*(2), 140–153. https://doi.org/10.1056/NEJMoa2020214

U.S. Department of Veterans Affairs & U.S. Department of Defense. (2021). *VA/DoD clinical practice guideline for the management of substance use disorders*. https://www.healthquality.va.gov/guidelines/MH/sud/

XI. SLEEP-WAKE DISORDERS

SECTION INTRODUCTION

Sleep-wake disorders comprise a group of conditions characterized by disturbances in sleep quality, sleep timing, sleep continuity, circadian regulation, or sleep-related behaviors that result in clinically significant distress, impaired daytime functioning, cognitive dysfunction, emotional dysregulation, occupational impairment, or reduced quality of life. Sleep disturbances are among the most common complaints encountered in psychiatric and primary care settings and frequently coexist with mood disorders, anxiety disorders, trauma-related conditions, substance use disorders, neurodevelopmental disorders, and chronic medical illness. When antidepressants (e.g., doxepin, trazodone, mirtazapine) are used for sleep, note the class boxed warning for an increased risk of suicidal thoughts and behaviors in patients aged 24 years and younger; monitor for clinical worsening and emergent suicidality, especially early in treatment and after dose changes.

Insomnia disorder represents the most prevalent sleep-related condition within outpatient psychiatric practice and is commonly associated with difficulty initiating sleep, maintaining sleep, early morning awakening, or nonrestorative sleep despite adequate opportunity for rest. Excessive daytime sleepiness, circadian rhythm disruption, parasomnias, restless legs syndrome, and sleep-related breathing disorders may also contribute significantly to psychiatric symptoms, emotional instability, impaired concentration, irritability, fatigue, and functional decline. Chronic sleep disturbance may worsen psychiatric illness severity, increase relapse risk, impair treatment response, and contribute to long-term medical morbidity.

The relationship between sleep and psychiatric illness is highly bidirectional. Sleep disturbances may emerge as primary disorders, prodromal symptoms, and consequences of psychiatric illness, medication side effects, or manifestations of underlying neurologic or medical conditions. Insomnia commonly precedes depressive and anxiety disorders, while decreased need for sleep may signal emerging mania or mixed states in bipolar disorder. Trauma-related nightmares, hyperarousal, circadian disruption, stimulant use, chronic pain, and substance withdrawal may also substantially impair sleep architecture and daytime functioning.

Comorbidity is extremely common among patients with sleep-wake disorders. Major depressive disorder, bipolar disorder, anxiety disorders, PTSD, ADHD, substance use disorders, chronic pain syndromes, neurocognitive disorders, obesity, cardiovascular disease, and obstructive sleep apnea frequently coexist and may complicate both diagnosis and treatment planning. Because sleep symptoms may overlap with fatigue, cognitive impairment, low motivation, or emotional dysregulation, careful longitudinal assessment is essential to identify underlying contributors and avoid oversimplified treatment approaches.

Sleep disorders are associated with increased risk of psychiatric decompensation, suicidality, accidents, impaired occupational performance, cognitive dysfunction, and reduced adherence to psychiatric treatment. Chronic insomnia and severe sleep deprivation may contribute to emotional instability, panic symptoms, psychotic experiences, impulsivity, substance misuse, and worsening mood symptoms. Comprehensive psychiatric evaluation should therefore include assessment of sleep duration, sleep hygiene, circadian patterns, medication effects, substance use, nocturnal behaviors, respiratory symptoms, and daytime impairment.

Although pharmacotherapy may provide symptomatic benefit in selected patients, nonpharmacologic interventions remain foundational components of treatment for many sleep-wake disorders. Cognitive behavioral therapy for insomnia (CBT-I), sleep hygiene optimization, circadian stabilization, behavioral modification, stimulus control, and treatment of underlying psychiatric or medical conditions frequently provide substantial long-term benefit. Sedative-hypnotic medications, benzodiazepines, melatonin agonists, orexin receptor antagonists, antidepressants, and wake-promoting agents may be considered depending on the clinical presentation, symptom severity, comorbidity profile, and safety considerations.

Clinicians should remain attentive to medication-related risks including tolerance, physiologic dependence, cognitive impairment, falls, respiratory suppression, parasomnias, next-day sedation, misuse potential, and drug interactions. Particular caution is warranted in elderly populations, patients with substance use disorders, individuals with obstructive sleep apnea, and patients receiving concurrent sedating medications. Sleep medications should generally be used within a broader longitudinal treatment framework emphasizing functional recovery and stabilization of underlying psychiatric or medical contributors.

The following sections provide a structured, evidence-informed framework for the evaluation and treatment of sleep-wake disorders within outpatient psychiatric practice. Recommendations are intended to support safe, individualized, and clinically consistent care while recognizing the importance of longitudinal reassessment, behavioral intervention, interdisciplinary collaboration, and professional clinical judgment throughout the course of illness.

1. INSOMNIA DISORDER

A. OVERVIEW

Aspect	Detail	Evidence Source
Definition	Persistent difficulty initiating or maintaining sleep, or early awakening with daytime impairment despite adequate sleep opportunity	DSM-5-TR (APA, 2022)
Core clinical patterns	Sleep-onset, sleep-maintenance, and early-morning awakening patterns help guide treatment selection	DSM-5-TR (APA, 2022); AASM (2017)
Functional impact	Associated with fatigue, impaired concentration, mood symptoms, occupational dysfunction, and reduced quality of life	DSM-5-TR (APA, 2022); AASM (2021)
First-line treatment	CBT-I is preferred first-line treatment; medications are generally adjunctive or time-limited	AASM (2021); AASM (2017)
Pharmacologic role	Medication choice should consider insomnia type, age, comorbidity, fall risk, and next-day impairment	AASM (2017); Beers Criteria (2023)

B. Diagnostic Considerations

Clinical Consideration	Clinical Notes	Evidence Source
Confirm insomnia phenotype	Differentiate sleep-onset, sleep-maintenance, and early-morning awakening patterns	DSM-5-TR (APA, 2022); AASM (2017)
Confirm chronicity and impairment	Assess frequency, duration, distress, and daytime impairment before diagnosing chronic insomnia disorder	DSM-5-TR (APA, 2022)
Evaluate psychiatric comorbidity	Assess for mood, anxiety, trauma-related, bipolar, and substance-related disorders	DSM-5-TR (APA, 2022); AASM (2021)
Screen for medical contributors	Evaluate pain, GERD, nocturia, cardiopulmonary, endocrine, neurologic, and medication-related causes	AASM (2017); Clinical consensus
Rule out primary sleep disorders	Screen for OSA, restless legs syndrome, circadian disorders, REM behavior disorder, and PLMD before long-term hypnotics	AASM (2017); Clinical consensus
Review substance and medication contributors	Assess caffeine, nicotine, alcohol, cannabis, stimulants, corticosteroids, and activating medications	AASM (2017); Clinical consensus

Clinical Consideration	Clinical Notes	Evidence Source
Assess sleep habits and environment	Evaluate schedule irregularity, naps, screen exposure, and environmental disruption; sleep hygiene alone is insufficient	AASM (2021)
DSM-5-TR diagnostic threshold	Dissatisfaction with sleep quantity or quality occurring ≥3 nights per week for ≥3 months despite adequate opportunity for sleep, with associated daytime impairment.	DSM-5-TR (APA, 2022)

C. First-Line Treatment

Treatment	Clinical Notes	Evidence Source
CBT-I	Preferred first-line treatment; improves sleep latency, sleep efficiency, and remission rates	AASM (2021); AASM Systematic Review (2021)
Stimulus control therapy	Reduces conditioned arousal and strengthens bed-sleep association	AASM (2021)
Sleep restriction therapy	Helps consolidate sleep and improve sleep efficiency when monitored carefully	AASM (2021)
Relaxation-based interventions	May reduce physiologic and cognitive hyperarousal, especially with anxiety	AASM (2021)
Sleep hygiene as adjunct only	Useful within broader treatment plans but insufficient as stand-alone therapy	AASM (2021)

D. Pharmacologic Treatment — FDA-Approved / Guideline-Supported Options

Generic	Brand	Dose Range	Clinical Notes	Evidence Source
Ramelteon	Rozerem	8 mg HS	Melatonin receptor agonist useful for sleep-onset insomnia; no known abuse liability	AASM (2017); FDA (2018)
Zaleplon	Sonata	5–20 mg HS	Very short-acting agent useful for sleep-onset insomnia or selected middle-of-night dosing	AASM (2017); FDA (2020)
Zolpidem	Ambien	5–10 mg HS	Useful for sleep-onset insomnia; monitor next-day impairment and complex sleep behaviors. Boxed warning: complex sleep behaviors (sleep-walking, sleep-driving)—discontinue if these occur	AASM (2017); FDA (2019)

Generic	Brand	Dose Range	Clinical Notes	Evidence Source
Zolpidem ER	Ambien CR	6.25–12.5 mg HS	More useful for sleep-maintenance insomnia; monitor sedation, falls, and cognitive effects. Boxed warning: complex sleep behaviors (sleep-walking, sleep-driving)—discontinue if these occur	AASM (2017); FDA (2019)
Eszopiclone	Lunesta	1–3 mg HS	Useful for sleep-onset and sleep-maintenance insomnia; may cause metallic taste or sedation. Boxed warning: complex sleep behaviors (sleep-walking, sleep-driving, other activities while not fully awake)—discontinue if these occur	AASM (2017); FDA (2019)
Doxepin	Silenor	3–6 mg HS	Low-dose formulation useful for sleep-maintenance and early awakening	AASM (2017); FDA (2010)
Temazepam	Restoril	7.5–30 mg HS	Benzodiazepine hypnotic effective short-term; dependence and fall risk limit use	AASM (2017); FDA (2016)
Estazolam	ProSom	1–2 mg HS	Benzodiazepine hypnotic reserved for selected short-term cases	AASM (2017); FDA (2021)
Suvorexant	Belsomra	10–20 mg HS	DORA useful for sleep-onset and maintenance insomnia; avoid in narcolepsy	AASM (2017); FDA (2014)
Lemborexant	Dayvigo	5–10 mg HS	DORA useful for sleep-onset and maintenance insomnia; monitor sedation and falls	AASM (2017); FDA (2019)
Daridorexant	Quviviq	25–50 mg HS	DORA useful for sleep-onset and maintenance insomnia; 50 mg preferred for greater efficacy; Schedule IV controlled substance; monitor for CNS depression and next-day impairment	FDA Labeling (2022); AASM (2017)

E. Pharmacologic Treatment — Off-Label / Selected-Use Options

Generic	Brand	Dose Range	Clinical Notes	Evidence Source
Trazodone	Desyrel	25–100 mg HS	Common off-label option when insomnia coexists with depression or anxiety; evidence for primary insomnia remains limited	AASM (2017); Limited evidence; Clinical consensus
Mirtazapine	Remeron	7.5–15 mg HS	May help selected patients with comorbid depression, anxiety, and insomnia; not guideline-supported for primary insomnia	Limited evidence; Clinical consensus
Hydroxyzine	Vistaril	25–100 mg HS PRN	Sometimes used short-term for sedation; anticholinergic burden and next-day sedation limit routine use	Clinical consensus; Beers Criteria (2023)

Clinical note

These agents may be encountered in routine practice, particularly when insomnia co-occurs with depression or anxiety, but they should not be interpreted as guideline-supported first-line pharmacologic treatments for primary chronic insomnia.

2. HYPERSOMNOLENCE DISORDER

A. OVERVIEW

Aspect	Detail	Evidence Source
Definition	Excessive sleepiness despite adequate sleep duration, with recurrent sleep episodes, prolonged sleep, or difficulty awakening	DSM-5-TR (APA, 2022)
Core clinical features	May include prolonged nocturnal sleep, daytime sleepiness, frequent naps, and sleep inertia	DSM-5-TR (APA, 2022); Gandhi et al. (2021)
Treatment principle	Management should first address underlying causes before considering wake-promoting agents	Gandhi et al. (2021); Clinical consensus

B. Diagnostic Considerations

Clinical Consideration	Clinical Notes	Evidence Source
Confirm adequate sleep opportunity	Exclude sleep deprivation, irregular schedules, shift work, and behavioral sleep restriction	DSM-5-TR (APA, 2022); Gandhi et al. (2021)
Rule out obstructive sleep apnea	OSA is a common cause of excessive daytime sleepiness and should be assessed first	Gandhi et al. (2021); Clinical consensus
Differentiate from narcolepsy	Assess for cataplexy, sleep paralysis, hypnagogic hallucinations, and REM-related findings	DSM-5-TR (APA, 2022); Gandhi et al. (202

C. First-Line Treatment

Treatment	Clinical Notes	Evidence Source
Address the underlying cause first	Evaluate sleep deprivation, OSA, circadian disruption, medications, medical illness, and psychiatric contributors before symptomatic treatment	Gandhi et al. (2021); Clinical consensus
Sleep medicine evaluation when central hypersomnolence is suspected	Formal sleep evaluation and objective testing may be needed before diagnosing primary hypersomnolence	DSM-5-TR (APA, 2022); Gandhi et al. (2021)

D. Off-Label Symptomatic Options After Diagnostic Clarification

Generic	Brand	Dose Range	Clinical Notes	Evidence Source
Modafinil	Provigil	100–400 mg/day	Off-label option sometimes used after specialist evaluation when significant daytime sleepiness persists. Warning: rare but serious rash, including Stevens-Johnson syndrome/TEN and DRESS — discontinue at the first sign of rash. May reduce the effectiveness of hormonal contraceptives; use an additional or alternative method during and for 1 month after discontinuation	Gandhi et al. (2021); Limited evidence; Clinical consensus
Armodafinil	Nuvigil	150–250 mg/day	Similar off-label role to modafinil; use cautiously with anxiety, insomnia, or cardiovascular risk. Warning: rare but serious rash (SJS/TEN, DRESS) — discontinue at the first sign of rash; may reduce hormonal contraceptive effectiveness (use additional/alternative contraception during and for 1 month after discontinuation)	Gandhi et al. (2021); Limited evidence; Clinical consensus
Methylphenidate	Ritalin, Concerta	Product-specific	Used selectively for central hypersomnolence after specialist evaluation	Gandhi et al. (2021); Limited evidence; Clinical consensus
Amphetamine formulations	Various	Product-specific	Sometimes used in refractory central hypersomnolence; evidence is less established for idiopathic hypersomnia	Gandhi et al. (2021); Limited evidence; Clinical consensus

Clinical note

These medications should be presented as off-label symptomatic options used in practice after specialist diagnostic clarification, not as formally established or broadly guideline-endorsed treatments for DSM hypersomnolence disorder.

3. NARCOLEPSY

A. OVERVIEW

Aspect	Detail	Evidence Source
Definition	Chronic neurologic disorder of sleep-wake regulation characterized by excessive daytime sleepiness and REM dysregulation	DSM-5-TR (APA, 2022); Barker et al. (2020)
Subtypes	Type 1 includes cataplexy and/or hypocretin deficiency; type 2 lacks cataplexy and usually has normal hypocretin levels	DSM-5-TR (APA, 2022); Gandhi et al. (2021)
Treatment principle	Management is symptom-targeted and may combine behavioral, wake-promoting, and cataplexy-directed treatments	Thorpy (2020); Clinical consensus

B. Diagnostic Considerations

Clinical Consideration	Clinical Notes	Evidence Source
Confirm excessive daytime sleepiness phenotype	Assess for sleep attacks, cataplexy, sleep paralysis, hypnagogic hallucinations, and fragmented sleep	DSM-5-TR (APA, 2022); Barker et al. (2020)
Differentiate type 1 vs type 2 narcolepsy	Cataplexy and/or hypocretin deficiency support narcolepsy type 1	DSM-5-TR (APA, 2022); Rémi et al. (2019)
Objective sleep testing	Polysomnography followed by MSLT is central to diagnostic clarification	Rémi et al. (2019); Clinical consensus

C. First-Line Treatment

Treatment	Clinical Notes	Evidence Source
Behavioral scheduling and sleep hygiene	Regular sleep schedules, strategic naps, and safety counseling are important adjuncts	Thorpy (2020); Clinical consensus
Wake-promoting treatment for excessive daytime sleepiness	Medication is often required when daytime sleepiness causes functional impairment	Thorpy (2020); Clinical consensus

D. Pharmacologic Treatment

Generic	Brand	Dose Range	Clinical Notes	Evidence Source
Modafinil	Provigil	100–400 mg/day	Common first-line wake-promoting option with lower misuse potential than traditional stimulants	Thorpy (2020); Clinical consensus

Generic	Brand	Dose Range	Clinical Notes	Evidence Source
Armodafinil	Nuvigil	150–250 mg/day	Longer-acting wake-promoting agent useful for sustained daytime alertness	Thorpy (2020); Clinical consensus
Solriamfetol	Sunosi	75–150 mg/day	Effective for excessive daytime sleepiness; monitor BP, pulse, anxiety, and insomnia	Thorpy (2020); Abad (2021)
Pitolisant	Wakix	8.9–35.6 mg QAM	H3 receptor antagonist/inverse agonist; monitor QTc and insomnia risk; may reduce hormonal contraceptive effectiveness	Thorpy (2020); FDA Labeling (2019)
Sodium oxybate	Xyrem	4.5–9 g/night in 2 divided doses	Effective for cataplexy, EDS, and sleep fragmentation; REMS program and boxed warning apply	Thorpy (2020); FDA Labeling
Sodium oxybate ER	Lumryz	4.5–9 g HS	Once-nightly extended-release formulation; same REMS and boxed warning requirements	Thorpy (2020); FDA Labeling (2023)
Mixed oxybate salts	Xywav	4.5–9 g/night in 2 divided doses	Low-sodium formulation preferred when sodium burden is a concern; REMS program and boxed warning apply	FDA Labeling (2020)

Clinical note

Sodium oxybate formulations (Xyrem, Lumryz, Xywav) are available only through restricted REMS programs. Prescribers must be certified and patients must be enrolled before dispensing. Consult current prescribing information and the applicable REMS program before initiating any oxybate therapy.

4. SLEEP-RELATED BREATHING DISORDERS (OBSTRUCTIVE SLEEP APNEA)

A. OVERVIEW

Aspect	Detail	Evidence Source
Definition	Repetitive upper airway collapse during sleep causing hypoxemia, sleep fragmentation, and nonrestorative sleep	Gandhi et al. (2021); Clinical consensus
Psychiatric relevance	OSA may mimic or worsen depression, cognitive symptoms, fatigue, irritability, and treatment-resistant insomnia or hypersomnolence	Gandhi et al. (2021); Clinical consensus

B. Diagnostic Considerations

Clinical Consideration	Clinical Notes	Evidence Source
Screen for snoring, witnessed apneas, gasping, and daytime sleepiness	Collateral history from a bed partner may improve detection	Gandhi et al. (2021); Clinical consensus
Assess risk factors	Obesity, sedatives, alcohol use, craniofacial anatomy, and cardiometabolic disease increase risk	Clinical consensus
Confirm with sleep testing	Polysomnography or home sleep apnea testing should guide diagnosis and severity assessment	Clinical consensus

C. First-Line Treatment

Treatment	Clinical Notes	Evidence Source
Positive airway pressure (PAP/CPAP)	First-line treatment for clinically significant OSA; improves sleepiness and nocturnal breathing abnormalities	Clinical consensus
Weight reduction when indicated	Important adjunctive strategy in overweight or obese patients	Clinical consensus
Oral appliance therapy	Reasonable alternative when PAP is not tolerated or preferred	Clinical consensus

5. CIRCADIAN RHYTHM SLEEP-WAKE DISORDERS

A. OVERVIEW

Aspect	Detail	Evidence Source
Definition	Persistent sleep disturbance caused by misalignment between the circadian system and the desired sleep-wake schedule	AASM (2017); Clinical consensus
Treatment principle	Management focuses on circadian realignment using timed light exposure, melatonin, and behavioral scheduling	AASM (2017); Clinical consensus

B. Diagnostic Considerations

Clinical Consideration	Clinical Notes	Evidence Source
Differentiate circadian misalignment from insomnia	Patients are often sleepy at biologically inappropriate times rather than unable to sleep	Selsick & O'Regan (2018); Clinical consensus

Clinical Consideration	Clinical Notes	Evidence Source
Identify phase pattern and environmental mismatch	Delayed phase, advanced phase, non-24-hour rhythm, jet lag, and shift-work patterns require different timing strategies	Clinical consensus

C. First-Line Treatment

Treatment	Clinical Notes	Evidence Source
Timed light therapy	Core circadian intervention; timing should match the specific phase pattern	Clinical consensus
Melatonin timed to circadian target	May help phase shifting, particularly in delayed phase and jet lag-related disturbance	Clinical consensus
Sleep schedule stabilization	Consistent sleep and wake timing are foundational interventions	Bjorvatn & Pallesen (2021); Clinical consensus

6. PARASOMNIAS

A. OVERVIEW

Aspect	Detail	Evidence Source
Definition	Undesirable physical events or experiences occurring during sleep or sleep-wake transitions	Clinical consensus
Major categories	NREM parasomnias include sleepwalking and sleep terrors; REM parasomnias include REM sleep behavior disorder and nightmare disorder	Clinical consensus

B. Diagnostic Considerations

Clinical Consideration	Clinical Notes	Evidence Source
Differentiate NREM vs REM parasomnias	Sleepwalking and sleep terrors differ from REM sleep behavior disorder in timing and presentation	Rémi et al. (2019); Clinical consensus
Rule out nocturnal seizures and sleep-disordered breathing	Nocturnal seizures are an important differential; sleep studies may be needed in selected cases	Rémi et al. (2019); Clinical consensus
REM sleep behavior disorder as neurodegenerative marker	RBD may precede Parkinson's disease, Lewy body dementia, or multiple system atrophy by years	Rémi et al. (2019); Clinical consensus

C. First-Line Treatment

Treatment	Clinical Notes	Evidence Source
Safety and environmental protection	Protect the patient and bed partner; remove dangerous objects and address triggers	Clinical consensus
Treat underlying contributors	Address PTSD, anxiety, medications, OSA, or neurologic disease when relevant	Clinical consensus

D. Pharmacologic / Adjunctive Treatment

Generic / Strategy	Clinical Notes	Evidence Source
Melatonin	Commonly used in selected REM sleep behavior disorder cases, especially when sedative burden is a concern	Limited evidence; Clinical consensus
Clonazepam	Traditional option for selected REM sleep behavior disorder cases; use cautiously in older adults or fall-risk patients	Limited evidence; Clinical consensus
Nightmare-focused treatment	Treat underlying PTSD or anxiety rather than escalating sedatives alone	Clinical consensus

7. RESTLESS LEGS SYNDROME

A. OVERVIEW

Aspect	Detail	Evidence Source
Definition	Urge to move the legs with uncomfortable sensations that worsen at rest and at night and improve with movement	Clinical consensus
Treatment principle	Management focuses on reversible contributors, iron correction, and symptom-targeted treatment when indicated	Clinical consensus

B. Diagnostic Considerations

Clinical Consideration	Clinical Notes	Evidence Source
Confirm urge to move worse at rest and night	Symptoms typically improve with movement and worsen in the evening or at night	Aurora et al. (2012); Clinical consensus
Check reversible contributors	Iron deficiency, renal disease, pregnancy, medications, caffeine, alcohol, and antihistamines may worsen symptoms	Braley & Chervin (2015); Aurora et al. (2012); Clinical consensus

C. First-Line Treatment

Treatment	Clinical Notes	Evidence Source
Correct iron deficiency when present	Check serum ferritin and transferrin saturation. Consider oral iron repletion with ferrous sulfate 325 mg, providing approximately 65 mg elemental iron, once daily or every other day, preferably with vitamin C, when ferritin is ≤75 µg/L or TSAT is <20%, unless contraindicated or poorly tolerated. Monitor ferritin/TSAT and avoid iron overload. IV iron may be considered in selected cases with poor oral tolerance	Aurora et al. (2012); Clinical consensus
Reduce exacerbating agents	Avoid or minimize antihistamines and other symptom-worsening medications when possible	Braley & Chervin (2015); Clinical consensus

D. Pharmacologic Treatment

Generic	Brand	Dose Range	Clinical Notes	Evidence Source
Gabapentin	Neurontin	300–1800 mg/day; administered at bedtime or in divided doses	Commonly used when RLS coexists with insomnia, neuropathic pain, or nocturnal discomfort	Aurora et al. (2012); Clinical consensus
Pregabalin	Lyrica	75–450 mg/day; administered at bedtime or in divided doses	Useful for persistent symptoms; monitor sedation, dizziness, and weight gain	Aurora et al. (2012); Clinical consensus
Pramipexole	Mirapex	0.125–0.5 mg taken 2–3 hours before bedtime	Effective dopaminergic option; monitor for augmentation and impulse-control symptoms	Aurora et al. (2012); Clinical consensus
Ropinirole	Requip	0.25–4 mg taken 1–3 hours before bedtime	Alternative dopaminergic option; monitor augmentation, behavioral effects, and daytime sleepiness	Aurora et al. (2012); Clinical consensus

E. Off-Label / Adjunctive Considerations

Strategy	Clinical Notes	Evidence Source
Behavioral contributors	Review caffeine, nicotine, alcohol, and sleep deprivation	Clinical consensus
Medication review	SSRIs, SNRIs, antihistamines, dopamine antagonists, and lithium may worsen symptoms in susceptible patients	Braley & Chervin (2015); Clinical consensus

F. Practical Treatment Selection

Clinical Scenario	Preferred Treatment	Rationale	Avoid / Caution	Evidence Source
RLS with insomnia and neuropathic discomfort	Gabapentin or pregabalin	May improve sensory symptoms and sleep disruption	Monitor sedation and dizziness	—
Frequent classic RLS symptoms without major pain	Pramipexole or ropinirole	Dopaminergic benefit may be meaningful in selected patients	Monitor augmentation and impulse-control symptoms	—

G. Risks / Monitoring

Strategy / Risk Area	Clinical Notes	Evidence Source
Dopamine agonist augmentation	Symptoms may begin earlier, intensify, or spread with chronic dopaminergic exposure	Clinical consensus
Sedating medications	May worsen cognition, falls, and morning impairment, especially in older adults	Clinical consensus
Antihistamine exposure	May worsen RLS symptoms and sleep fragmentation in susceptible patients	Clinical consensus

REFERENCES

American Academy of Sleep Medicine. (2017). Clinical practice guideline for the pharmacologic treatment of chronic insomnia in adults. *Journal of Clinical Sleep Medicine, 13*(2), 307–349. https://doi.org/10.5664/jcsm.6470

American Academy of Sleep Medicine. (2021). Behavioral and psychological treatments for chronic insomnia disorder in adults: An American Academy of Sleep Medicine clinical practice guideline. *Journal of Clinical Sleep Medicine, 17*(2), 255–262. https://doi.org/10.5664/jcsm.8986

American Academy of Sleep Medicine. (2021). Behavioral and psychological treatments for chronic insomnia disorder in adults: An American Academy of Sleep Medicine systematic review, meta-analysis, and GRADE assessment. *Journal of Clinical Sleep Medicine, 17*(2), 263–298. https://doi.org/10.5664/jcsm.8988

American Geriatrics Society Beers Criteria® Update Expert Panel. (2023). American Geriatrics Society 2023 updated AGS Beers Criteria® for potentially inappropriate medication use in older adults. *Journal of the American Geriatrics Society, 71*(7), 2052–2081. https://doi.org/10.1111/jgs.18372

American Psychiatric Association. (2022). *Diagnostic and statistical manual of mental disorders* (5th ed., text rev.; DSM-5-TR). American Psychiatric Publishing.

Abad, V. C. (2021). Profile of solriamfetol in the management of excessive daytime sleepiness associated with narcolepsy or obstructive sleep apnea: Focus on patient selection and perspectives. *Nature and Science of Sleep, 13*, 75–91. https://doi.org/10.2147/NSS.S227867

Aurora, R. N., Kristo, D. A., Bista, S. R., Rowley, J. A., Zak, R. S., Casey, K. R., Lamm, C. I., Tracy, S. L., Rosenberg, R. S., & American Academy of Sleep Medicine. (2012). The treatment of restless legs syndrome and periodic limb movement disorder in adults—An update for 2012: Practice parameters with an evidence-based systematic review and meta-analyses. *Sleep, 35*(8), 1039–1062. https://doi.org/10.5665/sleep.1988

Barker, E. C., Flygare, J., & Paruthi, S. (2020). Living with narcolepsy: Current management strategies, future prospects, and overlooked real-life concerns. *Nature and Science of Sleep, 12*, 453–466. https://doi.org/10.2147/NSS.S162758

Bjorvatn, B., & Pallesen, S. (2021). Circadian rhythm sleep disorders. In C. Bassetti, Z. Dogas, & P. Peigneux (Eds.), *Sleep Medicine Textbook* (2nd ed.). European Sleep Research Society (ESRS).

Braley, T. J., & Chervin, R. D. (2015). A practical approach to the diagnosis and management of sleep disorders in patients with multiple sclerosis. *Therapeutic Advances in Neurological Disorders, 8*(6), 294–310. https://doi.org/10.1177/1756285615601509

Gandhi, K., Mansukhani, M. P., & Silber, M. H. (2021). Excessive daytime sleepiness: A clinical review. *Mayo Clinic Proceedings, 96*(5), 1288–1301. https://doi.org/10.1016/j.mayocp.2020.08.033

Rémi, J., Pollmächer, T., & Spiegelhalder, K. (2019). Sleep-related disorders in neurology and psychiatry. *Deutsches Ärzteblatt International, 116*(41), 681–688. https://doi.org/10.3238/arztebl.2019.0681

Selsick, H., & O'Regan, D. (2018). Sleep disorders in psychiatry. *BJPsych Advances, 24*(4), 273–283. https://doi.org/10.1192/bja.2018.8

Thorpy, M. J. (2020). Recently approved and upcoming treatments for narcolepsy. *CNS Drugs, 34*(1), 9–27. https://doi.org/10.1007/s40263-019-00689-1

U.S. Food and Drug Administration. (2010). *Silenor (doxepin) prescribing information*. https://www.accessdata.fda.gov

U.S. Food and Drug Administration. (2014). *Belsomra (suvorexant) prescribing information*. https://www.accessdata.fda.gov

U.S. Food and Drug Administration. (2016). *Restoril (temazepam) prescribing information*. https://www.accessdata.fda.gov

U.S. Food and Drug Administration. (2018). *Rozerem (ramelteon) prescribing information*. https://www.accessdata.fda.gov

U.S. Food and Drug Administration. (2019). *Dayvigo (lemborexant) prescribing information*. https://www.accessdata.fda.gov

U.S. Food and Drug Administration. (2019). *Ambien (zolpidem tartrate) prescribing information*. https://www.accessdata.fda.gov

U.S. Food and Drug Administration. (2019). *Lunesta (eszopiclone) prescribing information*. https://www.accessdata.fda.gov

U.S. Food and Drug Administration. (2020). *Sonata (zaleplon) prescribing information.* https://www.accessdata.fda.gov

U.S. Food and Drug Administration. (2020). *Xywav (calcium, magnesium, potassium, and sodium oxybates) prescribing information*. Jazz Pharmaceuticals. https://www.accessdata.fda.gov

U.S. Food and Drug Administration. (2021). *ProSom (estazolam) prescribing information*. https://www.accessdata.fda.gov

U.S. Food and Drug Administration. (2022). Quviviq (daridorexant) prescribing information. https://www.accessdata.fda.gov

U.S. Food and Drug Administration. (2023). Lumryz (sodium oxybate extended-release) prescribing information. https://www.accessdata.fda.gov

XII. ADVERSE EFFECT MANAGEMENT

SECTION INTRODUCTION

Adverse effects associated with psychopharmacologic treatment represent a major contributor to medication nonadherence, treatment discontinuation, functional impairment, emergency medical presentations, and reduced quality of life in psychiatric patients. Effective identification, prevention, monitoring, and management of medication-related adverse effects are therefore essential components of safe outpatient psychiatric practice and long-term treatment success. Clinicians must balance therapeutic efficacy with tolerability, medical safety, patient preference, and overall functional outcomes when selecting and managing psychiatric medications.

Psychotropic medications may affect multiple organ systems and produce a broad spectrum of adverse effects ranging from mild and transient symptoms to severe, life-threatening medical emergencies. Common adverse effects include sedation, gastrointestinal symptoms, sexual dysfunction, weight gain, metabolic abnormalities, extrapyramidal symptoms (EPS), tremor, cognitive impairment, orthostasis, insomnia, emotional blunting, and cardiovascular effects. Serious complications such as neuroleptic malignant syndrome (NMS), serotonin syndrome, agranulocytosis, severe drug interactions, seizures, hepatotoxicity, lithium toxicity, QT prolongation, and metabolic syndrome require early recognition and prompt intervention to reduce morbidity and mortality.

Medication tolerability plays a central role in adherence and long-term psychiatric stabilization. Many patients discontinue otherwise effective treatment because of adverse effects involving weight gain, sexual dysfunction, sedation, emotional numbing, akathisia, gastrointestinal intolerance, or cognitive slowing. Inadequately addressed side effects may worsen depressive symptoms, anxiety, social functioning, occupational performance, self-esteem, and therapeutic alliance. Routine adverse effect assessment should therefore be incorporated into every stage of psychiatric treatment, including initiation, titration, maintenance, switching strategies, and polypharmacy management.

Certain psychiatric populations may demonstrate increased vulnerability to medication-related complications. Elderly patients, medically complex individuals, children and adolescents, pregnant patients, individuals with substance use disorders, and patients receiving multiple psychotropic or nonpsychiatric medications require particularly careful monitoring. Comorbid cardiovascular disease, obesity, diabetes, renal impairment, hepatic dysfunction, neurologic illness, and sleep-disordered breathing may substantially alter medication safety profiles and influence treatment selection.

Metabolic complications associated with second-generation antipsychotics remain a major clinical concern within psychiatric practice. Weight gain, dyslipidemia, insulin resistance, and diabetes risk contribute significantly to long-term cardiovascular morbidity and reduced life expectancy among psychiatric populations. Likewise, extrapyramidal symptoms—including akathisia, dystonia, parkinsonism, and tardive dyskinesia—may cause substantial distress, impaired adherence, and functional deterioration if inadequately recognized or treated. Routine metabolic monitoring and movement disorder assessment are therefore critical components of psychopharmacologic management.

Clinicians must also remain attentive to medication interactions, withdrawal syndromes, and discontinuation phenomena. Abrupt discontinuation of antidepressants, benzodiazepines, mood stabilizers, stimulants, or antipsychotics may produce clinically significant rebound symptoms, withdrawal syndromes, relapse, or medical instability. Polypharmacy further increases the risk of pharmacokinetic and pharmacodynamic interactions, particularly in patients receiving multiple serotonergic, sedating, anticholinergic, or QT-prolonging agents.

Management of adverse effects should remain individualized and clinically pragmatic. Strategies may include dose reduction, slower titration, schedule adjustment, switching medications, targeted adjunctive treatment, behavioral interventions, laboratory monitoring, or referral for medical evaluation when indicated. Shared decision-making and patient education are essential to improve adherence, reduce fear regarding medication treatment, and promote early reporting of concerning symptoms or medical complications.

The following sections provide a structured, evidence-informed framework for the recognition, monitoring, prevention, and management of psychotropic medication adverse effects within outpatient psychiatric practice. Recommendations are intended to support safe, clinically individualized, and longitudinal psychopharmacologic care while recognizing the importance of ongoing reassessment, interdisciplinary collaboration, patient education, and professional clinical judgment throughout treatment.

1. WEIGHT GAIN AND METABOLIC CHANGES

A. OVERVIEW

Highest-risk agents	Olanzapine and clozapine carry the greatest risk of clinically significant weight gain and metabolic disturbance; quetiapine and valproate carry intermediate risk; mirtazapine may also contribute to weight gain	NICE (2022); De Hert et al. (2011)
Clinical importance	Weight gain may impair adherence and increase long-term risk of diabetes, dyslipidemia, hypertension, and cardiovascular disease	NICE (2022); De Hert et al. (2011); Stroup & Gray (2018)
Required monitoring	Weight, BMI, waist circumference, blood pressure, fasting glucose or HbA1c, and lipid profile should be monitored systematically	NICE (2022); ADA/APA Consensus (2004); De Hert et al. (2024)
Monitoring timing	Assess at baseline, during early titration, at 3 months, and periodically thereafter according to agent and patient risk	NICE (2022); ADA/APA Consensus (2004); De Hert et al. (2024)

B. Diagnostic Considerations

Clinical Consideration	Clinical Notes	Evidence Source
Identify early rapid weight gain	Early increase in weight often predicts longer-term metabolic burden and should trigger prompt intervention	NICE (2022); Stroup & Gray (2018)
Review baseline metabolic risk	Pre-existing obesity, diabetes, dyslipidemia, sedentary lifestyle, and family history increase vulnerability	NICE (2022); De Hert et al. (2011)
Distinguish agent effect from lifestyle contributors	Medication burden, diet, sleep disruption, and reduced physical activity often interact and should all be addressed	Clinical consensus

C. First-line Treatment

Clinical Scenario	Preferred Treatment	Rationale	Avoid / Caution	Evidence Source
Early psychotropic-related weight gain	Lifestyle intervention + metabolic monitoring	Early intervention may improve long-term outcomes and adherence	Avoid delaying intervention until severe gain occurs	NICE (2022); Stroup & Gray (2018)
Ongoing antipsychotic-related weight gain	Switch to a lower-risk antipsychotic when feasible	May reduce metabolic burden while maintaining treatment	Avoid switching if relapse risk is high	NICE (2022); De Hert et al. (2011); Speyer et al. (2021)

D. Second-line / Augmentation

Base Treatment	Add-On Agent	Dose Range	Clinical Notes	Evidence Source
Lifestyle intervention or continued antipsychotic treatment	Metformin	500–2000 mg/day	Best-supported adjunct; greater benefit when started early	De Silva et al. (2016); Bak et al. (2024); De Hert et al. (2024)
Lifestyle intervention or continued antipsychotic treatment	Topiramate	25–300 mg/day	May reduce weight; cognitive adverse effects may limit use	Zheng et al. (2016); Kameg & Champion (2021)
Lifestyle intervention or continued antipsychotic treatment	Semaglutide or other GLP-1 receptor agonists	Per prescribing guidelines	Effective adjunctive option for antipsychotic-induced weight gain; growing evidence base; requires metabolic coordination and insurance/access consideration	Bak et al. (2024); Larsen et al. (2024)

E. Risks / Monitoring

Clinical Risk	Clinical Notes	Evidence Source
Delayed intervention	Failure to address early gain increases long-term metabolic burden and reduces treatment acceptance	NICE (2022); Stroup & Gray (2018)
Metformin tolerability	Monitor gastrointestinal tolerability and overall clinical response; assess renal function according to standard metformin prescribing precautions	De Silva et al. (2016); Clinical consensus
Topiramate cognitive burden	Cognitive slowing, word-finding difficulty, and poor tolerability may limit benefit	Generali & Cada (2014)

2. NAUSEA AND GASTROINTESTINAL DISTRESS

A. OVERVIEW

Aspect	Detail	Evidence Source
Common causative agents	SSRIs, SNRIs, bupropion IR, and some antipsychotics commonly cause early nausea or GI discomfort	NICE (2022)
Typical course	Symptoms are often transient and improve within the first 1-2 weeks	NICE (2022); Clinical consensus
Clinical importance	Persistent GI intolerance may impair adherence and justify dose adjustment or switch	NICE (2022)

B. First-line Treatment

Clinical Scenario	Preferred Treatment	Rationale	Avoid / Caution	Evidence Source
Mild early nausea after initiation	Take with food or dose at bedtime when feasible	May reduce GI intolerance and improve adherence	Avoid abrupt discontinuation for mild early symptoms	NICE (2022)
Persistent but tolerable nausea	Reduce dose or slow titration	May improve tolerability while maintaining treatment	Avoid excessive dose reduction if efficacy declines	NICE (2022)

C. Practical Treatment Selection

Clinical Scenario	Preferred Treatment	Rationale	Avoid / Caution	Evidence Source
Persistent nausea despite adjustment	Switch to a better-tolerated agent or formulation	Some patients do not adapt despite dose modification	Reassess for non-medication GI causes	NICE (2022)

Clinical Scenario	Preferred Treatment	Rationale	Avoid / Caution	Evidence Source
Short-term symptomatic relief needed	Ondansetron 4–8 mg PRN (preferred); avoid metoclopramide and prochlorperazine in patients on antipsychotics or with Parkinson's disease risk. Ondansetron may prolong the QT interval. Rare reports describe serotonin syndrome with 5-HT3 antagonists, generally in combination with other serotonergic agents; a causal role is uncertain. Use the lowest effective dose and avoid unnecessary QT-risk stacking	May improve adherence during early treatment	Avoid metoclopramide and prochlorperazine with antipsychotics or in Parkinson's patients — dopamine antagonism may worsen symptoms or cause EPS; avoid routine long-term antiemetic use	Clinical consensus

3. CONSTIPATION

A. OVERVIEW

Aspect	Detail	Evidence Source
Common causative agents	Clozapine, olanzapine, TCAs, and other anticholinergic agents commonly contribute to constipation	NICE (2022); Every-Palmer et al. (2017); Stroup & Gray (2018)
Clinical importance	Constipation ranges from mild discomfort to severe ileus, particularly with clozapine-associated GI hypomotility	Every-Palmer et al. (2017); Stroup & Gray (2018)
High-risk group	Patients treated with clozapine require proactive bowel monitoring	Every-Palmer et al. (2017)

B. First-line Treatment

Clinical Scenario	Preferred Treatment	Rationale	Avoid / Caution	Evidence Source
Mild constipation	Increase fiber, hydration, activity, and review bowel habits	First-line conservative management	Avoid relying on intermittent PRN treatment if symptoms are recurrent	NICE (2022)

Clinical Scenario	Preferred Treatment	Rationale	Avoid / Caution	Evidence Source
Persistent constipation	Polyethylene glycol (MiraLax) or senna; for clozapine patients consider scheduled rather than PRN regimen	Standard escalation when conservative measures fail	Tailor regimen to severity, age, and medical comorbidity	Every-Palmer et al. (2017)

C. Practical Treatment Selection

Clinical Scenario	Preferred Treatment	Rationale	Avoid / Caution	Evidence Source
High anticholinergic burden	Reduce anticholinergic load or switch to a lower-burden agent when feasible	Addresses the pharmacologic driver	Avoid destabilizing the primary psychiatric regimen without a replacement plan	NICE (2022)
Clozapine-associated constipation	Scheduled/ prophylactic laxative therapy from clozapine initiation, plus proactive monitoring and early intervention	Conservative measures alone may be insufficient; clozapine-related hypomotility can be life-threatening, and absence of reported constipation does not exclude dangerous GI hypomotility	Do not minimize reduced bowel frequency, abdominal pain, or distention	Every-Palmer et al. (2017); Stroup & Gray (2018)

D. Risks / Monitoring

Clinical Risk	Clinical Notes	Evidence Source
Clozapine-related GI hypomotility	May progress to ileus, bowel obstruction, sepsis, or fatal complications if not recognized early	Every-Palmer et al. (2017)

4. SEXUAL DYSFUNCTION

A. OVERVIEW

Aspect	Detail	Evidence Source
Common causative agents	SSRIs, SNRIs, and prolactin-elevating antipsychotics are frequent causes	NICE (2022); Clayton et al. (2014); Stroup & Gray (2018)
Clinical importance	Sexual adverse effects are underreported and may significantly reduce adherence and quality of life	Clayton et al. (2014); Stroup & Gray (2018)
Assessment focus	Ask directly about libido, arousal, orgasm, erectile function, and prolactin-related symptoms when relevant	Clinical consensus

B. First-line Treatment

Clinical Scenario	Preferred Treatment	Rationale	Avoid / Caution	Evidence Source
Dose-related antidepressant sexual dysfunction	Reduce dose if clinically feasible	Symptoms may improve with lower exposure	Avoid dose reduction if relapse risk is substantial	NICE (2022)
SSRI-related sexual dysfunction	Switch to bupropion or consider mirtazapine in selected cases	Lower sexual adverse effect burden than many SSRIs	Balance against anxiety, insomnia, or weight effects depending on the alternative	Clayton et al. (2014)

C. Second-line / Augmentation

Base Treatment	Add-On Agent	Dose Range	Clinical Notes	Evidence Source
SSRI treatment with sexual dysfunction	Bupropion	150-300 mg/day	May improve sexual function while preserving antidepressant response	Clayton et al. (2014)
Serotonergic treatment with erectile dysfunction	Sildenafil	25-100 mg PRN	Symptomatic strategy when clinically appropriate	NICE (2022)

Clinical note

When sexual dysfunction persists despite dose reduction or medication switch, referral to primary care or urology is recommended for further evaluation. PDE5 inhibitors (e.g., sildenafil, tadalafil) may be considered by the managing physician after cardiovascular assessment. Clayton et al. (2014); Clinical consensus.

D. Risks / Monitoring

Clinical Risk	Clinical Notes	Evidence Source
Underrecognition	Many patients do not report sexual side effects unless asked directly	Clayton et al. (2014)
Prolactin-mediated dysfunction	Evaluate galactorrhea, amenorrhea, gynecomastia, and reduced libido when prolactin-elevating agents are used	NICE (2022); Clinical consensus

5. SEDATION

A. OVERVIEW

Aspect	Detail	Evidence Source
Common causative agents	Mirtazapine, quetiapine, trazodone, clozapine, and olanzapine commonly cause sedation	NICE (2022); Stroup & Gray (2018)
Clinical importance	Sedation may impair functioning, adherence, cognition, and fall safety	NICE (2022); Stroup & Gray (2018)

B. First-line Treatment

Clinical Scenario	Preferred Treatment	Rationale	Avoid / Caution	Evidence Source
Daytime sedation after starting a sedating agent	Move dosing to bedtime	Reduces daytime impairment	Ensure bedtime dosing does not worsen morning carryover	NICE (2022)
Persistent sedation	Reduce dose if feasible	Sedation is often dose-related	Avoid compromising efficacy without reassessing symptoms	NICE (2022)

Clinical Scenario	Preferred Treatment	Rationale	Avoid / Caution	Evidence Source
Ongoing functional impairment	Switch to a less sedating alternative	Improves daytime cognition and tolerability	Consider whether sedation was therapeutically useful for insomnia or agitation	NICE (2022); Stroup & Gray (2018)

C. Risks / Monitoring

Clinical Risk	Clinical Notes	Evidence Source
Falls and cognitive slowing	Risk increases in older adults, medical comorbidity, and polypharmacy	NICE (2022); Stroup & Gray (2018)

6. MEDICATION-INDUCED INSOMNIA

A. OVERVIEW

Aspect	Detail	Evidence Source
Common activating agents	Fluoxetine, bupropion, venlafaxine, stimulants, and aripiprazole may worsen insomnia	NICE (2022)
Clinical importance	Persistent activation may reduce adherence and worsen anxiety, fatigue, and daytime function	Clinical consensus

B. First line Treatment

Clinical Scenario	Preferred Treatment	Rationale	Avoid / Caution	Evidence Source
Activation after initiation	Morning dosing and sleep hygiene optimization	Reduces evening stimulation	Avoid late-day dosing of activating agents	NICE (2022)
Persistent but manageabl e insomnia	Reduce dose if feasible	Addresses the underlying cause	Avoid layering multiple sedatives before optimizing the primary regimen	NICE (2022)

C. Practical Treatment Selection

Clinical Scenario	Preferred Treatment	Rationale	Avoid / Caution	Evidence Source
Continued insomnia despite schedule optimization	Consider melatonin or low-dose trazodone when clinically appropriate	Symptomatic relief may support continuation of the primary medication in selected patients	Use trazodone cautiously because of orthostasis and next-day sedation; avoid reflexive sedative polypharmacy before optimizing the causative regimen	Stroup & Gray (2018); Clinical consensus
Ongoing activating adverse effect	Switch to a less activating alternative	Removes the pharmacologic driver	Avoid chronic compensatory polypharmacy without reassessment	NICE (2022)

7. AKATHISIA

A. OVERVIEW

Aspect	Detail	Evidence Source
Common causative agents	Haloperidol, risperidone, aripiprazole, and metoclopramide are common triggers	Barnes (2014); Stroup & Gray (2018)
Clinical importance	Akathisia is often misidentified as anxiety or agitation and may markedly increase distress	Barnes (2014); Stroup & Gray (2018)

B. Diagnostic Considerations

Clinical Consideration	Clinical Notes	Evidence Source
Differentiate from agitation	Ask specifically about inner restlessness and urge to move; pacing alone is not sufficient	Barnes (2014)
Review dose relationship	Higher dose and rapid dose escalation increase risk	Stroup & Gray (2018)

C. First-line Treatment

Clinical Scenario	Preferred Treatment	Rationale	Avoid / Caution	Evidence Source
Suspected medication-induced akathisia	Reduce dose or switch to a lower-risk agent	Directly addresses the cause	Avoid escalating the offending agent when restlessness is medication-related	NICE (2022); Stroup & Gray (2018)
Persistent akathisia	Propranolol when tolerated	Best-established symptomatic option; typical dose 20–40 mg BID–TID; titrate based on response and heart rate tolerance	Avoid in clinically significant asthma, bradycardia, or hypotension	Barnes (2014); Stroup & Gray (2018)

D. Second-line / Augmentation

Base Treatment	Add-On Agent	Dose Range	Clinical Notes	Evidence Source
Dose reduction or switch strategy	Lorazepam	Short-term only	May reduce acute distress; avoid long-term dependence	Clinical consensus
Dose reduction or switch strategy	Mirtazapine	Variable	Consider in selected cases when beta-blockers are not suitable	Stroup & Gray (2018); Clinical consensus

E. Practical Treatment Selection

Clinical Scenario	Preferred Treatment	Rationale	Avoid / Caution	Evidence Source
Persistent need for antipsychotic treatment with severe akathisia	Consider lower-EPS agents such as quetiapine or clozapine when clinically appropriate	These agents carry lower akathisia risk than high-potency alternatives	Clozapine requires full monitoring infrastructure and is not a routine first-line solution for akathisia alone	Stroup & Gray (2018); NICE (2022)

8. TARDIVE DYSKINESIA

A. OVERVIEW

Aspect	Detail	Evidence Source
Risk setting	Long-term dopamine receptor blocking exposure is the main risk context; both FGAs and SGAs can cause tardive dyskinesia	APA (2020); Stroup & Gray (2018); Ricciardi et al. (2019)
Clinical importance	Early recognition improves the likelihood of limiting progression and treatment burden	APA (2020); Ricciardi et al. (2019)

B. First-line Treatment

Clinical Scenario	Preferred Treatment	Rationale	Avoid / Caution	Evidence Source
Suspected tardive dyskinesia	Reassess antipsychotic exposure and reduce dopamine-blocking burden when feasible	Continued exposure may worsen symptoms	Avoid confusing tardive dyskinesia with acute EPS syndromes	APA (2020); NICE (2022); Ricciardi et al. (2019)
Need for ongoing antipsychotic treatment	Consider switch to clozapine	Clozapine has the lowest tardive liability among antipsychotics	Requires full risk-benefit review and monitoring capacity	APA (2020); Ricciardi et al. (2019)

C. Second-line / Augmentation

Base Treatment	Add-On Agent	Dose Range	Clinical Notes	Evidence Source
Persistent clinically significant tardive dyskinesia	Valbenazine (Ingrezza)	40-80 mg/day	Evidence-supported VMAT2 inhibitor option	APA (2020); Ricciardi et al. (2019)
Persistent clinically significant tardive dyskinesia	Deutetrabenazine (Austedo)	6-24 mg BID	Evidence-supported VMAT2 inhibitor option	APA (2020); Ricciardi et al. (2019)

D. Risks / Monitoring

Clinical Risk	Clinical Notes	Evidence Source
Delayed recognition	Perform periodic structured abnormal involuntary movement assessment during long-term antipsychotic treatment	APA (2020)

9. HYPERPROLACTINEMIA

A. OVERVIEW

Aspect	Detail	Evidence Source
Common causative agents	Risperidone, paliperidone, and haloperidol commonly elevate prolactin	NICE (2022); Haddad & Wieck (2004); Stroup & Gray (2018)
Clinical importance	May cause galactorrhea, amenorrhea, sexual dysfunction, gynecomastia, infertility concerns, and bone health consequences over time	Haddad & Wieck (2004); Stroup & Gray (2018)
Monitoring uncertainty	Monitoring and management approaches vary because high-quality consensus standards remain limited	Stroup & Gray (2018); Clinical consensus

B. First-line Treatment

Clinical Scenario	Preferred Treatment	Rationale	Avoid / Caution	Evidence Source
Symptomatic hyperprolactinemia	Switch to aripiprazole or quetiapine when feasible	Lower prolactin liability than risperidone- or paliperidone-like strategies	Avoid destabilizing a uniquely effective regimen without psychiatric reassessment	NICE (2022); Haddad & Wieck (2004); Stroup & Gray (2018)

C. Second-line / Augmentation

Base Treatment	Add-On Agent	Dose Range	Clinical Notes	Evidence Source
Ongoing antipsychotic treatment with persistent hyperprolactinemia	Aripiprazole	2-15 mg/day adjunct in selected cases	May reduce prolactin while preserving antipsychotic efficacy	Clinical consensus

D. Practical Treatment Selection

Clinical Scenario	Preferred Treatment	Rationale	Avoid / Caution	Evidence Source
Specialist-managed refractory case	Dopamine agonist; may normalize prolactin but carries risk of cardiac valvular abnormalities and psychosis exacerbation; use only in exceptional circumstances under specialist supervision	Can reduce prolactin but may worsen psychosis risk	Avoid routine use outside specialist supervision	Melmed et al. (2011); Haddad & Wieck (2004); Clinical consensus

E. Risks / Monitoring

Clinical Risk	Clinical Notes	Evidence Source
Symptom underrecognition	Ask directly about menstrual changes, libido, galactorrhea, erectile dysfunction, and breast symptoms	Haddad & Wieck (2004); Clinical consensus

10. ORTHOSTATIC HYPOTENSION

A. OVERVIEW

Aspect	Detail	Evidence Source
Common causative agents	Quetiapine, clozapine, TCAs, and other alpha-adrenergic blocking agents may cause orthostasis	NICE (2022); Stroup & Gray (2018); Kameg & Champion (2021)
Clinical importance	Orthostasis increases fall risk, treatment intolerance, and functional impairment	NICE (2022); Stroup & Gray (2018)

B. First-line Treatment

Clinical Scenario	Preferred Treatment	Rationale	Avoid / Caution	Evidence Source
Early orthostasis during titration	Slow titration, hydration, and dose reduction if needed	Reduces autonomic burden and fall risk	Use extra caution in older adults and medically frail patients	NICE (2022); Stroup & Gray (2018)

Clinical Scenario	Preferred Treatment	Rationale	Avoid / Caution	Evidence Source
Persistent symptoms	Review all contributing medications and consider switch	Addresses cumulative hypotensive burden	Avoid attributing all dizziness to psychotropics without medical review	Clinical consensus

C. Practical Treatment Selection

Clinical Scenario	Preferred Treatment	Rationale	Avoid / Caution	Evidence Source
Refractory orthostatic symptoms	Consider nonpharmacologic supports such as compression stockings when appropriate	May reduce venous pooling and symptom burden	Assess cardiovascular status before adding salt-loading strategies	Clinical consensus

11. QT PROLONGATION

A. OVERVIEW

Aspect	Detail	Evidence Source
Common high-risk agents	Ziprasidone, haloperidol, methadone, and high-dose citalopram are notable QT-risk agents. The FDA maximum for citalopram is 40 mg/day; limit to 20 mg/day in patients older than 60 years, with hepatic impairment, who are CYP2C19 poor metabolizers, or taking CYP2C19 inhibitors	Stroup & Gray (2018); Rochester et al. (2018); Clinical consensus
Clinical importance	QT prolongation increases risk of Torsades de pointes and sudden cardiac death in susceptible patients	Stroup & Gray (2018); Clinical consensus

B. Diagnostic Considerations

Clinical Consideration	Clinical Notes	Evidence Source
Identify risk factors	Cardiac disease, electrolyte abnormalities, high doses, interacting medications, and rapid administration increase risk	Stroup & Gray (2018); Rochester et al. (2018)
Review full medication list	Risk often reflects cumulative QT burden rather than a single agent alone	Stroup & Gray (2018); Clinical consensus

Clinical Consideration	Clinical Notes	Evidence Source
High-risk QT threshold	QTc greater than 500 ms or an increase of 60 ms above baseline should prompt urgent reassessment, discontinuation or reduction of the offending agent, and cardiology referral	Stroup & Gray (2018)

C. First-line Treatment

Clinical Scenario	Preferred Treatment	Rationale	Avoid / Caution	Evidence Source
Starting a higher-risk QT agent	Obtain baseline ECG when clinically indicated and review cardiac risk	Helps identify preexisting vulnerability	Do not rely on medication list review alone	Stroup & Gray (2018); Rochester et al. (2018)
Multiple QT-risk factors or interacting drugs	Avoid QT-prolonging combinations whenever possible	Reduces arrhythmic risk	Use special caution with ziprasidone, haloperidol, methadone, and high-dose citalopram	Stroup & Gray (2018); Rochester et al. (2018)
Correctable contributors present	Replete potassium and magnesium and address reversible causes	Electrolyte correction reduces risk	Persistent QTc prolongation requires broader regimen reassessment	Clinical consensus

12. HYPONATREMIA

A. OVERVIEW

Aspect	Detail	Evidence Source
Common causative agents	SSRIs, venlafaxine, carbamazepine, and oxcarbazepine may cause hyponatremia, often via SIADH	NICE (2022)
High-risk group	Older adults and patients with prior hyponatremia, low body weight, or medical comorbidity are at greater risk. Evaluate severity based on sodium level, symptom burden, acuity, trajectory, and medical risk factors. Symptomatic, severe, rapidly falling, or medically unstable hyponatremia requires urgent medical evaluation	NICE (2022); Clinical consensus

B. First-line Treatment

Clinical Scenario	Preferred Treatment	Rationale	Avoid / Caution	Evidence Source
High-risk patient starting a causative medication	Check sodium at baseline and follow-up when clinically indicated	Improves early detection	Avoid missing subtle symptoms such as fatigue, confusion, or gait change	NICE (2022)
Confirmed medication-related hyponatremia	Discontinue or replace the offending agent based on severity	Removes the likely cause	Severe or symptomatic hyponatremia requires urgent medical referral; do not manage in outpatient setting without medical clearance	NICE (2022)
SIADH pattern present	Fluid restriction and medical management as indicated	Standard supportive approach	Refer to primary care or emergency services if sodium <125 mEq/L or neurologic symptoms present; do not manage severe SIADH in outpatient psychiatric setting alone	Clinical consensus

13. ELEVATED LIVER FUNCTION TESTS (LFTs)

A. OVERVIEW

Aspect	Detail	Evidence Source
Common causative agents	Valproate, carbamazepine, and duloxetine may increase hepatic monitoring burden	NICE (2022); Clinical consensus
Clinical importance	Most mild elevations are transient, but clinically significant hepatotoxicity must be recognized early	Clinical consensus

B. First-line Treatment

Clinical Scenario	Preferred Treatment	Rationale	Avoid / Caution	Evidence Source
Starting hepatically relevant medication	Obtain baseline LFTs and repeat according to agent and patient risk	Establishes baseline and detects early toxicity	Do not ignore malaise, nausea, jaundice, or abdominal pain	NICE (2022); Clinical consensus
Mild asymptomatic elevation	Repeat testing and assess trend, symptoms, and alternative causes	Not all mild elevations require discontinuation	Avoid reflexive discontinuation without clinical context	Clinical consensus
Significant elevation or hepatotoxic symptoms	Discontinue the suspected agent, refer to gastroenterology or hepatology, and pursue medical evaluation	Prevents progression of injury	Refer to gastroenterology or hepatology for LFTs >3x upper limit of normal or hepatotoxic symptoms; valproate requires particular caution given known hepatotoxicity risk; do not re-challenge without specialist guidance	Clinical consensus

14. COGNITIVE BLUNTING

A. OVERVIEW

Aspect	Detail	Evidence Source
Common contributors	TCAs, paroxetine, benzodiazepines, sedating agents, and cumulative anticholinergic burden commonly impair cognition	NICE (2022); Clinical consensus
Clinical importance	Cognitive blunting may reduce adherence, occupational function, and quality of life	Clinical consensus

B. First-line Treatment

Clinical Scenario	Preferred Treatment	Rationale	Avoid / Caution	Evidence Source
Cognitive slowing with sedating or anticholinergic treatment	Reduce dose when feasible	Adverse cognitive effects are often dose-related	Avoid worsening psychiatric control without a replacement strategy	NICE (2022)
High anticholinergic burden	Switch to a lower anticholinergic burden alternative (e.g., sertraline or escitalopram instead of paroxetine or TCAs; aripiprazole or lurasidone instead of olanzapine or quetiapine)	Reduces medication-related cognitive impairment	Review the full regimen, not only the primary psychotropic	Clinical consensus

C. Practical Treatment Selection

Clinical Scenario	Preferred Treatment	Rationale	Avoid / Caution	Evidence Source
[illegible]	[illegible]	[illegible]	[illegible]	[illegible]

D. Risks / Monitoring

Clinical Risk	Clinical Notes	Evidence Source
Cumulative anticholinergic burden	Commonly worsens cognition, especially in older adults and polypharmacy	Clinical consensus

REFERENCES

American Diabetes Association, American Psychiatric Association, American Association of Clinical Endocrinologists, & North American Association for the Study of Obesity.

(2004). Consensus development conference on antipsychotic drugs and obesity and diabetes. *Diabetes Care, 27*(2), 596–601. https://doi.org/10.2337/diacare.27.2.596

American Psychiatric Association. (2020). *The American Psychiatric Association practice guideline for the treatment of patients with schizophrenia* (3rd ed.). American Psychiatric Association Publishing.

Bak, M., Campforts, B., Domen, P., et al. (2024). Glucagon-like peptide agonists for weight management in antipsychotic-induced weight gain: A systematic review and meta-analysis. *Acta Psychiatrica Scandinavica, 150*(6), 516–529. https://doi.org/10.1111/acps.13734

Barnes, T. R. E. (2014). Rating scales for antipsychotic-induced movement disorders. *Journal of Clinical Psychiatry, 75*(10), e01. https://doi.org/10.4088/JCP.13049tx1c

Christensen, M. C., Florea, I., Lindsten, A., & Baldwin, D. S. (2018). Efficacy of vortioxetine on the physical symptoms of major depressive disorder. *Journal of Psychopharmacology, 32*(10), 1086–1097. https://doi.org/10.1177/0269881118790014

Clayton, A. H., Croft, H. A., & Handiwala, L. (2014). Antidepressants and sexual dysfunction: Mechanisms and clinical implications. *Postgraduate Medicine, 126*(2), 91–99. https://doi.org/10.3810/pgm.2014.03.2744

De Hert, M., Detraux, J., van Winkel, R., Yu, W., & Correll, C. U. (2011). Metabolic and cardiovascular adverse effects associated with antipsychotic drugs. *Nature Reviews Endocrinology, 8*(2), 114–126. https://doi.org/10.1038/nrendo.2011.156

De Hert, M., Coppens, V., Lehman, R., Correll, C. U., Detraux, J., & Stubbs, B. (2024). Monitoring and management of metabolic adverse effects of antipsychotics: An update. *European Neuropsychopharmacology, 84*, 1–17.

De Silva, V. A., Suraweera, C., Ratnatunga, S. S., Dayabandara, M., Wanniarachchi, N., Hanwella, R., & de Silva, H. J. (2016). Metformin in prevention and treatment of antipsychotic-induced weight gain: A systematic review and meta-analysis. *BMC Psychiatry, 16*, 341. https://doi.org/10.1186/s12888-016-1049-5

Every-Palmer, S., Newton-Howes, G., & Clarke, M. J. (2017). Pharmacological treatment for antipsychotic-related constipation. *Cochrane Database of Systematic Reviews, 2017*(1), CD011128. https://doi.org/10.1002/14651858.CD011128.pub2

Generali, J. A., & Cada, D. J. (2014). Topiramate: Antipsychotic-induced weight gain. Hospital Pharmacy, 49(4), 345–347. https://doi.org/10.1310/hpj4904-345

Haddad, P. M., & Wieck, A. (2004). Antipsychotic-induced hyperprolactinaemia: Mechanisms, clinical features and management. *Drugs, 64*(20), 2291–2314. https://doi.org/10.2165/00003495-200464200-00003

Kameg, B., & Champion, C. (2021). Atypical antipsychotics: Managing adverse effects. *Perspectives in Psychiatric Care, 58*(2), 691–695. https://doi.org/10.1111/ppc.12837

Larsen, J. R., Vedtofte, L., Jakobsen, M. S. L., Jespersen, H. R., Jakobsen, M. I., Svensson, C. K., Koyuncu, K., Schjerning, O., Oturai, P., Vilsbøll, T., Fink-Jensen, A., & Correll, C. U. (2024). Effect of liraglutide treatment on prediabetes and obesity in clozapine- or olanzapine-treated patients: 3-year follow-up. *Acta Psychiatrica Scandinavica, 149*(1), 60–70.

Melmed, S., Casanueva, F. F., Hoffman, A. R., Kleinberg, D. L., Montori, V. M., Schlechte, J. A., & Wass, J. A. H. (2011). Diagnosis and treatment of hyperprolactinemia: An

Endocrine Society clinical practice guideline. *Journal of Clinical Endocrinology & Metabolism*, 96(2), 273–288. https://doi.org/10.1210/jc.2010-1692

National Institute for Health and Care Excellence. (2022). *Psychosis and schizophrenia in adults: Prevention and management*. NICE. https://www.nice.org.uk/guidance/cg178

Pan, Z., Park, C., Brietzke, E., Rosenblat, J. D., Lee, Y., Musial, N., Zuckerman, H., Ragguett, R. M., Rong, C., Fus, D., Brietzke, S., Lin, K., & McIntyre, R. S. (2018). Cognitive impairment in major depressive disorder. *CNS Spectrums*, *24*(1), 22–29. https://doi.org/10.1017/S1092852918001207

Ricciardi, L., Pringsheim, T., Barnes, T. R. E., Martino, D., Gardner, D., Remington, G., & Prasad, S. (2019). Treatment recommendations for tardive dyskinesia. *Canadian Journal of Psychiatry*, *64*(6), 388–399. https://doi.org/10.1177/0706743718816068

Rochester, M. P., Kane, A. M., & Linnebur, S. A. (2018). Evaluating the risk of QTc prolongation associated with antidepressant use in older adults: A review of the evidence. *Therapeutic Advances in Drug Safety*, *9*(6), 297–308. https://doi.org/10.1177/2042098618772975

Speyer, H., Westergaard, C., Albert, N., Karlsen, M., Stürup, A. E., Nordentoft, M., & Hjorthøj, C. (2021). Reversibility of antipsychotic-induced weight gain: A systematic review and meta-analysis. *Frontiers in Endocrinology*, *12*, 577919. https://doi.org/10.3389/fendo.2021.577919

Stroup, T. S., & Gray, N. (2018). Management of common adverse effects of antipsychotic medications. *World Psychiatry*, *17*(3), 341–356. https://doi.org/10.1002/wps.20567

Zheng, W., Xiang, Y.-T., Xiang, Y., et al. (2016). Efficacy and safety of adjunctive topiramate for schizophrenia: A meta-analysis of randomized controlled trials. Acta Psychiatrica Scandinavica, 134(5), 385–398. https://doi.org/10.1111/acps.12631

XIII. SPECIAL POPULATIONS AND MEDICAL COMORBIDITIES

SECTION INTRODUCTION

Psychiatric evaluation and treatment frequently require modification when caring for special populations or patients with significant medical comorbidities. Age-related physiologic changes, pregnancy, neurologic illness, chronic medical disease, polypharmacy, developmental considerations, and altered pharmacokinetics may substantially influence psychiatric presentation, medication tolerability, safety risk, and treatment response. Comprehensive and individualized treatment planning is therefore essential to ensure safe, effective, and clinically appropriate psychiatric care across diverse patient populations.

Patients with significant medical comorbidity often present with complex interactions between psychiatric symptoms and underlying medical illness. Cardiovascular disease, diabetes mellitus, obesity, chronic pain syndromes, renal impairment, hepatic dysfunction, endocrine disorders, neurologic disease, autoimmune conditions, and sleep-disordered breathing may both mimic and exacerbate psychiatric symptoms while simultaneously increasing vulnerability to medication adverse effects and drug interactions. Careful medical assessment, laboratory monitoring, and interdisciplinary coordination are therefore critical components of psychiatric management in medically complex patients.

Elderly patients represent a particularly high-risk population within psychiatric practice due to age-related changes in metabolism, increased medication sensitivity, cognitive vulnerability, fall risk, polypharmacy, and medical frailty. Psychiatric symptoms in geriatric populations may present atypically and frequently overlap with neurocognitive disorders, delirium, medical illness, or medication effects. Sedation, orthostasis, anticholinergic burden, extrapyramidal symptoms, metabolic complications, and QT prolongation may occur more readily in older adults, requiring conservative dosing strategies and careful longitudinal monitoring.

Children and adolescents require developmentally informed psychiatric assessment and treatment approaches. Neurodevelopmental stage, family environment, academic functioning, psychosocial stressors, and evolving cognitive and emotional regulation capacities may significantly influence symptom presentation and treatment planning. Pediatric populations may also demonstrate increased sensitivity to activation, behavioral disinhibition, appetite suppression, growth effects, suicidality warnings, and long-term developmental implications associated with psychotropic medication use.

Pregnancy and the postpartum period present unique psychiatric and medical challenges requiring careful balancing of maternal psychiatric stability with fetal and neonatal safety considerations. Untreated psychiatric illness during pregnancy may itself contribute to significant maternal, fetal, and developmental risk, including poor prenatal care, substance use, suicide risk, impaired bonding, preterm birth, and obstetric complications. Treatment planning should therefore incorporate individualized risk-benefit assessment, reproductive counseling, breastfeeding considerations, teratogenicity risk, and close coordination with obstetric providers whenever possible.

Patients with neurologic disorders—including epilepsy, traumatic brain injury, Parkinson's disease, multiple sclerosis, stroke, dementia, and movement disorders—may demonstrate substantial overlap between neurologic and psychiatric symptoms. Cognitive impairment, emotional dysregulation, psychosis, impulsivity, depression, anxiety, sleep disturbance, and behavioral changes frequently coexist and may complicate diagnosis and treatment. Certain psychotropic medications may additionally lower seizure threshold, worsen cognition, impair motor functioning, or interact with neurologic therapies.

Substance use disorders and chronic medical illness further complicate psychiatric treatment across many patient populations. Hepatic disease, renal impairment, obesity, respiratory disease, cardiovascular risk factors, and chronic pain syndromes may significantly alter medication metabolism, increase adverse effect burden, and limit available pharmacologic options. Clinicians should therefore remain attentive to organ function, medication interactions, overdose risk, respiratory suppression, metabolic burden, and cumulative sedative exposure when managing medically complex individuals.

Treatment planning within special populations should remain highly individualized and longitudinal. Important clinical considerations include physiologic vulnerability, cognitive status, developmental stage, medical burden, reproductive considerations, social support, functional capacity, caregiver involvement, adherence challenges, and access to multidisciplinary care. Conservative dosing strategies, slower titration schedules, careful laboratory monitoring, and enhanced patient education may be necessary in selected populations to optimize both safety and clinical outcomes.

The following sections provide a structured, evidence-informed framework for the psychiatric management of special populations and medically complex patients within outpatient psychiatric practice. Recommendations are intended to support safe, compassionate, and clinically individualized care while recognizing the importance of interdisciplinary collaboration, longitudinal reassessment, medical-psychiatric integration, and professional clinical judgment throughout treatment.

1. PREGNANCY AND LACTATION

A. OVERVIEW

Aspect	Key notes	Evidence Source
Core principle	Balance maternal psychiatric stability with fetal and neonatal safety	ACOG (2023); NICE (2022)
First-line approach	Prefer nonpharmacologic interventions when feasible, but avoid undertreating moderate-to-severe illness	ACOG (2023); NICE (2022)
If medication is necessary	Use the lowest effective dose and avoid unnecessary polypharmacy	ACOG (2023); NICE (2022)
Clinical priority	Untreated maternal mental illness also carries obstetric and neonatal risk	ACOG (2023); NICE (2022)
Emergency principle	Severe symptoms or postpartum psychosis require urgent psychiatric assessment and possible hospitalization	Rodríguez-Cabezas & Clark (2018); Perry et al. (2021)

B. Medication / Pharmacologic Considerations

Medication / Class	Main Perinatal Use	Clinical Notes	Avoid / Caution	Evidence Source
Sertraline	Severe anxiety, panic disorder, major depression	Often preferred SSRI in pregnancy and lactation	Not for rapid control of agitation or psychosis	ACOG (2023); NICE (2022)
Escitalopram	Severe anxiety or depression	Reasonable alternative when previously effective or better tolerated	Lactation preference less established than sertraline	ACOG (2023); Clinical consensus
Lorazepam	Severe panic, acute anxiety, agitation	Useful for short-term symptom control	Avoid prolonged routine use	Clinical consensus
Haloperidol	Acute psychosis or severe agitation	Common option for rapid symptom control	Monitor EPS and QT-related risk	Rodríguez-Cabezas & Clark (2018); Clinical consensus
Olanzapine	Psychosis, mania, severe agitation	Useful when sedation is beneficial	Monitor metabolic burden	ACOG (2023); Clinical consensus

Medication / Class	Main Perinatal Use	Clinical Notes	Avoid / Caution	Evidence Source
Quetiapine	Bipolar-spectrum illness, psychosis, mood instability	Often used when prior response exists	Monitor sedation and metabolic effects	ACOG (2023); Clinical consensus
Lithium	Bipolar relapse, postpartum psychosis, severe mania	Important option in selected high-risk patients; monitor levels closely	Requires perinatal coordination	ACOG (2023); Clinical consensus
Valproate	Bipolar disorder	Generally avoid during pregnancy because of teratogenic risk	Not a routine pregnancy option	ACOG (2023)
ECT	Severe depression, psychosis, catatonia, postpartum psychosis	Important option when rapid response is required	Requires procedural coordination	Frieder et al. (2019); Rodríguez-Cabezas & Clark (2018)
Zuranolone (Zurzuvae)	Moderate-to-severe postpartum depression	FDA-approved oral neuroactive steroid; 14-day course	Avoid in pregnancy; monitor CNS depression	FDA labeling (2023); Deligiannidis et al. (2023)

C. Lactation-Specific Considerations

Medication / Class	Preferred / Use With Caution	Clinical Notes	Avoid / Caution	Evidence Source
Sertraline	Often preferred	Low infant exposure; commonly preferred SSRI during lactation	Monitor infant irritability, feeding, or sedation if concerns arise	McAllister-Williams et al. (2017); Clinical consensus

Medication / Class	Preferred / Use With Caution	Clinical Notes	Avoid / Caution	Evidence Source
Paroxetine	Often low-exposure option	Low reported infant exposure; prior maternal response still matters. Low infant exposure in lactation is not a general perinatal preference: in pregnancy or pregnancy planning, paroxetine is generally avoided when reasonable alternatives exist (sertraline is commonly preferred), though it is not contraindicated	Consider maternal tolerability and discontinuation concerns	McAllister-Williams et al. (2017); Clinical consensus
Olanzapine / Quetiapine	Often usable with caution	Available data suggest relatively low infant exposure	Monitor infant sedation, feeding, and weight gain if indicated	McAllister-Williams et al. (2017); Clinical consensus
Lithium	Specialist-guided use only	Consider only in selected high-risk cases	Requires infant monitoring for lithium toxicity	McAllister-Williams et al. (2017); Petrosellini et al. (2024)
Long-acting benzodiazepines	Generally avoid routine use	Longer half-life increases infant exposure risk	Avoid prolonged or high-dose use when possible	Clinical consensus

D. Practical Treatment Selection

Clinical Scenario	Preferred Treatment	Rationale	Avoid / Caution	Evidence Source
Mild depression or anxiety in pregnancy	Psychotherapy first when feasible	Minimizes fetal exposure while addressing symptoms	Avoid undertreating worsening illness	NICE (2022); ACOG (2023)

Clinical Scenario	Preferred Treatment	Rationale	Avoid / Caution	Evidence Source
Severe anxiety with panic and functional impairment	Sertraline; consider short-term lorazepam rescue if necessary	Severe panic may require more than supportive therapy	Avoid relying on psychotherapy alone during decompensation	ACOG (2023); Clinical consensus
Psychosis during pregnancy	Haloperidol, olanzapine, or quetiapine	Untreated psychosis may compromise maternal and fetal safety	Avoid outpatient-only management in severe cases	ACOG (2023); Clinical consensus
Postpartum psychosis	Hospitalization, antipsychotic, ± lithium or ECT	Psychiatric emergency with high maternal-infant risk	Avoid delayed referral or routine outpatient follow-up	Perry et al. (2021); Frieder et al. (2019); Clinical consensus
Breastfeeding patient needing an SSRI	Sertraline often preferred	Lower infant exposure and broad clinical familiarity	Avoid unnecessary switching from an effective agent	McAllister-Williams et al. (2017); Clinical consensus
Breastfeeding patient on lithium	Specialist coordination with pediatric monitoring	May be appropriate in selected high-risk cases	Avoid presenting lithium as routine lactation first-line treatment	McAllister-Williams et al. (2017); Petrosellini et al. (2024)

2. GERIATRICS

A. OVERVIEW

Aspect	Detail	Evidence Source
Core principle	Favor lower-burden regimens, slower titration, and close monitoring for falls, cognition, orthostasis, and anticholinergic effects	Beers Criteria (2023); Clinical consensus

B. Medication / Pharmacologic Considerations

Medication / Class	Preferred / Use With Caution	Clinical Notes	Evidence Source
Sertraline, escitalopram	Often preferred first-line options	Lower anticholinergic burden; commonly recommended SSRIs in older adults	Beers Criteria (2023); Clinical consensus
Duloxetine	Appropriate first-line option	Useful when pain comorbidity is present; monitor blood pressure and fall risk	Beers Criteria (2023); Clinical consensus
Bupropion	Appropriate option	Useful when fatigue or low energy predominate; lower anticholinergic burden; monitor seizure threshold	Clinical consensus
Mirtazapine	Appropriate option with caution	Useful when insomnia or weight loss are prominent; sedation and weight gain may occur	Clinical consensus
Venlafaxine	Use with caution	Monitor blood pressure; taper gradually to reduce discontinuation symptoms	Clinical consensus
Fluoxetine	Use with caution; generally not preferred in older adults	Long half-life and CYP2D6 inhibition may increase prolonged adverse effects, activation, insomnia, and drug–drug interactions; consider sertraline or escitalopram when feasible	Beers Criteria (2023); Clinical consensus
Aripiprazole, lurasidone	Useful when antipsychotic is necessary	Prefer lower metabolic and cognitive burden in older adults	Clinical consensus
Benzodiazepines	Generally avoid routine use	Falls, sedation, cognitive impairment, and delirium vulnerability are major concerns	Beers Criteria (2023)
TCAs, diphenhydramine, paroxetine, fluoxetine	Avoid or minimize	High anticholinergic burden; paroxetine and fluoxetine are generally not preferred in older adults	Beers Criteria (2023)

C. Practical Treatment Selection

Clinical Scenario	Preferred Treatment	Rationale	Avoid / Caution	Evidence Source
Older adult with insomnia and anxiety	Address sleep hygiene and psychotherapy first; if pharmacotherapy needed: low-dose trazodone, mirtazapine, or ramelteon	Reduces fall and delirium burden	Avoid reflexive benzodiazepine prescribing	AASM (2017); Clinical consensus
Older adult with depression and pain comorbidity	Duloxetine at lower starting dose	Addresses both mood and pain; monitor blood pressure and falls	Avoid TCAs and paroxetine	Beers Criteria (2023); Clinical consensus
Older adult with depression and insomnia or weight loss	Mirtazapine at low starting dose	Sedating properties may help sleep and appetite	Monitor sedation and falls	Clinical consensus
Older adult with depression and fatigue	Bupropion at lower starting dose	Activating profile may help energy and motivation; lower anticholinergic burden	Avoid in seizure history or eating disorders	Clinical consensus
Older adult needing antipsychotic	Aripiprazole or lurasidone when clinically appropriate	Lower metabolic and anticholinergic burden preferred in older adults	Avoid olanzapine and clozapine as first choice; dementia-related psychosis carries boxed warning	Beers Criteria (2023); Clinical consensus
Older adult on multiple medications	Review full regimen for anticholinergic burden and interactions	Polypharmacy is a major contributor to adverse outcomes in geriatric patients	Avoid passive continuation without periodic reassessment	Beers Criteria (2023); Clinical consensus

D. Risks / Monitoring

Risk / Issue	Monitoring Focus	Clinical Notes	Evidence Source
Falls and orthostasis	Vitals, gait, recent falls, sedation burden	Polypharmacy review is essential	Beers Criteria (2023); Clinical consensus

3. CARDIAC AND QTc RISK

A. OVERVIEW

Aspect	Detail	Evidence Source
Core principle	Match psychotropic choice to baseline QT risk, comorbidity burden, interacting drugs, and ECG context	FDA labeling; Clinical consensus

B. Medication / Pharmacologic Considerations

Agent / Pattern	Use With Caution / Preferred	Clinical Notes	Evidence Source
Ziprasidone, thioridazine, IV haloperidol	Higher caution	Commonly regarded as higher concern in clinical practice; risk rises further with interacting drugs, female sex, bradycardia, electrolyte abnormalities, higher doses, and structural heart disease	FDA labeling; Clinical consensus
High-dose citalopram	Higher caution	Respect dose limits and patient-specific risk factors including female sex, hypokalemia, hypomagnesemia, bradycardia, and polypharmacy	FDA labeling
Aripiprazole, lurasidone	Often lower-QT-burden options	Useful in higher-risk settings when clinically appropriate, though cumulative risk still matters	Clinical consensus
Multiple QT-prolonging drugs	Avoid combinations when possible	Review full medication list before adding new psychotropics	FDA labeling; Clinical consensus

C. Risk Factors

Risk Factor	Clinical Impact	Evidence Source
Female sex, bradycardia, structural heart disease	Increase vulnerability to QT prolongation	Clinical consensus
Hypokalemia, hypomagnesemia	Increase arrhythmia risk and should be corrected promptly	Clinical consensus
High doses and polypharmacy	Raise cumulative QT burden	FDA labeling; Clinical consensus

D. Practical Treatment Selection

Clinical Scenario	Preferred Treatment	Rationale	Avoid / Caution	Evidence Source
Patient with baseline prolonged QTc needing antipsychotic	Prefer lower-QT-burden options when clinically appropriate	May reduce additive arrhythmia risk	Avoid stacking QT-prolonging agents without review	Clinical consensus

4. HIV AND ANTIRETROVIRAL INTERACTIONS

A. OVERVIEW

Aspect	Detail	Evidence Source
Core principle	Review CYP interactions, sedation burden, and regimen-specific effects before starting psychotropics	DHHS (2024); Goodlet et al. (2019)

B. Medication / Pharmacologic Considerations

Psychotropic Class	Preferred Options	Use With Caution / Avoid	Clinical Notes	Evidence Source
Benzodiazepines	Lorazepam, oxazepam, temazepam	Midazolam, triazolam	Prefer agents with minimal CYP metabolism; monitor sedation and respiratory depression	DHHS (2024); Goodlet et al. (2019)
SSRIs	Sertraline, escitalopram	Higher-interaction strategies may require more caution	Start low and monitor efficacy and tolerability	DHHS (2024); Goodlet et al. (2019)
Antipsychotics	Aripiprazole with dose awareness	Quetiapine and other CYP3A4-sensitive agents may require more caution	Dose adjustment and close monitoring may be required	DHHS (2024); Goodlet et al. (2019)
Mood stabilizers	Lamotrigine often favored	Carbamazepine generally problematic in many ARV regimens	Avoid strong inducers when possible	DHHS (2024); Clinical consensus

C. Practical Treatment Selection

Clinical Scenario	Preferred Treatment	Rationale	Avoid / Caution	Evidence Source
Patient on boosted antiretroviral regimen needing anxiolytic	Prefer lorazepam, oxazepam, or temazepam	Reduces CYP-driven interaction burden	Avoid routine use of interaction-prone benzodiazepines	DHHS (2024); Goodlet et al. (2019)

D. Monitoring

Monitoring Focus	Clinical Notes	Evidence Source
Drug-drug interaction review	Check full ARV regimen and recent changes before psychotropic adjustments	DHHS (2024); Goodlet et al. (2019)

5. RENAL IMPAIRMENT

A. OVERVIEW

Aspect	Detail	Evidence Source
Core principle	Match drug choice and dose to renal function, frailty, and toxicity risk	Clinical consensus

B. Medication / Pharmacologic Considerations

Medication	Preferred / Use With Caution	Clinical Notes	Evidence Source
Lithium	Use with major caution or avoid depending on severity	High toxicity risk; close level and renal monitoring required	Clinical consensus
Gabapentin / Pregabalin	Dose adjust	Renally cleared and prone to accumulation	FDA labeling
Duloxetine	Avoid in severe renal impairment	Exposure may increase and tolerability may worsen	FDA labeling
Sertraline, escitalopram	Often practical options in renal impairment	Suitability still depends on overall medical context, comorbidity burden, and monitoring needs	Clinical consensus
Many antipsychotics	Often usable with caution	Many are not primarily renally cleared, but dose selection should still reflect frailty, sedation risk, orthostasis, and overall medical burden	Clinical consensus

C. Practical Treatment Selection

Clinical Scenario	Preferred Treatment	Rationale	Avoid / Caution	Evidence Source
CKD patient on lithium	Reassess urgently	Toxicity risk is substantial	Avoid routine continuation without clear monitoring plan	Clinical consensus
Severe renal impairment needing antidepressant	Sertraline or escitalopram may be practical with monitoring	Often manageable choices when renal handling is less problematic than with some alternatives	Avoid duloxetine in severe renal impairment	FDA labeling; Clinical consensus
CKD patient with insomnia and neuropathic pain	Renally adjusted gabapentin may be reasonable	Symptom-targeted benefit is possible if dosing is adjusted appropriately	Avoid full standard doses	FDA labeling; Clinical consensus

D. Monitoring

Monitoring Focus	Clinical Notes	Evidence Source
Renal function and accumulation risk	Reassess after clinical deterioration, dehydration, or dose change	Clinical consensus

6. END-STAGE RENAL DISEASE (ESRD) AND DIALYSIS

A. OVERVIEW

Aspect	Detail	Evidence Source
Core principle	Anticipate altered clearance, dialysis effects, sedation burden, and frailty	Clinical consensus

B. Medication / Pharmacologic Considerations

Medication / Class	Preferred / Use With Caution	Clinical Notes	Evidence Source
Lithium	Generally avoid	Narrow therapeutic index and unstable handling make use difficult in ESRD	Clinical consensus

Medication / Class	Preferred / Use With Caution	Clinical Notes	Evidence Source
Gabapentin / Pregabalin	Dose reduce; dialysis-aware timing	Dialyzable and prone to accumulation	FDA labeling; Clinical consensus
Sertraline	Commonly used in practice because of a relatively manageable profile	Close clinical monitoring remains necessary in ESRD	Clinical consensus
SNRIs	More caution needed	Duloxetine is generally avoided in severe renal impairment; venlafaxine may require dose reduction and closer monitoring	Clinical consensus
Antipsychotics	Many are usable with careful monitoring	Sedation and orthostasis remain important	Clinical consensus
Benzodiazepines	Use cautiously and only when clearly necessary	Frailty and dialysis-related instability increase adverse-effect risk	Beers Criteria (2023); Clinical consensus

C. Practical Treatment Selection

Clinical Scenario	Preferred Treatment	Rationale	Avoid / Caution	Evidence Source
Dialysis patient with depression	Sertraline is often a practical option with monitoring	Commonly used because of a relatively manageable profile in practice	Avoid accumulation-prone strategies without review	Clinical consensus
Dialysis patient with neuropathic symptoms and insomnia	Renally adjusted gabapentinoid only if clearly indicated	May still help if dosed correctly and timed appropriately	Avoid standard daily dosing	FDA labeling; Clinical consensus
ESRD patient on lithium	Reassess urgently	Toxicity risk and unstable levels are major concerns	Avoid routine continuation	Clinical consensus

D. Monitoring

Monitoring Focus	Clinical Notes	Evidence Source
Dialysis timing and dose review	Reassess dosing schedule when symptoms or dialysis plans change	Clinical consensus

7. HEPATIC IMPAIRMENT

A. OVERVIEW

Aspect	Detail	Evidence Source
Core principle	Account for hepatic metabolism, sedation burden, and severity of liver disease when selecting psychotropics	Clinical consensus

B. Medication / Pharmacologic Considerations

Medication	Preferred / Use With Caution	Clinical Notes	Evidence Source
Valproate	Use with great caution or avoid in active liver disease	Hepatotoxicity risk is clinically important	FDA labeling
Carbamazepine	Monitor carefully	Hepatic metabolism and adverse hepatic effects require caution	FDA labeling
Sertraline, escitalopram	May be used cautiously with lower starting doses and slower titration in significant hepatic impairment; severity assessment such as Child-Pugh class should inform selection	Suitability depends on severity of liver disease, tolerability, and need for slower titration	Clinical consensus
Aripiprazole, risperidone	May require dose adjustment and slower titration; severity assessment such as Child-Pugh class should guide use	Sedation and exposure may increase	Clinical consensus

C. Child-Pugh Severity Framework

Severity Context	General Approach	Evidence Source
Child-Pugh A	Use cautiously; many agents remain usable with conservative titration	Clinical consensus
Child-Pugh B	Use lower starting doses and slower titration with closer monitoring	Clinical consensus
Child-Pugh C	Avoid when safer alternatives exist or use only with specialist oversight	Clinical consensus

D. Practical Treatment Selection

Clinical Scenario	Preferred Treatment	Rationale	Avoid / Caution	Evidence Source
Active liver disease with mood instability	Use the lowest-hepatotoxic reasonable strategy	Reduces added hepatic burden	Avoid valproate when possible	FDA labeling; Clinical consensus
Significant hepatic impairment needing antidepressant	Sertraline or escitalopram may be practical at reduced starting dose	Exposure may be increased even with common agents, so slower titration is often needed	Avoid standard aggressive titration	Clinical consensus
Patient with rising LFTs on psychotropics	Reassess regimen promptly	May reflect drug effect, illness, or interaction	Avoid passive continuation without review	Clinical consensus

8. SEIZURE DISORDERS

A. OVERVIEW

Aspect	Detail	Evidence Source
Core principle	Consider seizure threshold, anti seizure drug interactions, and reproductive implications when relevant	Vora & Citrome (2017); Clinical consensus

B. Medication / Pharmacologic Considerations

Medication	Lower / Higher Risk	Clinical Notes	Evidence Source
Sertraline, escitalopram	Generally lower risk at therapeutic doses	Often practical antidepressant options in seizure-prone patients	Vora & Citrome (2017); Clinical consensus
Bupropion	Higher, dose-related risk	Avoid high doses and other threshold-lowering combinations when possible	FDA labeling
Clozapine	Higher risk	Risk is dose-related and clinically important	FDA labeling; Vora & Citrome (2017)
Most other antipsychotics	Usually low to moderate at therapeutic doses	Clozapine remains the standout higher-risk antipsychotic	Vora & Citrome (2017); Clinical consensus

C. Antiseizure Drug Interactions Relevant to Psychopharmacology

Antiseizure Medication / Pattern	Psychopharmacology Relevance	Clinical Notes	Avoid / Caution	Evidence Source
Carbamazepine / phenytoin and other enzyme-inducing regimens	May lower concentrations of some antipsychotics, antidepressants, and hormonal contraceptives	Review for loss of efficacy and interaction-driven dose changes	Avoid assuming psychiatric nonresponse without checking interactions	Clinical consensus
Lamotrigine plus estrogen-containing oral contraceptives	Bidirectional interaction concern	Estrogen-containing contraceptives can lower lamotrigine levels; changes in contraceptive use may alter lamotrigine exposure	Avoid unmonitored dose changes when contraceptives are started, stopped, or changed	Clinical consensus
Valproate co-therapy	Interaction burden and teratogenicity matter	May complicate reproductive counseling and combination treatment decisions	Avoid routine reproductive-age use in pregnancy-prone patients when safer alternatives exist	Clinical consensus

D. Practical Treatment Selection

Clinical Scenario	Preferred Treatment	Rationale	Avoid / Caution	Evidence Source
Patient with epilepsy needing antidepressant	Sertraline or escitalopram is often practical	Lower relative seizure risk at therapeutic doses	Avoid threshold-lowering combinations when possible	Vora & Citrome (2017); Clinical consensus

9. OBESITY AND METABOLIC SYNDROME

A. OVERVIEW

Aspect	Detail	Evidence Source
Core principle	Prefer lower-burden options when baseline metabolic risk is high, while balancing illness severity and prior response	De Hert et al. (2011); Clinical consensus

B. Medication / Pharmacologic Considerations

Issue	Preferred / Higher-Risk Options	Clinical Notes	Evidence Source
Lower metabolic burden choices	Aripiprazole, lurasidone, ziprasidone, lamotrigine, bupropion	Often preferred when baseline metabolic risk is high; lower relative burden does not mean metabolically neutral	De Hert et al. (2011); Clinical consensus
Higher metabolic burden choices	Olanzapine, clozapine, quetiapine, mirtazapine, valproate	Use when clinically needed, but recognize higher burden	De Hert et al. (2011); Clinical consensus
Metformin adjunct	Consider in selected cases of antipsychotic-associated weight gain	May help when benefit-risk profile is favorable	De Silva et al. (2016); Clinical consensus
GLP-1 receptor agonist adjunct	Semaglutide or other GLP-1 agents in selected patients	Effective adjunctive option for antipsychotic-associated weight gain in metabolically high-risk patients; not yet formally incorporated into psychiatric guidelines but supported by clinical trial evidence; requires metabolic specialist coordination	Bak et al. (2024); Larsen et al. (2024)

C. Practical Treatment Selection

Clinical Scenario	Preferred Treatment	Rationale	Avoid / Caution	Evidence Source
Patient with severe obesity starting antipsychotic	Favor lower relative metabolic burden options when clinically appropriate	May reduce added cardiometabolic burden	Avoid ignoring prior antipsychotic response and illness severity	De Hert et al. (2011); Clinical consensus

D. Monitoring

Monitoring Focus	Clinical Notes	Evidence Source
Weight, waist, glucose, lipids	Track baseline and follow-up metabolic parameters systematically	De Hert et al. (2011); Clinical consensus

10. RESPIRATORY DISORDERS (FOCUS: OBSTRUCTIVE SLEEP APNEA)

A. OVERVIEW

Aspect	Detail	Evidence Source
Core principle	Limit avoidable respiratory depressants and reassess untreated OSA before escalating sedative strategies	AASM (2017); Clinical consensus

B. Medication / Pharmacologic Considerations

Medication / Class	Preferred / Use With Caution	Clinical Notes	Evidence Source
Benzodiazepines	Avoid or minimize when possible	May worsen respiratory compromise and sedation burden	AASM (2017); Clinical consensus
Opioids	Avoid or minimize	High respiratory risk, especially in combination regimens	CDC (2022)
Sedating antipsychotics	Use caution	Sedation and weight effects may worsen respiratory vulnerability	Clinical consensus
Z-drugs	Use cautiously and selectively	Do not assume benign respiratory impact in high-risk patients	AASM (2017); Clinical consensus
Lower-sedation antidepressant strategies	May be preferable when clinically feasible	May reduce cumulative respiratory burden compared with sedative stacking	Clinical consensus

C. Practical Treatment Selection

Clinical Scenario	Preferred Treatment	Rationale	Avoid / Caution	Evidence Source
Patient with suspected OSA needing insomnia treatment	Screen and treat OSA before escalating sedatives	OSA may be driving or worsening symptoms	Avoid reflexive sedative prescribing	AASM (2017); Clinical consensus
Patient on opioids plus benzodiazepines with OSA risk	Reassess regimen urgently	Combined respiratory burden may be dangerous	Avoid additive sedative prescribing	CDC (2022)

Clinical Scenario	Preferred Treatment	Rationale	Avoid / Caution	Evidence Source
Psychiatric patient with poor CPAP adherence and residual symptoms	Coordinate sleep and psychiatric care; consider sleep-medicine referral for CPAP desensitization, mask refit, or alternative interfaces	Better sleep treatment may improve psychiatric and cognitive outcomes	Avoid assuming medication failure alone	Winkelman et al. (2016); Clinical consensus

D. Monitoring

Monitoring Focus	Clinical Notes	Evidence Source
Sedation stack and adherence review	Check opioids, benzodiazepines, hypnotics, CPAP use, and daytime somnolence regularly	Clinical consensus

11. PEDIATRICS

A. OVERVIEW

Aspect	Detail	Evidence Source
Core principle	Use age-appropriate diagnosis, psychotherapy when indicated, and conservative psychopharmacology	AACAP; Clinical consensus
Monitoring priority	Track weight, height, sleep, appetite, activation, suicidality, and behavioral change	AACAP; Clinical consensus

B. Medication / Pharmacologic Considerations

Medication / Class	Preferred / Use With Caution	Clinical Notes	Evidence Source
SSRIs	Use selectively when clinically indicated	Fluoxetine, sertraline, and escitalopram are commonly used depending on age and diagnosis	AACAP (2022); AACAP (2020); Clinical consensus
Antipsychotics	Use only when indication is clear	Monitor weight, metabolic burden, and extrapyramidal effects	AACAP; Clinical consensus
Benzodiazepines	Generally avoid routine long-term use	Sedation, paradoxical disinhibition, and dependence concerns apply	Clinical consensus

Medication / Class	Preferred / Use With Caution	Clinical Notes	Evidence Source
Stimulants (methylphenidate, amphetamine formulations)	Use when ADHD diagnosis is confirmed	First-line pharmacotherapy for ADHD in school-age children and adolescents; monitor appetite, weight, sleep, heart rate, and blood pressure; start low and titrate; use with behavioral interventions	AAP (2019); Clinical consensus
Non-stimulant options (atomoxetine, guanfacine, clonidine)	Consider when stimulants are not tolerated or contraindicated	Useful alternatives in ADHD with comorbid anxiety, tics, or substance-use concern; slower onset than stimulants	AAP (2019); Clinical consensus

C. Practical Treatment Selection

Clinical Scenario	Preferred Treatment	Rationale	Avoid / Caution	Evidence Source
Child or adolescent with mild anxiety or depression	Psychotherapy first when feasible	Reduces medication exposure and addresses family/system contributors	Avoid premature polypharmacy	AACAP (2022); AACAP (2020); Clinical consensus
Youth started on antidepressant	Close follow-up early in treatment	Behavioral activation and suicidality monitoring are essential	Avoid dose escalation without reassessment	AACAP (2022); Clinical consensus
Child or adolescent with confirmed ADHD	Stimulant medication plus behavioral interventions	Best-supported combined approach for ADHD in pediatric patients	Avoid stimulants without diagnostic clarification; monitor for appetite suppression, insomnia, and cardiovascular effects	AAP (2019); Clinical consensus

D. Monitoring

Monitoring Focus	Clinical Notes	Evidence Source
Growth, activation, suicidality, family feedback	Early follow-up and caregiver education are essential	AACAP (2022); AACAP (2020); AAP (2019); Clinical consensus

REFERENCES

American Academy of Pediatrics. (2019). Clinical practice guideline for the diagnosis, evaluation, and treatment of attention-deficit/hyperactivity disorder in children and adolescents. *Pediatrics*, *144*(4), e20192528. https://doi.org/10.1542/peds.2019-2528

American Academy of Child and Adolescent Psychiatry. (2020). Clinical practice guideline for the assessment and treatment of children and adolescents with anxiety disorders. Journal of the American Academy of Child and Adolescent Psychiatry, 59(10), 1107–1124.

American Academy of Child and Adolescent Psychiatry. (2022). Clinical practice guideline for the assessment and treatment of children and adolescents with major and persistent depressive disorders. Journal of the American Academy of Child and Adolescent Psychiatry, 62(5), 479–502.

American Academy of Sleep Medicine. (2017). Clinical practice guideline for the pharmacologic treatment of chronic insomnia in adults. Journal of Clinical Sleep Medicine, 13(2), 307–349.

American College of Obstetricians and Gynecologists. (2023). Treatment and management of mental health conditions during pregnancy and postpartum (ACOG Clinical Practice Guideline).

American Geriatrics Society Beers Criteria Update Expert Panel. (2023). American Geriatrics Society 2023 updated AGS Beers Criteria for potentially inappropriate medication use in older adults. Journal of the American Geriatrics Society, 71(7), 2052–2081.

Centers for Disease Control and Prevention. (2022). CDC clinical practice guideline for prescribing opioids for pain. CDC.

De Hert, M., Detraux, J., van Winkel, R., Yu, W., & Correll, C. U. (2011). Metabolic and cardiovascular adverse effects associated with antipsychotic drugs. Nature Reviews Endocrinology, 8(2), 114–126.

De Silva, V. A., Suraweera, C., Ratnatunga, S. S., et al. (2016). Metformin in prevention and treatment of antipsychotic induced weight gain: A systematic review and meta-analysis. BMC Psychiatry, 16, 341.

Deligiannidis, K. M., Meltzer-Brody, S., Gunduz-Bruce, H., et al. (2023). Effect of zuranolone vs placebo in postpartum depression: A randomized clinical trial. *JAMA Psychiatry*, *80*(9), 883–891.

Department of Health and Human Services. (2024). Guidelines for the use of antiretroviral agents in adults and adolescents with HIV. Panel on Antiretroviral Guidelines for Adults and Adolescents.

Frieder, A., Fersh, M. E., Hainline, R., & Deligiannidis, K. M. (2019). Pharmacotherapy of postpartum depression: Current approaches and novel drug development. CNS Drugs, 33(3), 265–282.

Larsen, J. R., Vedtofte, L., Jakobsen, M. S. L., et al. (2024). Effect of liraglutide treatment on prediabetes and obesity in clozapine- or olanzapine-treated patients: 3-year follow-up. *Acta Psychiatrica Scandinavica, 149*(1), 60–70.

McAllister-Williams, R. H., Baldwin, D. S., Cantwell, R., et al. (2017). British Association for Psychopharmacology consensus guidance on the use of psychotropic medication preconception, in pregnancy and postpartum. Journal of Psychopharmacology, 31(5), 519–552.

National Institute for Health and Care Excellence. (2022). Antenatal and postnatal mental health: Clinical management and service guidance.

Perry, A., Gordon-Smith, K., Jones, L., & Jones, I. (2021). Phenomenology, epidemiology and aetiology of postpartum psychosis: A review. Brain Sciences, 11(1), 47.

Petrosellini, C., McAlpine, L., & Protti, O. (2024). The use of psychotropic medication in the perinatal period. The Obstetrician & Gynaecologist, 26(3), 127–138.

Rodríguez-Cabezas, L., & Clark, C. T. (2018). Psychiatric emergencies in pregnancy and postpartum. Clinical Obstetrics and Gynecology, 61(3), 615–627.

U.S. Food and Drug Administration. (2023). *Zurzuvae (zuranolone) prescribing information*. Sage Therapeutics/Biogen.

Vora, J., & Citrome, L. (2017). Neuropsychiatric considerations for patients with seizure disorders: A therapeutic dilemma. Expert Opinion on Pharmacotherapy, 18(9), 879–887.

Winkelman, J. W., Finn, L., Young, T., & Bhatt, D. L. (2016). Psychiatry and obstructive sleep apnea: Implications for diagnosis and treatment. *Current Psychiatry Reports, 18*(6), 64.

XIV. LABORATORY AND MONITORING

SECTION INTRODUCTION

Laboratory assessment and clinical monitoring represent essential components of safe and effective psychopharmacologic treatment. Appropriate baseline evaluation, ongoing laboratory surveillance, metabolic monitoring, and clinical reassessment help identify medical contraindications, reduce adverse effects, improve medication safety, detect treatment-related complications early, and support evidence-informed psychiatric decision-making. Monitoring practices should remain individualized according to medication selection, patient-specific risk factors, medical comorbidity, age, reproductive status, and overall clinical complexity.

Psychotropic medications may significantly affect metabolic, cardiovascular, endocrine, hepatic, renal, hematologic, and neurologic functioning. Second-generation antipsychotics may contribute to weight gain, dyslipidemia, insulin resistance, and diabetes mellitus. Mood stabilizers such as lithium and valproate require ongoing monitoring because of risks involving renal dysfunction, thyroid abnormalities, hepatotoxicity, hematologic effects, and toxicity syndromes. Antidepressants, stimulants, benzodiazepines, and other psychotropic agents may also require selective laboratory evaluation or physiologic monitoring depending on patient characteristics and medication profile.

Baseline medical assessment is particularly important prior to initiating medications associated with significant metabolic burden, cardiovascular risk, teratogenicity, hematologic complications, or drug-specific safety requirements. Important components of evaluation may include weight and body mass index (BMI), blood pressure, heart rate, fasting glucose or hemoglobin A1c, lipid profile, renal function, liver function testing, thyroid studies, complete blood count (CBC), pregnancy testing, electrocardiography (ECG), and therapeutic drug monitoring when clinically indicated. Comprehensive medication reconciliation and assessment of over-the-counter medications, supplements, and substance use are also critical to reduce drug interaction risk.

Ongoing monitoring should extend beyond laboratory testing alone and include structured assessment of adverse effects, treatment response, medication adherence, movement disorders, sedation, suicidality, substance use, cognitive functioning, sleep disturbance, and overall functional status. Routine clinical follow-up provides an opportunity to identify early warning signs of relapse, toxicity, medication intolerance, metabolic deterioration, or emerging psychiatric instability before severe complications occur.

Patients receiving antipsychotic medications require particular attention to metabolic and neurologic monitoring because of increased risks of obesity, diabetes, dyslipidemia, extrapyramidal symptoms, tardive dyskinesia, hyperprolactinemia, and cardiovascular disease.

Clozapine requires specialized hematologic monitoring because of the risk of agranulocytosis, while lithium treatment requires serial serum levels and monitoring of renal and thyroid function because of its narrow therapeutic index and toxicity potential.

Special populations may require enhanced monitoring strategies. Elderly patients, pregnant individuals, medically complex patients, patients with substance use disorders, and individuals receiving polypharmacy are often at increased risk of adverse effects, altered drug metabolism, falls, electrolyte abnormalities, cardiovascular complications, and medication interactions. Children and adolescents may additionally require monitoring of growth parameters, appetite changes, blood pressure, and behavioral activation depending on treatment regimen.

Clinicians should also remain attentive to medical conditions and laboratory abnormalities that may mimic psychiatric illness or contribute to worsening psychiatric symptoms. Thyroid dysfunction, vitamin deficiencies, anemia, electrolyte abnormalities, hepatic dysfunction, renal impairment, sleep apnea, inflammatory conditions, neurologic disease, and substance-related complications may significantly affect psychiatric presentation and treatment response. Comprehensive psychiatric care therefore requires ongoing integration of psychiatric and medical assessment throughout treatment.

Monitoring practices should remain evidence-informed while also balancing clinical necessity, patient burden, cost considerations, and individualized risk assessment. Shared decision-making and patient education regarding laboratory testing, medication risks, and monitoring rationale are essential to improve adherence, reduce anxiety regarding treatment, and promote early reporting of adverse effects or concerning symptoms.

The following sections provide a structured, evidence-informed framework for laboratory assessment, physiologic monitoring, and safety surveillance within outpatient psychiatric practice. Recommendations are intended to support safe, clinically individualized, and longitudinal psychopharmacologic care while recognizing the importance of medical integration, preventive monitoring, patient education, and professional clinical judgment throughout treatment.

1. BASELINE LABORATORY PARAMETERS

A. OVERVIEW

Aspect	Detail	Evidence Source
Purpose	Establish medical safety before initiating psychotropic treatment and identify baseline abnormalities that may affect drug selection, dosing, or monitoring intensity	Clinical consensus
Timing	Obtain baseline studies before treatment initiation or as early as possible at the time of initiation when clinically necessary	Clinical consensus
Documentation	Review, interpret, and document clinically relevant baseline results in the medical record before or during early treatment planning	Clinical consensus

B. Baseline Laboratory Tests

Test	Rationale	Clinical Notes	Evidence Source
Complete blood count (CBC)	Detect anemia, infection, and hematologic abnormalities	Particularly relevant before clozapine, carbamazepine, or valproate	Clinical consensus
Comprehensive metabolic panel (CMP)	Assess renal function, liver function, and electrolytes	Especially important before lithium, valproate, and carbamazepine	Clinical consensus
Fasting lipid panel	Establish baseline metabolic risk	Recommended before antipsychotic initiation, especially second-generation agents	ADA/APA CONSENSUS (2004)
Fasting glucose or HbA1c	Assess baseline diabetes risk	Supports future metabolic comparison during antipsychotic treatment	ADA/APA CONSENSUS (2004)
Thyroid function (TSH, free T4 if indicated)	Establish baseline thyroid status	Particularly important before lithium	Clinical consensus
Pregnancy test when indicated	Identify pregnancy before exposure to potentially teratogenic agents	Relevant for lithium, valproate, carbamazepine, and other agents when applicable	Clinical consensus
Prolactin when indicated	Establish baseline for comparison if prolactin-elevating antipsychotics are planned	Most relevant when symptoms are present or risperidone/paliperidone is anticipated	Clinical consensus

Test	Rationale	Clinical Notes	Evidence Source
ECG when indicated	Assess baseline cardiac risk before QT-liability or conduction-risk medications	Consider for patients with cardiac history, electrolyte risk, older age, or QT-risk agents	Clinical consensus

Clinical note

Vitamin D and B12 levels may be considered in selected patients, including older adults, vegetarians, patients on metformin, or those with atypical treatment response or cognitive symptoms. Routine screening is not universally recommended. *Clinical consensus.*

C. Practical Treatment Selection

Clinical Scenario	Preferred Monitoring Strategy	Rationale	Avoid / Caution	Evidence Source
Lithium initiation planned	Obtain renal function, electrolytes, thyroid function, and other lithium-relevant baseline studies before starting	Lithium has a narrow therapeutic index and important renal and thyroid implications	Avoid starting without baseline renal and thyroid assessment unless urgent circumstances clearly justify it	Clinical consensus
Valproate or carbamazepine initiation planned	Obtain baseline CBC and liver-related studies	These agents may affect hematologic and hepatic safety	Avoid overlooking reproductive counseling and pregnancy risk where relevant	Clinical consensus
Second-generation antipsychotic initiation planned	Obtain baseline weight/BMI, blood pressure, glucose/HbA1c, and lipids	Enables structured metabolic monitoring over time	Avoid relying on symptom-based recognition of metabolic adverse effects alone	ADA/APA CONSENSUS (2004)

2. GENERAL FOLLOW-UP MONITORING SCHEDULE

A. OVERVIEW

Aspect	Detail	Evidence Source
Purpose	Detect emerging laboratory abnormalities early and support safe long-term psychotropic prescribing	Clinical consensus
Principle	Monitoring frequency should be individualized according to medication class, comorbidity burden, age, and prior abnormalities	Clinical consensus
Escalation	Increase monitoring intensity when abnormal results, dose changes, interacting medications, or medical instability are present	Clinical consensus

B. General Monitoring Schedule

Parameter	Initial Follow-Up	Chronic Monitoring	Clinical Notes	Evidence Source
CBC	As indicated by agent	Periodic or agent-specific	Required more intensively for clozapine and relevant hematologic-risk agents	Clinical consensus
CMP	Within early treatment phase if indicated	At least annually for many long-term treatments; more often if risk is high	Frequency depends on agent and baseline abnormalities	Clinical consensus
Lipid panel	Around 3 months after antipsychotic initiation	Annually thereafter or more often if abnormal	Most relevant for metabolic-risk antipsychotics	ADA/APA CONSENSUS (2004)
Glucose or HbA1c	Around 3 months after antipsychotic initiation	Annually thereafter or more often if abnormal	Supports diabetes screening and longitudinal metabolic tracking	ADA/APA CONSENSUS (2004)
Thyroid function	Within 6–12 months when lithium is used	Annually thereafter or more often if abnormal	Particularly important during lithium treatment	Bosi et al. (2023)
Drug serum level when applicable	After dose changes and early titration	Periodically according to agent and stability	Especially important for lithium	Nederlof et al. (2018)
Prolactin	Recheck when symptoms emerge or when clinically indicated	Routine universal repeated testing is less standardized than symptom-guided monitoring	Especially relevant with risperidone and paliperidone	FDA labeling, Clinical consensus
ECG	Reassess when risk factors or symptoms emerge	Periodic follow-up only when clinically indicated	Not required routinely for all patients on all psychotropics	Clinical consensus

C. Risks / Monitoring

Clinical Risk	Clinical Notes	Evidence Source
Monitoring drift over time	Adherence to recommended laboratory monitoring often decreases over time, particularly in long-term lithium treatment and other chronic psychopharmacologic care	Bosi et al. (2023); Clinical consensus
Under-monitoring in stable patients	Long-term treatment can create false reassurance even when cumulative toxicity risk remains clinically relevant	Clinical consensus
Over-standardization	Not every patient requires identical monitoring intervals; agent-specific and patient-specific tailoring is appropriate	Clinical consensus

3. METABOLIC MONITORING FOR ANTIPSYCHOTIC TREATMENT

A. OVERVIEW

Aspect	Detail	Evidence Source
Purpose	Detect early weight gain, dysglycemia, dyslipidemia, and cardiometabolic risk during antipsychotic treatment	ADA/APA CONSENSUS (2004)
Highest relevance	Particularly important for olanzapine, clozapine, and other metabolically burdensome antipsychotics	ADA/APA CONSENSUS (2004); Stroup & Gray (2018)
Clinical priority	Early weight gain should prompt intervention because it predicts longer-term metabolic burden	ADA/APA CONSENSUS (2004); Stroup & Gray (2018)

B. Standard Metabolic Monitoring Schedule

Measure	Timing	Goal / Notes	Evidence Source
Weight / BMI	Baseline; 4, 8, and 12 weeks; then quarterly	Detect early gain and guide intervention	ADA/APA CONSENSUS (2004); De Hert et al. (2024)
Waist circumference	Baseline; then annually	Assess central adiposity	ADA/APA CONSENSUS (2004); De Hert et al. (2024)
Blood pressure	Baseline; then periodically	Assess cardiovascular risk	ADA/APA CONSENSUS (2004); De Hert et al. (2024)
Fasting glucose or HbA1c	Baseline; around 12 weeks; then annually	Screen for diabetes and glycemic change	ADA/APA CONSENSUS (2004); De Hert et al. (2024)
Lipid profile	Baseline; around 12 weeks; then annually	Screen for dyslipidemia	ADA/APA CONSENSUS (2004); De Hert et al. (2024)

C. Metabolic Monitoring Flow

Time Point	Assessments	Evidence Source
Baseline	Weight/BMI, waist circumference, blood pressure, fasting glucose or HbA1c, fasting lipids	ADA/APA CONSENSUS (2004); De Hert et al. (2024)
4 weeks	Weight/BMI	ADA/APA CONSENSUS (2004); De Hert et al. (2024)
8 weeks	Weight/BMI	ADA/APA CONSENSUS (2004); De Hert et al. (2024)

Time Point	Assessments	Evidence Source
12 weeks	Weight/BMI, glucose or HbA1c, lipids	ADA/APA CONSENSUS (2004); De Hert et al. (2024)
Quarterly	Weight/BMI	ADA/APA CONSENSUS (2004); De Hert et al. (2024)
Annually	Waist circumference, blood pressure, glucose or HbA1c, lipids, and overall metabolic review	ADA/APA CONSENSUS (2004); De Hert et al. (2024)

D. Practical Treatment Selection

Clinical Scenario	Preferred Monitoring Strategy	Rationale	Avoid / Caution	Evidence Source
Olanzapine or clozapine initiated	Follow full metabolic schedule strictly	Highest metabolic-risk antipsychotics require close tracking	Avoid waiting for symptoms of diabetes or dyslipidemia before testing	ADA/APA CONSENSUS (2004); Stroup & Gray (2018)
Rapid early weight gain	Intensify counseling and reassess treatment plan promptly	Early gain predicts persistent metabolic burden	Avoid labeling early gain as trivial or self-limited without reassessment	ADA/APA CONSENSUS (2004); Stroup & Gray (2018)

4. LITHIUM MONITORING PROTOCOL

A. OVERVIEW

Aspect	Detail	Evidence Source
Indications	Bipolar disorder and selected treatment-resistant depression augmentation settings	CANMAT/ISBD (2018)
Core safety issue	Lithium has a narrow therapeutic index and requires ongoing serum and organ-function monitoring	Nederlof et al. (2018)
Maintenance target range	Common maintenance targets often fall in the 0.6–0.8 mmol/L range, although higher levels may be appropriate in selected clinical contexts. Acute mania commonly targets 0.8–1.2 mmol/L; older adults a lower 0.4–0.6 mmol/L because of higher nephrotoxicity risk. Express all targets in mmol/L (numerically equal to mEq/L for lithium)	CANMAT/ISBD (2018); Nederlof et al. (2018)

B. Baseline and Ongoing Monitoring

Parameter	Frequency	Clinical Notes	Evidence Source
Serum lithium level	5–7 days after initiation or dose change; then every 3–6 months once stable	Draw as a trough level using consistent timing relative to last dose	Nederlof et al. (2018)
Renal function / creatinine	Baseline; then every 6–12 months	Increase frequency if renal risk or abnormal results are present	Bosi et al. (2023)
Thyroid function	Baseline; then every 6–12 months	Monitor for hypothyroidism over time	Bosi et al. (2023)
Calcium	Baseline and periodically during long-term treatment	Hypercalcemia and hyperparathyroid effects may emerge over time	Bosi et al. (2023); Clinical consensus
Electrolytes	Baseline; then periodically as clinically indicated	Sodium shifts can alter lithium levels	Clinical consensus
ECG when indicated	Baseline in older adults or cardiac-risk patients; repeat as clinically indicated	Not required universally in all patients	Clinical consensus

C. Reproductive Safety

Cardiac teratogenicity	Ebstein's anomaly risk was historically overstated but remains clinically relevant; absolute risk is low	ACOG (2023); Clinical consensus
First-trimester exposure	Greatest cardiac malformation concern occurs during first-trimester organogenesis	ACOG (2023)
Fetal echocardiography	Consider fetal echocardiography after first-trimester lithium exposure	ACOG (2023)
Neonatal effects	Neonatal toxicity, including hypotonia, cyanosis, and bradycardia, may occur near delivery	ACOG (2023); McAllister-Williams et al. (2017)
Lithium levels near delivery	Monitor closely; dose adjustment may be needed as renal clearance changes during pregnancy and postpartum	ACOG (2023); Clinical consensus
Breastfeeding	Lithium passes into breast milk; infant monitoring is required if breastfeeding is continued	McAllister-Williams et al. (2017); Petrosellini et al. (2024)
Contraception counseling	Discuss reliable contraception in women of reproductive age receiving lithium	Clinical consensus
Pregnancy planning	If pregnancy is planned, individualized risk-benefit discussion is essential; abrupt discontinuation may increase relapse risk	ACOG (2023); Clinical consensus

D. Factors That Increase Lithium Levels

Factor	Mechanism	Management	Evidence Source
Dehydration	Reduces lithium clearance and increases serum concentration variability	Maintain hydration and reassess lithium level if clinically relevant	Clinical consensus
NSAIDs	May reduce renal lithium clearance and raise serum lithium levels	Avoid routine use when possible or monitor lithium more closely if required	Clinical consensus
Thiazide diuretics	Increase renal lithium reabsorption and may significantly raise lithium levels	Avoid when possible or adjust dose and monitoring carefully	Clinical consensus
ACE inhibitors / ARBs	May reduce lithium clearance and increase toxicity risk	Monitor lithium level and renal function closely if co-prescribed	Clinical consensus
Renal impairment	Reduces lithium elimination and increases toxicity risk	Use lower doses and more frequent monitoring	Bosi et al. (2023)

E. Risks / Monitoring

Clinical Risk	Clinical Notes	Evidence Source
Early toxicity	Early signs include tremor, nausea, diarrhea, blurred vision, worsening coordination, and slurred speech	Clinical consensus
Severe toxicity	Severe toxicity may include marked neurologic dysfunction, seizures, coma, and death	Clinical consensus
Monitoring deterioration over time	Real-world adherence to lithium monitoring often declines during long-term treatment	Bosi et al. (2023); Nederlof et al. (2018)

F. Practical Treatment Selection

Clinical Scenario	Preferred Monitoring Strategy	Rationale	Avoid / Caution	Evidence Source
New lithium start	Obtain full baseline labs and repeat level after dose stabilization	Early level confirmation improves safety and dosing precision	Avoid relying only on symptom response without serum monitoring	CANMAT/ISBD (2018)

Clinical Scenario	Preferred Monitoring Strategy	Rationale	Avoid / Caution	Evidence Source
Interacting medication added	Recheck lithium level and renal status earlier than routine schedule	Drug interactions may raise lithium exposure unexpectedly	Avoid assuming clinical stability protects against toxicity	Clinical consensus
Suspected toxicity	Hold lithium and urgently reassess clinical status and serum level	Toxicity can escalate quickly	Avoid waiting for the next routine monitoring interval	Clinical consensus

5. VALPROATE / DIVALPROEX MONITORING PROTOCOL

A. OVERVIEW

Aspect	Detail	Evidence Source
Indications	Bipolar mania, mixed states, rapid cycling, and seizure disorders	CANMAT/ISBD (2018); FDA labeling
Core safety issue	Hepatotoxicity, thrombocytopenia, teratogenicity, and drug interactions require structured monitoring	FDA labeling; Clinical consensus
Maintenance target range	Serum level 50–125 µg/mL; higher levels may be needed in acute mania	CANMAT/ISBD (2018)

B. Baseline and Ongoing Monitoring

Parameter	Frequency	Clinical Notes	Evidence Source
Serum valproate level	After initiation and dose changes; then every 6–12 months once stable	Draw as trough level	CANMAT/ISBD (2018); FDA labeling
CBC with platelets	Baseline; then every 6–12 months	Monitor for thrombocytopenia	FDA labeling
Liver function tests (LFTs)	Baseline; then every 6–12 months	Hepatotoxicity risk is highest in first 6 months	FDA labeling

Parameter	Frequency	Clinical Notes	Evidence Source
Weight / BMI	Baseline; then periodically	Weight gain is common	Clinical consensus
Pregnancy test when indicated	Before initiation in women of reproductive age	High teratogenic risk, including neural tube defects	FDA labeling; ACOG (2023)
Ammonia level when indicated	When encephalopathy symptoms emerge	Valproate-induced hyperammonemia can occur without LFT elevation	FDA labeling; Clinical consensus

C. Reproductive Safety

Consideration	Clinical Notes	Evidence Source
Neural tube defects	High teratogenic risk (approximately 10% major congenital malformations and dose-related reduction in childhood IQ): avoid in ALL persons of childbearing potential, not only during pregnancy, unless other options have failed and effective pregnancy prevention is in place; counsel and document a contraception plan before prescribing	FDA labeling; ACOG (2023)
Folic acid supplementation	Recommend in women of reproductive age on valproate	Clinical consensus
Contraception counseling	Discuss reliable contraception in women of reproductive age	FDA labeling; ACOG (2023)

D. Practical Treatment Selection

Clinical Scenario	Preferred Monitoring Strategy	Rationale	Avoid / Caution	Evidence Source
Valproate initiation	Obtain CBC with platelets, LFTs, and serum valproate level at baseline	Establishes hematologic, hepatic, and therapeutic baseline before treatment	Avoid initiating without hepatic and hematologic baseline	FDA labeling
Women of reproductive age	Provide reproductive counseling and obtain pregnancy test before initiation	High teratogenic risk requires explicit risk discussion and informed consent	Avoid initiating without documented reproductive risk discussion	FDA labeling; ACOG (2023)
Suspected hepatotoxicity	Hold valproate and reassess LFTs urgently	Hepatotoxicity can progress rapidly and requires prompt evaluation	Avoid passive continuation if LFTs are significantly elevated	FDA labeling
Encephalopathy symptoms	Check ammonia level urgently	Hyperammonemia can occur even without LFT abnormalities	Avoid attributing confusion to psychiatric illness alone	FDA labeling; Clinical consensus

6. CLOZAPINE MONITORING PROTOCOL

A. OVERVIEW

Aspect	Detail	Evidence Source
Indication	Treatment-resistant schizophrenia and selected severe psychotic illness contexts	APA (2020)
Core safety issue	Clozapine requires structured hematologic monitoring and broader medical safety surveillance	FDA labeling (2025)
REMS update	The Clozapine REMS program was eliminated effective June 13, 2025. ANC monitoring is no longer mandatory for dispensing but remains recommended per FDA prescribing information	FDA (2025)

Aspect	Detail	Evidence Source
Additional major risks	Constipation/GI hypomotility, myocarditis, metabolic burden, sedation, and tachycardia require active monitoring	Stroup & Gray (2018); Leung et al. (2023)

B. Hematologic Monitoring

Parameter	Frequency	Clinical Notes	Evidence Source
Baseline ANC	Before initiation	Confirm eligibility before starting clozapine	FDA labeling (2025)
ANC during first 6 months	Weekly	Intensive early monitoring reduces agranulocytosis risk	FDA labeling (2025)
ANC during months 6–12	Every 2 weeks	Applies after acceptable early hematologic course	FDA labeling (2025)
ANC after 12 months	Monthly	Continue while treatment is maintained, per FDA prescribing information (REMS program discontinued June 13, 2025)	FDA labeling (2025)

C. ANC Monitoring Actions

ANC Level	Action	Evidence Source
ANC ≥ 1500/μL	Continue treatment under standard monitoring schedule	FDA labeling (2025)
ANC 1000–1499/μL	Continue treatment; increase monitoring frequency and reassess clinically	FDA labeling (2025)
ANC 500–999/μL	Interrupt treatment; obtain urgent reassessment and intensified ANC monitoring	FDA labeling (2025)
ANC < 500/μL	Discontinue treatment and manage according to FDA prescribing information for severe neutropenia; do not rechallenge unless a compelling specialist rationale exists	FDA labeling (2025)

D. Other Required Monitoring

Parameter	Frequency	Clinical Notes	Evidence Source
Weight / BMI	Baseline; 4, 8, 12 weeks; then quarterly	Clozapine carries high metabolic risk	ADA/APA CONSENSUS (2004)
Glucose or HbA1c	Baseline; around 12 weeks; then annually	Diabetes risk is clinically significant	ADA/APA CONSENSUS (2004)

Parameter	Frequency	Clinical Notes	Evidence Source
Lipid profile	Baseline; around 12 weeks; then annually	Dyslipidemia risk is substantial	ADA/APA CONSENSUS (2004)
CMP / liver-related studies	Baseline; then periodically	Supports hepatic and metabolic safety review	Clinical consensus
Bowel-function assessment	Ongoing from initiation onward	Constipation must be identified early and managed proactively	Stroup & Gray (2018)
Early inflammatory / myocarditis vigilance. Obtain baseline and weekly CRP and troponin during the first ~4 weeks of clozapine treatment; evaluate promptly if cardiac symptoms occur	Highest in the first several weeks of titration	Review symptoms carefully and pursue targeted workup when clinically indicated; some settings use weekly troponin monitoring during the first month when this does not create an access barrier	Leung et al. (2023); Clinical consensus
ECG when indicated	Baseline in selected patients and as clinically indicated thereafter	Consider for cardiac history, symptoms, or abnormal findings	Clinical consensus
Clozapine serum level	When response is inadequate, toxicity is suspected, or adherence is uncertain	Target range generally 350–600 ng/mL for adequate response; levels above 1000 ng/mL associated with increased toxicity risk including seizures; useful to guide dose optimization	Yada et al. (2021); Clinical consensus

E. Patient Education

Topic		Evidence Source
Infection symptoms	Report fever, sore throat, or signs of infection urgently	U.S. Food and Drug Administration. Clozapine REMS program
Constipation	Constipation can become severe and requires early reporting and intervention	Stroup & Gray (2018)
Sedation	Use caution with driving or hazardous activities during early titration	FDA labeling; Clinical consensus
Tachycardia / chest symptoms	Report chest pain, palpitations, shortness of breath, or unexplained fatigue promptly	Leung et al. (2023); Clinical consensus
Adherence to blood monitoring	Ongoing ANC monitoring is strongly recommended per FDA prescribing information; REMS program enrollment is no longer required as of June 13, 2025	FDA labeling (2025)

F. Risks / Monitoring

Clinical Risk	Clinical Notes	Evidence Source
Agranulocytosis	Rare but potentially life-threatening; ANC monitoring remains strongly recommended per FDA prescribing information despite elimination of REMS program	FDA labeling (2025)
GI hypomotility	Constipation may progress to ileus or other severe complications if missed	Stroup & Gray (2018)
Early inflammatory reactions	Fever, eosinophilia, rising inflammatory markers, and myocarditis-related symptoms may emerge during early titration and should not be dismissed	Leung et al. (2023)
Myocarditis	Highest concern is during the first several weeks of titration; clinical suspicion remains essential because no universal evidence-based biomarker protocol fully replaces assessment	Leung et al. (2023); Clinical consensus
Restarting after interruption	Re-titration should be cautious after clinically significant interruption	Clinical consensus

G. Practical Treatment Selection

Clinical Scenario	Preferred Monitoring Strategy	Rationale	Avoid / Caution	Evidence Source
Clozapine initiation	Complete hematologic, metabolic, and medical baseline review before starting	Clozapine requires the most structured monitoring of common psychotropics	Avoid treating clozapine as a routine antipsychotic start without dedicated monitoring workflow	FDA labeling (2025)
First several weeks of titration	Intensify surveillance for infection, constipation, tachycardia, inflammatory symptoms, and myocarditis-related complaints	Early-treatment risk burden is highest	Avoid relying on ANC alone as the only safety screen	Leung et al. (2023)

Clinical Scenario	Preferred Monitoring Strategy	Rationale	Avoid / Caution	Evidence Source
Treatment interruption	Restart cautiously with re-titration rather than automatically resuming the prior full dose	Rapid resumption increases adverse effect risk	Avoid full-dose restart after clinically meaningful interruption	Clinical consensus

REFERENCES

American Diabetes Association, American Psychiatric Association, American Association of Clinical Endocrinologists, & North American Association for the Study of Obesity. (2004). Consensus development conference on antipsychotic drugs and obesity and diabetes. *Diabetes Care*, *27*(2), 596–601. https://doi.org/10.2337/diacare.27.2.596

American Psychiatric Association. (2020). *The American Psychiatric Association practice guideline for the treatment of patients with schizophrenia* (3rd ed.). American Psychiatric Association Publishing. https://doi.org/10.1176/appi.books.9780890424841

Bosi, A., Ceriani, L., Elinder, C.-G., et al. (2023). Quality of laboratory biomarker monitoring during treatment with lithium in patients with bipolar disorder. *Bipolar Disorders*, *25*(6), 499–506. https://doi.org/10.1111/bdi.13302

Yatham, L. N., Kennedy, S. H., Parikh, S. V., et al. (2018). Canadian Network for Mood and Anxiety Treatments (CANMAT) and International Society for Bipolar Disorders (ISBD) 2018 guidelines for the management of patients with bipolar disorder. Bipolar Disorders, 20(2), 97–170. https://doi.org/10.1111/bdi.12609

De Hert, M., Coppens, V., Lehman, R., et al. (2024). Monitoring and management of metabolic adverse effects of antipsychotics: An update. *European Neuropsychopharmacology*, *84*, 1–17.

Leung, J. G., Zhang, L., Markota, M., et al. (2023). A systematic review of clozapine-associated inflammation and related monitoring. *Pharmacotherapy*, *43*(12), 1364–1396. https://doi.org/10.1002/phar.2887

National Institute for Health and Care Excellence. (2014, updated 2025). *Bipolar disorder: Assessment and management* (NICE Guideline CG185). NICE. https://www.nice.org.uk/guidance/cg185

National Institute for Health and Care Excellence. (2014, updated 2019). *Psychosis and schizophrenia in adults: Prevention and management* (NICE Guideline CG178). NICE. https://www.nice.org.uk/guidance/cg178

Nederlof, M., Heerdink, E. R., Egberts, T. C. G., et al. (2018). Monitoring of patients treated with lithium for bipolar disorder: An international survey. *International Journal of Bipolar Disorders*, *6*(1), 12. https://doi.org/10.1186/s40345-018-0120-1

Ronaldson, K. J., Fitzgerald, P. B., Taylor, A. J., Topliss, D. J., & McNeil, J. J. (2011). A new monitoring protocol for clozapine-induced myocarditis based on an analysis of 75 cases and 94 controls. *Australian & New Zealand Journal of Psychiatry*, *45*(6), 458–465. https://doi.org/10.3109/00048674.2011.572852

U.S. Food and Drug Administration. (2025). *FDA removes risk evaluation and mitigation strategy (REMS) program for clozapine.* https://www.fda.gov/drugs/drug-safety-communications/fda-removes-risk-evaluation-and-mitigation-strategy-rems-program-antipsychotic-drug-clozapine

Yada, Y., Kitagawa, K., Sakamoto, S., et al. (2021). The relationship between plasma clozapine concentration and clinical outcome: A cross-sectional study. Acta Psychiatrica Scandinavica, 143(3), 227–237. https://doi.org/10.1111/acps.13264

XV. DRUG INTERACTIONS AND CYP SYSTEM

SECTION INTRODUCTION

Drug interactions represent a major source of adverse effects, treatment failure, toxicity, hospitalization, and medication nonadherence within psychiatric practice. Psychotropic medications frequently interact with one another as well as with nonpsychiatric medications, over-the-counter agents, herbal supplements, nicotine products, and substances of misuse. Understanding pharmacokinetic and pharmacodynamic interactions is therefore essential to support safe prescribing, minimize preventable complications, and optimize psychopharmacologic treatment outcomes.

The cytochrome P450 (CYP450) enzyme system plays a central role in the hepatic metabolism of many psychiatric medications. Variability in CYP450 activity may substantially influence serum drug concentrations, medication efficacy, adverse effect burden, withdrawal phenomena, and toxicity risk. Clinically significant interactions commonly occur when one medication inhibits or induces the metabolism of another agent, resulting in elevated or reduced plasma concentrations with corresponding changes in clinical response and tolerability.

Several CYP450 isoenzymes are particularly relevant within psychopharmacology, including CYP2D6, CYP3A4, CYP1A2, CYP2C19, and CYP2C9. Many antidepressants, antipsychotics, stimulants, mood stabilizers, benzodiazepines, and opioid medications are metabolized through these pathways. Potent enzyme inhibitors may increase medication exposure and toxicity risk, while enzyme inducers may lower serum concentrations and reduce therapeutic efficacy. Individual genetic variability in CYP metabolism may further contribute to unusual sensitivity, poor response, or adverse reactions in selected patients.

Psychiatric polypharmacy significantly increases interaction risk, particularly in patients receiving multiple serotonergic agents, sedating medications, anticholinergic drugs, stimulants, mood stabilizers, or QT-prolonging agents. Common clinically significant interactions include serotonin syndrome, excessive sedation, respiratory suppression, lithium toxicity, increased clozapine levels, elevated antipsychotic exposure, benzodiazepine accumulation, hypertensive crises involving monoamine oxidase inhibitors (MAOIs), and alterations in anticoagulant or cardiovascular medication metabolism. Clinicians should therefore routinely review medication combinations, recent medication changes, and nonprescription substance use during psychiatric evaluation and follow-up.

Substances outside traditional prescription medications may also substantially affect CYP metabolism and psychotropic drug exposure. Tobacco smoke induces CYP1A2 and may significantly lower serum concentrations of medications such as clozapine and olanzapine.

Abrupt smoking cessation may therefore unexpectedly increase antipsychotic levels and toxicity risk. Grapefruit juice, cannabidiol (CBD), St. John's Wort, caffeine, alcohol, and various herbal supplements may also alter psychotropic metabolism or increase pharmacodynamic adverse effects.

Certain patient populations are particularly vulnerable to clinically significant drug interactions. Elderly patients, medically complex individuals, patients with hepatic or renal impairment, pregnant individuals, and patients receiving multiple medications from different providers require especially careful medication reconciliation and monitoring. Reduced physiologic reserve, altered metabolism, and polypharmacy may substantially increase the risk of delirium, falls, cardiac complications, oversedation, cognitive impairment, and medication toxicity.

Although pharmacokinetic interactions involving the CYP450 system are critically important, pharmacodynamic interactions must also be considered. Medications with overlapping serotonergic, dopaminergic, anticholinergic, sedative, hypotensive, or QT-prolonging effects may produce additive toxicity even in the absence of direct metabolic interactions. Clinicians should therefore evaluate both metabolic pathways and cumulative physiologic burden when selecting medication combinations.

Effective management of drug interactions requires ongoing monitoring, patient education, conservative prescribing practices, and individualized risk assessment. Important strategies may include gradual dose titration, therapeutic drug monitoring, avoidance of high-risk combinations, ECG monitoring when appropriate, laboratory surveillance, and coordination with primary care providers, pharmacists, and specialty clinicians. Patients should also be educated regarding the risks associated with abrupt medication changes, self-medication, supplement use, and unsupervised discontinuation of psychiatric treatment.

The following sections provide a structured, evidence-informed framework for clinically relevant psychotropic drug interactions, CYP450 metabolism, and medication safety considerations within outpatient psychiatric practice. Recommendations are intended to support safe, clinically individualized, and pharmacologically informed psychiatric care while recognizing the importance of longitudinal reassessment, interdisciplinary collaboration, and professional clinical judgment throughout treatment.

1. CYP450

A. OVERVIEW

Aspect	Detail	Evidence Source
Definition	Cytochrome P450 enzymes mediate phase I metabolism of many psychotropic and nonpsychiatric medications	FDA labeling; Clinical consensus
Clinical relevance	Understanding CYP-mediated interactions helps reduce toxicity, treatment failure, and avoidable polypharmacy complications	FDA labeling; Preskorn (2013)
Major isoenzymes in psychiatry	CYP3A4, CYP2D6, CYP1A2, CYP2C19, and CYP2C9 are most clinically relevant for psychotropic prescribing	FDA labeling; Preskorn (2013)
Core interaction principle	Enzyme inhibition may increase drug exposure and toxicity risk; enzyme induction may reduce exposure and compromise efficacy	FDA labeling; Clinical consensus
Limitation of simple tables	Not every substrate–inhibitor or substrate–inducer pairing produces clinically meaningful change; magnitude depends on dose, route, therapeutic index, comorbidity, and competing pathways	Preskorn (2013); Clinical consensus

B. Diagnostic / Interaction Considerations

Clinical Consideration	Clinical Notes	Evidence Source
Identify the victim drug	The clinically affected drug is usually the substrate with narrow therapeutic range, active metabolite dependence, or dose-related toxicity	Preskorn (2013); Clinical consensus
Identify the perpetrator drug	Inhibitors and inducers differ in strength, onset, offset, and pathway selectivity	FDA labeling; Clinical consensus
Review full medication list	Important interactions often come from nonpsychiatric prescriptions, OTC products, supplements, smoking, and diet	FDA labeling; Boullata (2005)
Consider timing	Inhibition may appear relatively quickly; induction often evolves over days to weeks and may take days to weeks to reverse	FDA labeling; Nadkarni et al. (2012)
Distinguish smoking from nicotine	CYP1A2 induction is driven by polycyclic aromatic hydrocarbons in tobacco smoke rather than by nicotine itself	FDA labeling; Clinical consensus

C. Practical Interpretation Principles

Principle	Clinical Notes	Evidence Source
Do not use fixed dose-change rules universally	Dose changes must reflect the specific substrate, interaction strength, and patient response rather than a universal 25–50% rule	Preskorn (2013); Clinical consensus
Prioritize high-risk substrates	Clozapine, TCAs, methadone, warfarin, carbamazepine, and selected antipsychotics require greater caution	FDA labeling; Clinical consensus
Reassess after medication changes	New toxicity or loss of efficacy after adding or stopping a drug often reflects an interaction rather than treatment failure	Preskorn (2013); Clinical consensus

2. MAJOR CYP ISOENZYMES IN PSYCHIATRY CYP

A. Key Enzymes, Substrates, Inhibitors, and Inducers

Enzyme	Common Psychiatric Substrates	Common Inhibitors	Common Inducers	Clinical Notes	Evidence Source
CYP3A4	Quetiapine, buspirone, alprazolam, midazolam, zolpidem, aripiprazole (partly), iloperidone/ milsaperidone	Ketoconazole, itraconazole, ritonavir, grapefruit juice	Carbamazepine, phenytoin, rifampin, St. John's wort	Most broadly relevant pathway in psychopharmacology; interaction magnitude varies by substrate dependence	FDA labeling; Clinical consensus
CYP2D6	Risperidone, haloperidol, TCAs, atomoxetine, venlafaxine, fluoxetine, paroxetine, iloperidone/ milsaperidone	Fluoxetine, paroxetine, bupropion, quinidine	Not meaningfully inducible in routine clinical practice	Phenoconversion by strong inhibitors is clinically important. Fluoxetine and paroxetine are both substrates AND strong inhibitors of CYP2D6 — this dual role is clinically important	FDA labeling; Preskorn (2013)

Enzyme	Common Psychiatric Substrates	Common Inhibitors	Common Inducers	Clinical Notes	Evidence Source
CYP1A2	Clozapine, olanzapine, duloxetine, caffeine	Fluvoxamine, ciprofloxacin	Smoking, carbamazepine	Smoking changes may have major implications for clozapine and olanzapine dosing. Induction is caused by smoke hydrocarbons (not nicotine); after cessation, clozapine and olanzapine levels can rise within days, reaching a new steady state in about one week—consider dose reduction, toxicity monitoring, and a serum level	FDA labeling; Clinical consensus
CYP2C19	Citalopram, escitalopram, sertraline, diazepam	Fluvoxamine, omeprazole	Carbamazepine, rifampin	Genotype and inhibitor burden may both matter clinically Citalopram is a CYP2C19 substrate; in poor metabolizers or with strong CYP2C19 inhibitors, exposure and QT-prolongation risk rise, supporting the reduced 20 mg/day dose cap in these patients (see citalopram dosing/QT cautions). Sertraline undergoes multi-enzyme metabolism (CYP2B6, 2C19, 2C9, 2D6, 3A4) and is not a clean single-enzyme CYP2C19 example.	FDA labeling; Spina & de Leon (2015)
CYP2C9	Phenytoin, warfarin, selected NSAIDs	Fluconazole, valproate	Carbamazepine, rifampin	Most relevant when psychotropics interact with medical medications such as warfarin or phenytoin	FDA labeling; Nadkarni et al. (2012)

Clinical note

Pharmacogenomics: CYP2D6 and CYP2C19 are subject to clinically significant genetic variation. Poor metabolizers may experience elevated drug exposure and adverse effects at standard doses; ultrarapid metabolizers may have inadequate response. Phenoconversion — where a strong inhibitor converts a normal metabolizer to a functional poor metabolizer — is clinically important and does not require genetic testing to recognize. When unexpected toxicity or nonresponse occurs with CYP2D6 or CYP2C19 substrates, consider both genetic and drug-induced metabolic variation as contributing factors. *Spina & de Leon (2015)*

3. High-Risk Inducers

Inducer	Main Pathways	Commonly Affected Psychiatric Drugs	Clinical Notes	Evidence Source
Carbamazepine	CYP3A4, CYP1A2, CYP2C19 induction; also induces UGT (glucuronidation), with autoinduction; P-glycoprotein (P-gp) induction is commonly reported but supported less consistently — overall a broad enzyme inducer with potential transporter effects.	Antipsychotics, benzodiazepines, methadone, some antidepressants	Can substantially reduce serum exposure of susceptible drugs; interaction magnitude varies by substrate	FDA labeling; Clinical consensus
Phenytoin	CYP3A4, CYP2C19, CYP2C9 induction	Antidepressants, antipsychotics, benzodiazepines	Narrow therapeutic index complicates co-prescribing	FDA labeling
Rifampin	CYP3A4, CYP2C19, CYP2C9 induction	Many psychotropics	Strong inducer with broad interaction potential; often requires avoidance or close reassessment	FDA labeling
St. John's wort	CYP3A4 induction; may affect other pathways and transporters	SSRIs, SNRIs, antipsychotics, benzodiazepines, oral contraceptives, antiretrovirals	Commercial preparations vary substantially; clinically meaningful interactions are well documented	Borrelli & Izzo (2009); Barnes et al. (2001)

Inducer	Main Pathways	Commonly Affected Psychiatric Drugs	Clinical Notes	Evidence Source
Phenobarbital	CYP3A4, CYP2C19 induction	Antidepressants, antipsychotics, sedatives	Similar interaction framework to other strong enzyme inducers	FDA labeling

A. Practical Management of Inducers

Clinical Scenario	Preferred Strategy	Rationale	Avoid / Caution	Evidence Source
Adding a strong inducer to a stable psychotropic regimen	Reassess for loss of efficacy and consider dose adjustment or alternative agent	Induction may substantially lower exposure of susceptible substrates	Avoid assuming unchanged efficacy	FDA labeling; Clinical consensus
Stopping a strong inducer	Reassess for delayed toxicity as enzyme activity normalizes	Drug levels may rise after inducer removal	Avoid leaving prior high doses in place without follow-up	Nadkarni et al. (2012); Clinical consensus
Patient self-starts St. John's wort	Stop or avoid supplement and reassess interacting medications	Herbal preparation variability and CYP induction can cause clinically meaningful treatment failure	Avoid concurrent use with high-risk psychotropics or ARVs	Borrelli & Izzo (2009); Barnes et al. (2001)

4. High-Risk Inhibitors

Inhibitor	Main Pathways	Commonly Affected Psychiatric Drugs	Clinical Notes	Evidence Source
Fluoxetine	CYP2D6 inhibition; additional pathway effects may occur	TCAs, antipsychotics, atomoxetine, venlafaxine	Long half-life and active metabolite prolong inhibitory effect	FDA labeling
Paroxetine	CYP2D6 inhibition	Similar to fluoxetine for many CYP2D6 substrates	Strong CYP2D6 inhibition is clinically important	FDA labeling
Bupropion	CYP2D6 inhibition	TCAs, antipsychotics, atomoxetine, some beta-blockers	Inhibitory effect may be clinically meaningful even at common doses	FDA labeling

Inhibitor	Main Pathways	Commonly Affected Psychiatric Drugs	Clinical Notes	Evidence Source
Fluvoxamine	Strong CYP1A2 inhibition; additional CYP inhibition may occur	Clozapine, olanzapine, caffeine, some benzodiazepines	Particularly important for clozapine toxicity risk	FDA labeling
Ketoconazole / itraconazole	Strong CYP3A4 inhibition	Quetiapine, buspirone, alprazolam, other CYP3A4 substrates	Sedation, hypotension, or QT burden may rise depending on substrate	FDA labeling
Ritonavir	Potent CYP3A4 inhibition with complex interaction profile	Many psychotropics	Requires regimen-specific review; do not generalize dosing without checking the ARV combination	DHHS HIV Guidelines (2024); Goodlet et al. (2019)
Ciprofloxacin / enoxacin	CYP1A2 inhibition	Clozapine, olanzapine, caffeine	May markedly increase exposure of CYP1A2-sensitive substrates	FDA labeling
Grapefruit juice	Intestinal CYP3A4 inhibition	Selected CYP3A4 substrates	Effect is substrate-specific and not universal; highest concern when intestinal CYP3A4 contributes meaningfully to clearance	FDA labeling; Clinical consensus

A. Practical Management of Inhibitors

Clinical Scenario	Preferred Strategy	Rationale	Avoid / Caution	Evidence Source
Adding a strong inhibitor to a narrow-therapeutic-index substrate	Reassess for toxicity and consider dose reduction or alternative agent	Inhibition may rapidly increase exposure	Avoid fixed dose-change rules without monitoring	FDA labeling; Preskorn (2013)
Stopping a strong inhibitor	Reassess for loss of efficacy	Substrate exposure may fall after inhibitor removal	Avoid assuming prior dose remains effective	FDA labeling; Clinical consensus
Fluvoxamine added to clozapine	Use major caution and reduce clozapine dose if co-use is intentional	Clozapine exposure can rise substantially	Avoid casual co-prescribing without close monitoring	FDA labeling; Clinical consensus

5. SELECTED HIGH-RISK PSYCHIATRIC INTERACTION PAIRS

A. Common High-Risk Pairs

Interaction Pair	Expected Problem	Clinical Notes	Evidence Source
Fluvoxamine + clozapine	Major increase in clozapine exposure	May precipitate toxicity; monitor closely if intentional co-use	FDA labeling; Clinical consensus
Carbamazepine + quetiapine	Reduced quetiapine exposure	May produce marked efficacy loss in susceptible patients	FDA labeling; Clinical consensus
Carbamazepine + oral antipsychotics broadly	Reduced antipsychotic exposure	Magnitude varies by agent and pathway dependence	FDA labeling; Clinical consensus
Valproate + lamotrigine	Significantly increased lamotrigine levels	Valproate inhibits lamotrigine glucuronidation; lamotrigine dose must be reduced by approximately 50% when valproate is added	FDA labeling; Clinical consensus
Valproate + carbamazepine	Reduced valproate levels; carbamazepine toxicity risk	Bidirectional interaction; carbamazepine induces valproate metabolism while valproate inhibits carbamazepine epoxide clearance	FDA labeling; Clinical consensus
Valproate + aspirin	Increased free valproate levels	Aspirin displaces valproate from protein binding increasing free valproate and toxicity risk; use with caution	FDA labeling; Clinical consensus

Interaction Pair	Expected Problem	Clinical Notes	Evidence Source
Valproate + warfarin	Potential increased anticoagulant effect	Valproate may increase free warfarin fraction; evidence primarily in vitro but coagulation tests should be monitored if co-prescribed. Overall, clinical evidence for this interaction is limited.	FDA labeling; Nadkarni et al. (2012)
Valproate + CNS depressants	Additive sedation	Combined sedative burden may be clinically significant; monitor closely	FDA labeling; Clinical consensus
Valproate + topiramate	Hyperammonemia risk	Both agents impair the urea cycle; combination may cause encephalopathy even at therapeutic levels; monitor ammonia if encephalopathy symptoms emerge	FDA labeling; Clinical consensus
Fluoxetine / paroxetine / bupropion + beta-blockers	Increased beta-blocker exposure; bradycardia risk	CYP2D6 inhibition raises beta-blocker levels significantly; monitor heart rate and BP; consider atenolol as alternative (non-CYP2D6 substrate)	FDA labeling; Clinical consensus
Fluoxetine / paroxetine / bupropion + CYP2D6 substrates	Increased substrate exposure; toxicity risk	Potent CYP2D6 inhibition raises levels of TCAs, atomoxetine, and selected antipsychotics; dose reduction of substrate may be required; paroxetine and fluoxetine have long half-lives prolonging the interaction after discontinuation	FDA labeling; Clinical consensus
MAOI + any serotonergic agent	Serotonin syndrome risk	Potentially life-threatening; explicit washout periods required before and after MAOI use: at least 14 days for most serotonergic agents, and at least 5 weeks after discontinuing fluoxetine before starting an MAOI	FDA labeling; Clinical consensus
Lithium + NSAIDs or thiazide diuretics	Increased lithium levels and toxicity risk	NSAIDs reduce renal lithium clearance; monitor lithium level closely if co-prescribed. Lithium is renally eliminated and is not a CYP substrate, so these interactions (including ACE inhibitors and ARBs) are renal/pharmacokinetic, not CYP-mediated.	FDA labeling; Clinical consensus
Smoking cessation + clozapine or olanzapine	Rising drug exposure after CYP1A2 induction resolves	Dose may need reassessment after smoking reduction or cessation	FDA labeling; Clinical consensus

Interaction Pair	Expected Problem	Clinical Notes	Evidence Source
Ritonavir-boosted ARV + quetiapine or benzodiazepines	Excess exposure and sedation/toxicity risk	Interaction review should be regimen-specific	DHHS HIV Guidelines (2024); Goodlet et al. (2019)

6. QT-RELATED INTERACTION RISK

A. Higher-Risk QT Medications

Medication	Relative QT Concern	Clinical Notes	Evidence Source
Ziprasidone	Higher	Use caution in patients with other QT risk factors or interacting drugs	FDA labeling; CredibleMeds
Milsaperidone (Bysanti)	Higher	Iloperidone active metabolite; avoid with other QT-prolonging drugs; risk rises with CYP2D6/3A4 inhibitors or in CYP2D6 poor metabolizers; discontinue if QTc >500 ms	FDA labeling (2026)
Haloperidol, especially IV	Higher	IV route is of particular concern in medically ill patients	FDA labeling; CredibleMeds
Thioridazine	Higher	Historically recognized as a high-risk antipsychotic for QT prolongation	FDA labeling
Methadone	Higher	Risk increases with dose, interacting drugs, and cumulative vulnerability	FDA labeling; CredibleMeds
Citalopram	Moderate to higher at higher doses	Dose limits and patient risk factors matter	FDA labeling
Escitalopram	Moderate	Lower concern than citalopram in many contexts, but not risk-free	FDA labeling
TCAs	Moderate	Risk varies by agent and dose; more caution in overdose or cardiac disease	FDA labeling
Quetiapine	Moderate / context-dependent	QT concern is usually context-dependent and should be interpreted alongside dose, polypharmacy, electrolyte status, and medical comorbidity	FDA labeling; CredibleMeds
Ondansetron	Moderate to higher at higher doses	Commonly used antiemetic in psychiatric inpatient settings; additive QT risk when combined with antipsychotics, methadone, or other QT-prolonging agents; dose limits apply	FDA labeling; CredibleMeds

B. High-Risk QT Combinations

Combination	Risk	Preferred Alternative / Strategy	Evidence Source
Ziprasidone + methadone	Additive QT burden	Use lower-QT-burden alternative when feasible	FDA labeling; CredibleMeds
Citalopram above recommended dose + other QT-prolonging drugs	Additive QT burden and dose-related risk	Use safer dosing or alternative antidepressant	FDA labeling
IV haloperidol + other QT-prolonging agents such as ondansetron	Torsades risk increases in susceptible patients	Avoid combination when feasible and monitor medically ill patients closely	FDA labeling; Clinical consensus
Multiple QT-prolonging drugs	Cumulative risk	Reduce avoidable polypharmacy and correct reversible contributors	CredibleMeds; Clinical consensus

C. Practical QT Monitoring

Clinical Scenario	Preferred Strategy	Rationale	Avoid / Caution	Evidence Source
QTc >500 ms	Reassess psychotropic regimen, correct electrolytes, and obtain medical/cardiology input as indicated	High-risk threshold requiring action	Avoid passive continuation of multiple QT-risk drugs	FDA labeling; Clinical consensus
Patient with cardiac disease or syncope history starting a QT-risk psychotropic	Obtain baseline ECG when clinically appropriate	Helps identify pre-existing vulnerability	Avoid assuming average-risk prescribing applies	FDA labeling; Clinical consensus
Patient on methadone plus psychotropics	Review full medication list for cumulative QT burden	Combined pharmacodynamic risk can become clinically important	Avoid adding unnecessary QT-risk drugs	FDA labeling; Clinical consensus

7. HERBAL, OTC, AND LIFESTYLE INTERACTION RISKS

A. Higher-Relevance Supplements / OTC Products

Supplement / OTC / Lifestyle Factor	Interaction Concern	Clinical Notes	Evidence Source
St. John's wort	CYP induction; may reduce medication efficacy	Most clinically important herb–drug interaction in this chapter	Borrelli & Izzo (2009); Barnes et al. (2001)
Kava	CNS depression; hepatotoxicity concern	Evidence base is less standardized than for St. John's wort; use caution	FDA warnings; Clinical consensus
Valerian	Additive sedation	Most relevant when combined with sedatives or alcohol	Limited evidence; Clinical consensus
Diphenhydramine	Anticholinergic and sedative burden	Fall risk, cognitive impairment, and paradoxical confusion in vulnerable patients	Beers Criteria (2023)
Melatonin	Limited CYP interaction relevance	Usually lower interaction burden than many OTC sleep aids	Clinical consensus
CBD	CYP3A4 / CYP2C19 interaction potential and product variability	Interaction potential is plausible and may become clinically relevant at higher doses or with concentrated products, but product variability limits firm prediction	FDA labeling; Clinical consensus

Supplement / OTC / Lifestyle Factor	Interaction Concern	Clinical Notes	Evidence Source
Caffeine	CYP1A2 substrate; may worsen anxiety and insomnia	Also relevant when fluvoxamine or smoking changes alter exposure	FDA labeling
Grapefruit juice	Intestinal CYP3A4 inhibition	Interaction is substrate-specific but clinically important for some drugs	FDA labeling
Smoking	CYP1A2 induction via smoke exposure	Relevant for clozapine and olanzapine; cessation may increase levels	FDA labeling; Clinical consensus

B. Lower-Certainty Herbal Products

Supplement	Concern	Clinical Notes	Evidence Source
Ginkgo biloba	Potential CYP and bleeding interaction concerns	Clinical relevance appears less consistent than with St. John's wort	Limited evidence; Zhou et al. (2003)
Ginseng	Potential CYP modulation and glucose effects	Product variability and limited clinical data reduce certainty	Limited evidence; Clinical consensus

C. Patient Education Points

Topic	Key Message	Evidence Source
Always ask about supplements	OTC and herbal products can cause clinically meaningful interactions	Boullata (2005); Clinical consensus)
St. John's wort	Can reduce efficacy of many prescribed drugs	Borrelli & Izzo (2009); Clinical consensus
OTC sleep aids	Diphenhydramine is not a benign sleep aid, especially in older adults	Beers Criteria (2023)
CBD products	Product quality and interaction risk vary substantially	FDA labeling

Topic	Key Message	Evidence Source
Grapefruit juice	Ask specifically; patients often do not identify it as a medication interaction issue	FDA labeling
Smoking changes	Report smoking reduction or cessation promptly if taking clozapine or olanzapine	FDA labeling; Clinical consensus

8. MONITORING AND RISK REDUCTION

A. Monitoring Strategies

Strategy	Clinical Notes	Evidence Source
Review medication changes systematically	New prescriptions, discontinuations, supplements, and smoking changes should trigger interaction review	Preskorn (2013); Clinical consensus
Monitor for both toxicity and inefficacy	Drug interactions may present as oversedation, EPS, QT burden, relapse, or apparent treatment failure	FDA labeling; Clinical consensus
Use serum levels when available and clinically meaningful	Especially useful for clozapine, lithium, carbamazepine, valproate, and selected medical co-medications	FDA labeling; Clinical consensus
Document patient counseling	Interaction counseling is part of safe psychopharmacology practice	Clinical consensus

B. Practical Treatment Selection

Clinical Scenario	Preferred Strategy	Rationale	Avoid / Caution	Evidence Source
Patient on clozapine starts fluvoxamine or ciprofloxacin	Reassess urgently and reduce clozapine exposure if co-use is intentional	High toxicity risk	Avoid casual combination prescribing	FDA labeling; Clinical consensus

Clinical Scenario	Preferred Strategy	Rationale	Avoid / Caution	Evidence Source
Patient on quetiapine starts carbamazepine	Consider switching one agent or reassessing quetiapine efficacy closely	Induction may significantly reduce exposure	Avoid assuming standard quetiapine dose remains effective	FDA labeling; Clinical consensus
Patient on ritonavir-boosted ARV needs psychotropic	Choose lower-interaction agent and review regimen specifically	ARV interactions are often complex and high-impact	Avoid generalizing from non-boosted regimens	DHHS HIV Guidelines (2024); Goodlet et al. (2019)
Patient taking multiple QT-risk medications	Reduce avoidable QT burden and correct reversible risks	Cumulative risk matters more than single-drug labeling alone	Avoid unnecessary polypharmacy	FDA labeling; CredibleMeds
Patient uses St. John's wort or CBD without telling clinician	Stop, document, and reassess interacting prescriptions	Hidden supplements often explain unexpected instability	Avoid ignoring nonprescription products	Borrelli & Izzo (2009); FDA labeling

REFERENCES

American Academy of Sleep Medicine. (2017). Clinical practice guideline for the pharmacologic treatment of chronic insomnia in adults. *Journal of Clinical Sleep Medicine*, *13*(2), 307–349. https://doi.org/10.5664/jcsm.6470

American Geriatrics Society Beers Criteria® Update Expert Panel. (2023). American Geriatrics Society 2023 updated AGS Beers Criteria® for potentially inappropriate medication use in older adults. *Journal of the American Geriatrics Society*, *71*(7), 2052–2081. https://doi.org/10.1111/jgs.18372

Barnes, J., Anderson, L. A., & Phillipson, J. D. (2001). St John's wort (*Hypericum perforatum* L.): A review of its chemistry, pharmacology and clinical properties. *Journal of Pharmacy and Pharmacology*, *53*(5), 583–600. https://doi.org/10.1211/0022357011775910

Borrelli, F., & Izzo, A. A. (2009). Herb–drug interactions with St John's wort (*Hypericum perforatum*): An update on clinical observations. *The AAPS Journal*, *11*(4), 710–727. https://doi.org/10.1208/s12248-009-9146-8

Boullata, J. I. (2005). Natural health product interactions with medication. *Nutrition in Clinical Practice*, *20*(1), 33–51. https://doi.org/10.1177/011542650502000133

CredibleMeds. (n.d.). *QTdrugs list: Risk categories for drug-induced Torsades de pointes*. https://www.crediblemeds.org

Department of Health and Human Services. (2024). *Guidelines for the use of antiretroviral agents in adults and adolescents with HIV*. Panel on Antiretroviral Guidelines for Adults and Adolescents. https://clinicalinfo.hiv.gov/en/guidelines
Goodlet, K. J., Zmarlicka, M., & Peckham, A. M. (2019). Drug–drug interactions and clinical considerations with co-administration of antiretrovirals and psychotropic drugs. *CNS Spectrums, 24*(3), 287–312. https://doi.org/10.1017/S109285291800113X
Nadkarni, A., Oldham, M., & Howard, M. E. (2012). Drug–drug interactions between warfarin and psychotropics: Updated review of the literature. *Pharmacotherapy, 32*(10), 932–942. https://doi.org/10.1002/j.1875-9114.2012.01119
National Institute for Health and Care Excellence. (2014, updated 2019). *Psychosis and schizophrenia in adults: Prevention and management* (NICE Guideline CG178). NICE. https://www.nice.org.uk/guidance/cg178
Preskorn, S. H. (2013). Clinically relevant cytochrome P450 (CYP) enzyme interactions with psychotropic medications. *Journal of Psychiatric Practice, 19*(6), 441–454. https://doi.org/10.1097/01.pra.0000438188.14505.79
Spina, E., & de Leon, J. (2015). Clinical applications of CYP genotyping in psychiatry. *Journal of Neural Transmission, 122*(1), 5–28. https://doi.org/10.1007/s00702-014-1232-5
U.S. Food and Drug Administration. (2024). *Drug interactions: What you should know*. https://www.fda.gov/drugs/resources-drugs/drug-interactions-what-you-should-know
Zhou, S. F., Gao, Y., Jiang, W., Huang, M., Xu, A., & Paxton, J. W. (2003). Interactions of herbs with cytochrome P450. *Drug Metabolism Reviews, 35*(1), 35–98. https://doi.org/10.1081/DMR-120018248

XVI. MEDICATION COMPENDIUM

A. OVERVIEW

The Medication Compendium is a detailed resource summarizing key medications used in psychiatry and related medical fields. It organizes drugs by class, providing generic and brand names, indications, dosing ranges, key side effects, and important clinical notes. This compendium is designed to inform clinicians about safe and effective prescribing practices, including monitoring requirements, drug interactions, and special precautions for various populations.

B. How to Use This Section

- Reference Medication Classes: Use each medication class section to quickly identify drugs appropriate for specific conditions such as depression, bipolar disorder, anxiety, neurodevelopmental disorders, or substance use disorders.
- Review Dosing and Effects: Check the dose ranges and key effects to plan treatment and anticipate common side effects.
- Consider Clinical Notes: Pay close attention to the notes column for guidance on special populations, contraindications, necessary monitoring (e.g., ECG, blood levels), and drug interactions.
- Follow Prescribing Principles: Always start with the lowest effective dose and titrate slowly ("Start low, go slow"). Avoid polypharmacy when possible to minimize adverse effects and interactions.
- Monitor Metabolic and Other Risk Factors: Regularly assess metabolic parameters and watch for signs of toxicity or side effects related to the medication.
- Evaluate Drug - Drug Interactions: Consider potential interactions before initiating or changing medications to ensure patient safety.
- Use the Lowest Effective Dose: Employ the minimal dose that achieves therapeutic benefit to reduce risk and improve tolerability.

Dose ranges and recommendations represent typical adult outpatient psychiatric practice and may require modification for geriatric and pediatric patients, medical comorbidities, pregnancy, or hepatic/renal impairment.

Clinicians should always confirm dosing, contraindications, and monitoring requirements using current FDA labeling and institutional guidelines when initiating or adjusting therapy.

This compendium serves as a practical guide to support clinicians in making evidence-informed, safe, and patient-centered medication choices throughout the course of treatment.

1. SSRIs — CLINICAL PROFILE AND PRACTICAL USE

Generic	Brand	Indications	Dose Range	Key Adverse Effects	Clinical Notes	Evidence Source
Sertraline	Zoloft	MDD, OCD, PTSD, panic disorder, SAD, PMDD	50–200 mg/day	GI upset, sexual dysfunction	Usually well tolerated; start low in panic disorder	NICE (2022); FDA labeling
Escitalopram	Lexapro	MDD, GAD	10–20 mg/day	GI effects, sexual dysfunction	Generally well tolerated; QT caution at higher doses	NICE (2022); FDA labeling
Fluoxetine	Prozac	MDD, OCD, panic disorder, bulimia, PMDD	20–80 mg/day	Insomnia, activation, sexual dysfunction	Long half-life; requires longer MAOI washout	NICE (2022); FDA labeling
Paroxetine	Paxil	MDD, GAD, social anxiety disorder, PTSD, OCD, panic disorder	20–60 mg/day	Sexual dysfunction, weight gain, withdrawal symptoms	Difficult discontinuation; avoid in pregnancy when possible	NICE (2022); ACOG (2023); FDA labeling
Fluvoxamine	Luvox	OCD	100–300 mg/day	Sedation, GI upset, interactions	Significant CYP interaction burden; may increase clozapine levels	NICE (2022); FDA labeling
Citalopram	Celexa	MDD	10–40 mg/day	Nausea, dry mouth, QT prolongation	QT caution; avoid exceeding recommended limits — maximum 40 mg/day in adults; 20 mg/day in patients over 60 years, hepatic impairment, CYP2C19 poor metabolizers, or with concomitant CYP2C19 inhibitors	NICE (2022); FDA labeling

2. SNRIs — CLINICAL PROFILE AND PRACTICAL USE

Generic	Brand	Indications	Dose Range	Key Adverse Effects	Clinical Notes	Evidence Source
Venlafaxine XR	Effexor XR	MDD, GAD, panic disorder, SAD	75–225 mg/day	Nausea, withdrawal symptoms, BP elevation	More noradrenergic at higher doses; taper gradually	NICE (2022); FDA labeling

Generic	Brand	Indications	Dose Range	Key Adverse Effects	Clinical Notes	Evidence Source
Desvenlafaxine	Pristiq	MDD	50–100 mg/day	Nausea, sweating	Lower CYP interaction burden	FDA labeling
Duloxetine	Cymbalta	MDD, GAD, neuropathic pain, fibromyalgia	30–120 mg/day	Nausea, dry mouth, sweating	Useful with pain symptoms; avoid significant liver disease	NICE (2022); FDA labeling
Levomilnacipran	Fetzima	MDD	20–120 mg/day	Nausea, tachycardia, urinary hesitancy	More activating and noradrenergic	FDA labeling

3. NDRI — CLINICAL PROFILE AND PRACTICAL USE

Generic	Brand	Indications	Dose Range	Key Adverse Effects	Clinical Notes	Evidence Source
Bupropion XL	Wellbutrin XL	MDD, seasonal affective disorder, smoking cessation; ADHD off-label	150–450 mg/day	Insomnia, anxiety, seizure risk	Avoid in seizure/eating disorders; lower sexual adverse-effect burden	NICE (2022); FDA labeling

4. NaSSA — CLINICAL PROFILE AND PRACTICAL USE

Generic	Brand	Indications	Dose Range	Key Adverse Effects	Clinical Notes	Evidence Source
Mirtazapine	Remeron	MDD; commonly used for insomnia, anxiety, poor appetite	15–45 mg/day	Sedation, increased appetite, weight gain	Lower doses may be more sedating; useful with insomnia or weight loss	NICE (2022); FDA labeling

5. SARI — CLINICAL PROFILE AND PRACTICAL USE

Generic	Brand	Indications	Dose Range	Key Adverse Effects	Clinical Notes	Evidence Source
Trazodone	Desyrel	MDD; insomnia off-label	150–400 mg/day (depression); 25–100 mg HS (insomnia)	Sedation, orthostasis, rare priapism	Often used for sleep; antidepressant effects require higher doses	NICE (2022); FDA labeling

6. OTHER/MULTIMODAL ANTIDEPRESSANTS — CLINICAL PROFILE AND PRACTICAL USE

Generic	Brand	Indications	Dose Range	Key Adverse Effects	Clinical Notes	Evidence Source
Vilazodone	Viibryd	MDD	10–40 mg/day	GI upset, insomnia	Take with food; may cause less sexual dysfunction in some patients	FDA labeling
Vortioxetine	Trintellix	MDD	5–20 mg/day	Nausea, headache	Weight-neutral; possible cognitive benefit in selected MDD patients	NICE (2022); FDA labeling
Phenelzine	Nardil	Atypical depression, TRD, panic disorder	15–90 mg/day	Orthostasis, tyramine reaction risk, weight gain	Reserved for specialist management; strict dietary and interaction precautions	NICE (2022); Clinical consensus; FDA labeling
Clomipramine	Anafranil	OCD; depression off-label	25–250 mg/day	Anticholinergic effects, sedation, cardiac risk, seizure risk	Effective in OCD but generally less tolerated than SSRIs	NICE (2022); Fineberg et al. (2020); FDA labeling
Dextromethorphan-bupropion	Auvelity	MDD	Per prescribing schedule	Dizziness, nausea, interaction-related issues	Rapid-acting option; monitor interaction burden	FDA labeling
Zuranolone	Zurzuvae	Postpartum depression	50 mg HS for 14 days	Somnolence, dizziness, CNS depression	Oral neuroactive steroid; faster onset; avoid in pregnancy	FDA labeling (2023)

Generic	Brand	Indications	Dose Range	Key Adverse Effects	Clinical Notes	Evidence Source
Gepirone	Exxua	MDD	18.2–72.6 mg/day	Dizziness, nausea, insomnia, QT prolongation	Selective 5-HT1A agonist; ECG before and during treatment (avoid if QTc >450 ms); reduce 50% with moderate CYP3A4 inhibitors, contraindicated with strong inhibitors; 14-day MAOI washout; lower sexual-dysfunction and weight-gain burden	FDA labeling (2023)

7. MOOD STABILIZERS/ANTICONVULSANTS — CLINICAL PROFILE AND PRACTICAL USE

Generic	Brand	Indications	Therapeutic Dose / Level	Key Adverse Effects	Clinical Notes	Evidence Source
Lithium	Lithobid	Bipolar I/II disorder, maintenance, MDD augmentation, suicide risk reduction	0.6–0.8 mmol/L maintenance (0.8–1.0 if insufficient response; 0.8–1.2 acute mania; 0.4–0.6 in older adults)	Tremor, hypothyroidism, nephrotoxicity, polydipsia	Gold-standard mood stabilizer; monitor lithium, creatinine, TSH, calcium	CANMAT/ ISBD (2018); FDA labeling

Generic	Brand	Indications	Therapeutic Dose / Level	Key Adverse Effects	Clinical Notes	Evidence Source
Valproate	Depakote	Bipolar mania, mixed episodes, rapid cycling, seizure disorders	50–125 µg/mL	Weight gain, tremor, hepatotoxicity, thrombocytopenia	Useful in mania/mixed states; avoid in pregnancy when possible; monitor CBC/LFTs. Boxed warnings: hepatotoxicity (including fatal hepatic failure, highest risk in children under 2 years and with mitochondrial disease); teratogenicity (neural tube defects and reduced IQ — contraindicated in pregnancy for migraine/prophylaxis and avoided for psychiatric use when alternatives exist); and life-threatening pancreatitis (evaluate promptly for abdominal pain, nausea, or vomiting)	CANMAT/ ISBD (2018); FDA labeling

Generic	Brand	Indications	Therapeutic Dose / Level	Key Adverse Effects	Clinical Notes	Evidence Source
Lamotrigine	Lamictal	Bipolar depression prophylaxis, bipolar II disorder, seizure disorders	100–200 mg/day typical	Rash, dizziness, headache, nausea	Slow titration required; valproate increases and carbamazepine lowers levels Boxed warning: serious, potentially life-threatening rash (Stevens–Johnson syndrome, toxic epidermal necrolysis); risk increases with rapid titration, exceeding recommended starting/escalation doses, or concomitant valproate.	CANMAT/ ISBD (2018); FDA labeling

Generic	Brand	Indications	Therapeutic Dose / Level	Key Adverse Effects	Clinical Notes	Evidence Source
Carbamazepine	Tegretol	Bipolar mania, mixed states, seizure disorders, trigeminal neuralgia	4–12 µg/mL	Hyponatremia, rash, agranulocytosis, hepatotoxicity	Strong enzyme inducer; monitor CBC, CMP, sodium. Boxed warning: serious dermatologic reactions including Stevens-Johnson syndrome/toxic epidermal necrolysis (SJS/TEN); test for HLA-B*1502 in patients of at-risk (e.g., Southeast Asian) ancestry before initiation. Boxed warning: aplastic anemia and agranulocytosis. Undergoes autoinduction: serum levels decline over the first 2–4 weeks as carbamazepine induces its own metabolism, so re-titrate and recheck a level at 2–4 weeks even if	CANMAT/ ISBD (2018); FDA labeling

Generic	Brand	Indications	Therapeutic Dose / Level	Key Adverse Effects	Clinical Notes	Evidence Source
Oxcarbazepine	Trileptal	Bipolar disorder off-label, seizure disorders	600–2400 mg/day	Hyponatremia, dizziness, sedation, rash	Fewer interactions than carbamazepine; monitor sodium	Clinical consensus; FDA labeling
Topiramate	Topamax	Bipolar adjunctive use off-label, seizure disorders, migraine prevention	25–400 mg/day	Cognitive slowing, paresthesias, weight loss, kidney stones	Not first-line; may help when weight gain is a concern	Clinical consensus; FDA labeling

8. FIRST— GENERATION ORAL ANTIPSYCHOTICS — CLINICAL PROFILE AND PRACTICAL USE

Generic	Brand	Indications	Dose Range	Key Adverse Effects	Clinical Notes	Evidence Source
Haloperidol	Haldol	Schizophrenia, acute psychosis, agitation, Tourette's	2–20 mg/day	EPS, akathisia, QT prolongation	High-potency FGA; AIMS monitoring remains important	NICE (2022); FDA labeling
Perphenazine	Trilafon	Schizophrenia	8–64 mg/day	EPS, sedation, anticholinergic effects	Intermediate potency option	FDA labeling
Chlorpromazine	Thorazine	Schizophrenia, severe agitation	200–800 mg/day	Sedation, orthostasis, anticholinergic burden, QT risk	Low-potency FGA; more sedating and hypotensive	FDA labeling

Generic	Brand	Indications	Dose Range	Key Adverse Effects	Clinical Notes	Evidence Source
Thiothixene	Navane	Schizophrenia	5–60 mg/day	EPS, sedation, hyperprolactinemia	Used less often now	FDA labeling
Trifluoperazine	Stelazine	Schizophrenia	5–40 mg/day	EPS, prolactin elevation, sedation	Higher-potency FGA; less common contemporary use	FDA labeling

9. SECOND-GENERATION ORAL ANTIPSYCHOTICS — CLINICAL PROFILE AND PRACTICAL USE

Generic	Brand	Indications	Dose Range	Key Adverse Effects	Clinical Notes	Evidence Source
Risperidone	Risperdal	Schizophrenia, bipolar mania, autism irritability, OCD augmentation	1–6 mg/day	Hyperprolactinemia, EPS, weight gain	Common bridge before LAI transition	NICE (2022); APA (2020); FDA labeling
Paliperidone ER	Invega	Schizophrenia, schizoaffective disorder	3–12 mg/day	Similar to risperidone	Primarily renally cleared	FDA labeling
Olanzapine	Zyprexa	Schizophrenia, bipolar mania, IM agitation	5–20 mg/day	Weight gain, sedation, anticholinergic effects	High efficacy but major metabolic burden	NICE (2022); APA (2020); FDA labeling
Quetiapine	Seroquel	Schizophrenia, bipolar mania/depression, MDD adjunct	150–800 mg/day	Sedation, orthostasis, metabolic effects	Lower doses often more sedating	NICE (2022); FDA labeling
Ziprasidone	Geodon	Schizophrenia, bipolar mania	40–160 mg/day	QT prolongation, nausea, insomnia	Must be taken with food	NICE (2022); FDA labeling

Generic	Brand	Indications	Dose Range	Key Adverse Effects	Clinical Notes	Evidence Source
Aripiprazole	Abilify	Schizophrenia, bipolar disorder, MDD adjunct, autism irritability, Tourette's	10–30 mg/day	Akathisia, insomnia, nausea	Lower metabolic burden; partial D2 agonist	NICE (2022); FDA labeling
Lurasidone	Latuda	Schizophrenia, bipolar depression	20–160 mg/day	Akathisia, nausea	Take with food; avoid strong CYP3A4 modifiers	NICE (2022); FDA labeling
Cariprazine	Vraylar	Schizophrenia, bipolar mania/depression, MDD adjunct	1.5–6 mg/day	Akathisia, insomnia	Very long effective half-life	FDA labeling
Asenapine SL	Saphris	Schizophrenia, bipolar mania	10–20 mg/day	Sedation, oral hypoesthesia	Requires sublingual administration	FDA labeling
Asenapine TD	Secuado	Schizophrenia	Per patch strength	Application-site reactions, sedation, EPS	Rotate patch sites	FDA labeling
Iloperidone	Fanapt	Schizophrenia	6–24 mg/day	Orthostasis, sedation, QT risk	Slow titration required	FDA labeling
Milsaperidone	Bysanti	Schizophrenia; bipolar I (manic/mixed)	Schizophrenia 6–12 mg BID (7-day titration); bipolar I 12 mg BID (5-day titration)	Orthostasis, sedation, tachycardia, weight gain, QT risk	Active metabolite of iloperidone; titrate to reduce orthostasis; reduce dose in CYP2D6 poor metabolizers or with strong CYP2D6/3A4 inhibitors	FDA labeling (2026)

Generic	Brand	Indications	Dose Range	Key Adverse Effects	Clinical Notes	Evidence Source
Clozapine	Clozaril	Treatment-resistant schizophrenia, suicidality reduction	200–900 mg/day	Agranulocytosis, seizures, constipation, myocarditis	ANC monitoring recommended per FDA prescribing information; REMS eliminated June 13, 2025	NICE (2022); APA (2020); FDA labeling
Lumateperone	Caplyta	Schizophrenia, bipolar depression, MDD adjunctive (2025)	42 mg/day	Sedation, nausea, GI effects	Standard dose 42 mg once daily; no routine titration required; reduced doses (e.g., 21 mg) are used only for applicable hepatic impairment or drug-interaction circumstances per prescribing information; relatively lower metabolic burden	FDA labeling
Xanomeline/ trospium	Cobenfy	Schizophrenia	Per label	GI and cholinergic adverse effects	Novel non-D2 mechanism	FDA labeling

10. FIRST-GENERATION LAIs — CLINICAL PROFILE AND PRACTICAL USE

Generic	Brand	Dose / Frequency	Initiation	Advantages	Risks / Limitations	Clinical Notes	Evidence Source
Haloperidol decanoate	Haldol Decanoate	50–200 mg every 4 weeks	Oral conversion required	Low metabolic burden; long clinical experience	EPS, dysphoria, QT risk	Oral overlap often used initially; individualize conversion	FDA labeling; Clinical consensus

Generic	Brand	Dose / Frequency	Initiation	Advantages	Risks / Limitations	Clinical Notes	Evidence Source
Fluphenazine decanoate	Generic	12.5–25 mg every 3–4 weeks	Oral-to-LAI conversion individualized	Low cost; supports adherence	High EPS burden, dysphoria	Brand discontinued in U.S.; generic available	FDA labeling; Clinical consensus

11. SECOND-GENERATION LAIs — CLINICAL PROFILE AND PRACTICAL USE

Generic	Brand	Dose / Frequency	Initiation	Advantages	Risks / Limitations	Clinical Notes	Evidence Source
Risperidone IM	Risperdal Consta	Every 2 weeks	Oral overlap required	Established efficacy	Prolactin elevation, EPS, logistics	Slower-release IM option	FDA labeling
Risperidone SC	Uzedy	Monthly or q2 months	Oral tolerance first	No reconstitution	Injection-site effects, prolactin/EPS	Practical SC option; also FDA-approved for maintenance of bipolar I disorder (monotherapy or adjunct to lithium/valproate) — use the once-monthly regimen (q2-month not recommended for bipolar I)	FDA labeling
Paliperidone palmitate monthly	Invega Sustenna	Monthly	Loading strategy; no routine overlap	Simplified initiation	Injection burden, prolactin, cost	Base for longer-interval products	FDA labeling

Generic	Brand	Dose / Frequency	Initiation	Advantages	Risks / Limitations	Clinical Notes	Evidence Source
Paliperidone palmitate q3 months	Invega Trinza	Every 3 months	Stabilize on Sustenna first	Fewer visits	Reduced flexibility with adverse effects	Maintenance-only after stabilization	FDA labeling
Paliperidone palmitate q6 months	Invega Hafyera	Every 6 months	Prior stabilization required	Very long interval	Limited dose-adjustment flexibility	Use only after stable response	FDA labeling
Aripiprazole monohydrate	Abilify Maintena	Monthly	Oral overlap or bridge	Lower metabolic burden	Akathisia, initiation complexity	Also used in bipolar maintenance	FDA labeling
Aripiprazole 2-month	Abilify Asimtufii	960 mg IM every 2 months; 720 mg reduced dose	Oral initiation regimen or switch from Maintena per PI	Fewer visits	Akathisia, logistical issues	Can replace next scheduled Maintena dose after stabilization; use labeled initiation regimen if starting from oral therapy.	FDA labeling
Aripiprazole lauroxil	Aristada	Every 4–8 weeks	Initio or oral overlap	Flexible intervals	Complex initiation	Prodrug LAI formulation	FDA labeling

Generic	Brand	Dose / Frequency	Initiation	Advantages	Risks / Limitations	Clinical Notes	Evidence Source
Olanzapine pamoate	Zyprexa Relprevv	Every 2–4 weeks	Oral tolerability first	High efficacy	PDSS, metabolic effects, sedation	Post-injection delirium/sedation syndrome (PDSS) risk: mandatory 3-hour monitored observation after each injection, administered only through the restricted/registered facility program (Zyprexa Relprevv Patient Care Program)	FDA labeling

12. FIRST-GENERATION ANTIPSYCHOTICS IN EMERGENCY SETTINGS

Generic	Brand	Dose Range	Onset	Advantages	Risks / Limitations	Clinical Notes	Evidence Source
Haloperidol	Haldol	2.5–10 mg IM/PO	Moderate	Extensive experience, low cost	EPS, QT risk	Often combined with lorazepam; IV QT risk > IM	FDA labeling; ACEP (2024); Project BETA (2012)

Generic	Brand	Dose Range	Onset	Advantages	Risks / Limitations	Clinical Notes	Evidence Source
Chlorpromazine	Thorazine	25–50 mg IM typical	Moderate	Strong sedation	Orthostasis, anticholinergic burden, QT risk	Less favored due to hypotension and adverse-effect burden	FDA labeling

13. SECOND-GENERATION ANTIPSYCHOTICS IN EMERGENCY SETTINGS

Generic	Brand	Dose Range	Onset	Advantages	Risks / Limitations	Clinical Notes	Evidence Source
Olanzapine IM	Zyprexa IM	5–10 mg	Rapid	Effective monotherapy, lower EPS than FGAs	Sedation, hypotension	Avoid close IM benzodiazepine coadministration — concurrent IM olanzapine plus parenteral benzodiazepine is not recommended (risk of excessive sedation, cardiorespiratory depression, and hypotension); if sequential parenteral use is unavoidable, monitor closely	FDA labeling; Project BETA (2012)
Ziprasidone IM	Geodon IM	10–20 mg	Rapid	Lower EPS and metabolic burden	QT risk	Useful when metabolic burden is a concern	FDA labeling; Project BETA (2012)

Generic	Brand	Dose Range	Onset	Advantages	Risks / Limitations	Clinical Notes	Evidence Source
Aripiprazole IM	Abilify IM	5.25–15 mg	Slightly slower	Lower QT and metabolic burden	Less sedating	Useful when oversedation is undesirable	FDA labeling

14. ANXIOLYTICS AND HYPNOTICS — CLINICAL PROFILE AND PRACTICAL USE

Generic	Brand	Indications	Dose Range	Key Adverse Effects	Clinical Notes	Evidence Source
Buspirone	Buspar	GAD, anxiety adjunct	15–60 mg/day	Dizziness, nausea	Non-sedating; delayed onset; no abuse potential	NICE (2022); FDA labeling
Hydroxyzine	Vistaril	Short-term anxiety, sedation	25–100 mg PRN	Sedation, anticholinergic effects	Avoid routine use in older adults	FDA labeling; AGS Beers Criteria (2023)
Diazepam	Valium	Anxiety, alcohol withdrawal, seizures	2–10 mg BID–QID	Sedation, dependence, respiratory depression	Long half-life; boxed warnings apply	FDA labeling
Chlordiazepoxide	Librium	Anxiety, alcohol withdrawal	15–100 mg/day	Sedation, dependence, ataxia	Commonly used in alcohol withdrawal	FDA labeling
Clonazepam	Klonopin	Panic disorder, anxiety, seizures	0.5–2 mg/day	Sedation, dependence, withdrawal	Prefer short-term use when possible	FDA labeling
Lorazepam	Ativan	Panic, acute agitation, anxiety	0.5–4 mg/day	Sedation, dependence, withdrawal	Preferred in hepatic impairment	FDA labeling
Temazepam	Restoril	Insomnia	7.5–30 mg HS	Sedation, dependence	Avoid in older adults when possible	FDA labeling; AGS Beers Criteria (2023)
Estazolam	ProSom	Insomnia	1–2 mg HS	Sedation, dependence	Short-term use only	FDA labeling

Generic	Brand	Indications	Dose Range	Key Adverse Effects	Clinical Notes	Evidence Source
Zolpidem	Ambien	Insomnia	5–10 mg HS	Complex sleep behaviors, sedation	Boxed warning for sleep behaviors	FDA labeling
Eszopiclone	Lunesta	Insomnia	1–3 mg HS	Bitter taste, sedation	Intermediate half-life	FDA labeling
Zaleplon	Sonata	Sleep-onset insomnia	5–20 mg HS	Sedation, complex sleep behaviors	Very short half-life; useful for sleep onset	FDA labeling
Ramelteon	Rozerem	Sleep-onset insomnia	8 mg HS	Minimal adverse effects	Not controlled; no abuse potential	AASM (2017); FDA labeling
Propranolol	Inderal	Performance anxiety, akathisia, tremor	10–40 mg PRN or divided	Bradycardia, hypotension, bronchospasm	Avoid in asthma or heart block	FDA labeling
Atenolol	Tenormin	Performance anxiety off-label	25–50 mg PRN	Bradycardia, hypotension	More beta-1 selective than propranolol	FDA labeling
Suvorexant	Belsomra	Insomnia	10–20 mg HS	Next-day sedation, complex sleep behaviors	Avoid in narcolepsy; lower dose in older adults	AASM (2017); FDA labeling
Lemborexant	Dayvigo	Insomnia	5–10 mg HS	Next-day sedation, driving impairment	Start at 5 mg; avoid in narcolepsy	AASM (2017); FDA labeling
Daridorexant	Quviviq	Insomnia	25–50 mg HS	Next-day sedation, CNS depression	DORA; 50 mg preferred for greater efficacy; Schedule IV; avoid in narcolepsy	FDA labeling (2022)

Benzodiazepine class boxed warning: All benzodiazepines listed above (diazepam, chlordiazepoxide, clonazepam, lorazepam, temazepam, estazolam) carry FDA boxed warnings. Concomitant use with opioids may cause profound sedation, respiratory depression, coma, and death. Benzodiazepines also carry boxed warnings for the risks of abuse, misuse, addiction, physical dependence, and withdrawal reactions.

15. NEURODEVELOPMENTAL DISORDER MEDICATIONS

Generic	Brand	Indications	Dose Range	Key Adverse Effects	Clinical Notes	Evidence Source
Methylphenidate IR	Ritalin	ADHD	10–60 mg/day	Insomnia, appetite suppression, headache	Short duration; multiple daily doses often needed	NICE (2018); FDA labeling
Methylphenidate ER	Concerta	ADHD	18–72 mg/day	Similar to IR	Longer duration; do not crush or chew	NICE (2018); FDA labeling
Dexmethylphenidate	Focalin	ADHD	5–40 mg/day	Insomnia, appetite suppression	d-isomer formulation; IR and XR available	FDA labeling
Mixed amphetamine salts	Adderall	ADHD	5–40 mg/day	Insomnia, appetite suppression, cardiovascular effects	Higher misuse potential than lisdexamfetamine	NICE (2018); FDA labeling
Lisdexamfetamine	Vyvanse	ADHD, binge eating disorder	30–70 mg/day	Appetite suppression, insomnia, cardiovascular effects	Prodrug design may reduce misuse attractiveness	FDA labeling
Dextroamphetamine	Dexedrine	ADHD	5–40 mg/day	Similar to other amphetamines	IR and ER formulations available	FDA labeling
Atomoxetine	Strattera	ADHD	40–100 mg/day	GI effects, sedation, mood changes	Non-stimulant; slower onset; suicidality warning in youth	NICE (2018); FDA labeling

Generic	Brand	Indications	Dose Range	Key Adverse Effects	Clinical Notes	Evidence Source
Viloxazine XR	Qelbree	ADHD	200–600 mg/day	Somnolence, decreased appetite, nausea, irritability	First novel non-stimulant approved for adults in 20 years; once-daily; no abuse potential; avoid with MAOIs; boxed warning for suicidal thoughts and behaviors	FDA labeling (2022)
Guanfacine XR	Intuniv	ADHD, tics	1–7 mg/day	Sedation, hypotension, dry mouth	Useful with tics or sleep problems	FDA labeling
Clonidine XR	Kapvay	ADHD	0.1–0.4 mg/day	Sedation, hypotension	Helpful with hyperarousal or sleep disturbance	FDA labeling
Bupropion XL	Wellbutrin XL	ADHD off-label, depression	150–450 mg/day	Insomnia, seizure risk	Consider with comorbid depression; not first-line ADHD monotherapy	Clinical consensus

Generic	Brand	Indications	Dose Range	Key Adverse Effects	Clinical Notes	Evidence Source
Modafinil	Provigil	Narcolepsy; ADHD off-label	100–200 mg/day	Headache, insomnia, rare rash	Limited ADHD role; interaction burden matters. Serious rash, including Stevens-Johnson syndrome/toxic epidermal necrolysis (SJS/TEN), reported; discontinue at first sign of rash. Reduces effectiveness of hormonal contraceptives; use additional or alternative non-hormonal contraception during treatment and for one month after discontinuation	FDA labeling

16. OCD AND RELATED DISORDER MEDICATIONS — CLINICAL PROFILE AND PRACTICAL USE

Generic	Class	Brand	Indications	Dose Range	Key Adverse Effects	Clinical Notes	Evidence Source
Fluoxetine	SSRI	Prozac	OCD, BDD	20–80 mg/day	Typical SSRI adverse effects	Higher doses often needed in OCD-spectrum disorders	Fineberg et al. (2020)

Generic	Class	Brand	Indications	Dose Range	Key Adverse Effects	Clinical Notes	Evidence Source
Fluvoxamine	SSRI	Luvox	OCD	100–300 mg/day	Sedation, interactions	BID dosing may help at higher doses	Fineberg et al. (2020)
Paroxetine	SSRI	Paxil	OCD, BDD	20–60 mg/day	Sexual dysfunction, withdrawal, sedation	Higher withdrawal burden than some SSRIs	Fineberg et al. (2020)
Sertraline	SSRI	Zoloft	OCD, BDD	50–200 mg/day	Typical SSRI adverse effects	Common first-line option	Fineberg et al. (2020)
Clomipramine	TCA	Anafranil	OCD	25–250 mg/day	Anticholinergic effects, sedation, cardiac risk	Effective but less tolerated than SSRIs	Fineberg et al. (2020)
Venlafaxine XR	SNRI	Effexor XR	OCD off-label	75–225 mg/day	Nausea, BP effects, withdrawal	Usually reserved for refractory cases	Fineberg et al. (2020); Clinical consensus
N-acetylcysteine	Glutamatergic adjunct	OTC	Trichotillomania, excoriation	1200–2400 mg/day	GI upset	Better evidence in BFRBs than classic OCD	Fineberg et al. (2020)
Quetiapine XR	SGA	Seroquel XR	OCD augmentation	50–300 mg/day	Sedation, metabolic effects	Use lowest effective dose	Fineberg et al. (2020)
Risperidone	SGA	Risperdal	OCD augmentation	0.5–4 mg/day	EPS, prolactin elevation, weight gain	Strong augmentation evidence	Fineberg et al. (2020)

Generic	Class	Brand	Indications	Dose Range	Key Adverse Effects	Clinical Notes	Evidence Source
Aripiprazole	SGA	Abilify	OCD augmentation	10–30 mg/day	Akathisia, insomnia	Lower metabolic burden; akathisia may limit use	Fineberg et al. (2020)
Olanzapine	SGA	Zyprexa	OCD augmentation	2.5–10 mg/day	Sedation, metabolic effects	Reserve for refractory cases	Fineberg et al. (2020)

17. NEUROCOGNITIVE AND PARKINSON'S DISEASE AGENTS

Generic	Class	Brand	Indications	Dose Range	Key Adverse Effects	Clinical Notes	Evidence Source
Donepezil	Acetylcholinesterase inhibitor	Aricept	Alzheimer's disease	5–23 mg/day	GI upset, bradycardia, insomnia	Titrate gradually; monitor bradycardia/syncope. The 23 mg/day dose is reserved for moderate-to-severe Alzheimer's disease and only after at least 3 months of stability on 10 mg/day	NICE (2018); FDA labeling
Rivastigmine patch	Acetylcholinesterase inhibitor	Exelon Patch	Alzheimer's disease, Parkinson's disease dementia	4.6–13.3 mg/24 h	Rash, GI effects	Useful in Parkinson's disease dementia	NICE (2018); FDA labeling

Generic	Class	Brand	Indications	Dose Range	Key Adverse Effects	Clinical Notes	Evidence Source
Galantamine ER	Acetylcholinesterase inhibitor	Razadyne ER	Alzheimer's disease	8–24 mg/day	GI effects, bradycardia	ER daily or IR BID options. Reduce the dose in moderate renal or hepatic impairment (maximum 16 mg/day) and avoid in severe impairment (CrCl <9 mL/min or Child-Pugh C)	NICE (2018); FDA labeling
Memantine	NMDA antagonist	Namenda	Moderate to severe Alzheimer's disease	5–20 mg/day	Dizziness, confusion, headache	Can combine with cholinesterase inhibitors	NICE (2018); FDA labeling
Brexpiprazole	Dopamine-serotonin modulator	Rexulti	Agitation associated with Alzheimer's dementia	0.5–3 mg/day	Weight gain, sedation, akathisia	Boxed warning applies; use cautiously	FDA labeling

Generic	Class	Brand	Indications	Dose Range	Key Adverse Effects	Clinical Notes	Evidence Source
Pimavanserin	5-HT2A inverse agonist	Nuplazid	Parkinson's disease psychosis	34 mg/day	QT prolongation, edema, nausea	Avoids dopamine blockade and motor worsening; boxed warning for increased mortality in elderly patients with dementia-related psychosis; not approved for dementia-related psychosis unrelated to Parkinson's disease psychosis	FDA labeling
Amantadine	Dopaminergic/NMDA modulator	Symmetrel, Gocovri, Osmolex	Parkinson's disease, dyskinesia	Agent-specific	Confusion, hallucinations, livedo reticularis	May worsen psychosis; adjust for renal function	FDA labeling

18. SUBSTANCE USE DISORDER MEDICATIONS — CLINICAL PROFILE AND PRACTICAL USE

Generic	Class	Brand	Indications	Dose Range	Key Adverse Effects	Clinical Notes	Evidence Source
Naltrexone oral	Opioid antagonist	Revia	AUD	50 mg/day	GI upset, headache, hepatic caution	Avoid with active opioid use; review LFTs	NICE (2022); FDA labeling
Naltrexone XR IM	Opioid antagonist LAI	Vivitrol	AUD, OUD	380 mg IM every 4 weeks	Injection-site reaction, nausea, hepatic caution	Requires opioid-free interval	SAMHSA TIP 63 (2021); FDA labeling
Acamprosate	Glutamatergic modulator	Campral	AUD	666 mg TID	Diarrhea, headache	Renal dosing matters; useful after abstinence	NICE (2022); FDA labeling
Disulfiram	Aversive agent	Antabuse	AUD	125–500 mg/day	Hepatotoxicity, neuropathy, metallic taste	Best with supervised abstinence	NICE (2022); FDA labeling
Topiramate	Anticonvulsant off-label	Topamax	AUD off-label	25–300 mg/day	Cognitive slowing, paresthesias, weight loss	Off-label option; titrate slowly	Clinical consensus
Gabapentin	GABA analog off-label	Neurontin	AUD off-label, withdrawal adjunct	300–1800 mg/day	Sedation, dizziness, edema	Consider misuse risk in vulnerable patients	Clinical consensus

Generic	Class	Brand	Indications	Dose Range	Key Adverse Effects	Clinical Notes	Evidence Source
Buprenorphine/naloxone SL	Partial agonist + antagonist	Suboxone	OUD	8–24 mg/day typical	Precipitated withdrawal, constipation, sedation	Start during withdrawal; first-line MOUD	SAMHSA TIP 63 (2021); FDA labeling
Buprenorphine ER IM	Partial agonist LAI	Sublocade	OUD	Per label	Injection-site reaction, sedation, constipation	Usually after SL stabilization	SAMHSA TIP 63 (2021); FDA labeling
Methadone	Full opioid agonist	—	OUD in OTP setting	Individualized	QT prolongation, sedation, respiratory depression	OTP only; ECG caution in selected patients. Boxed warnings: QT prolongation/torsades de pointes, life-threatening respiratory depression, and addiction, abuse, and misuse	SAMHSA TIP 63 (2021); FDA labeling
Naloxone nasal spray	Opioid antagonist rescue	Narcan	Opioid overdose reversal	4 mg/spray	Acute withdrawal symptoms	Standard rescue treatment in OUD risk	SAMHSA TIP 63 (2021); FDA labeling

Generic	Class	Brand	Indications	Dose Range	Key Adverse Effects	Clinical Notes	Evidence Source
Hydroxyzine	Antihistamine adjunct	Vistaril	Anxiety symptom adjunct	25–100 mg PRN	Sedation, anticholinergic burden	Not a primary SUD treatment	FDA labeling
Propranolol	Beta-blocker adjunct	Inderal	Autonomic symptom adjunct	10–40 mg BID–TID	Bradycardia, hypotension	Not a primary SUD treatment	FDA labeling
N-acetylcysteine	Adjunctive supplement	OTC	Cannabis-related adjunctive use off-label	1200–2400 mg/day	GI upset	Limited and adjunctive evidence	Clinical consensus

19. CLASS ABBREVIATIONS LEGEND

Abbreviation	Full Name	Evidence Source
SSRI	Selective serotonin reuptake inhibitor	Clinical consensus
SNRI	Serotonin-norepinephrine reuptake inhibitor	Clinical consensus
NDRI	Norepinephrine-dopamine reuptake inhibitor	Clinical consensus
NaSSA	Noradrenergic and specific serotonergic antidepressant	Clinical consensus
SARI	Serotonin antagonist and reuptake inhibitor	Clinical consensus
TCA	Tricyclic antidepressant	Clinical consensus
MAOI	Monoamine oxidase inhibitor	Clinical consensus
FGA	First-generation antipsychotic	Clinical consensus
SGA	Second-generation antipsychotic	Clinical consensus
BZD	Benzodiazepine	Clinical consensus

REFERENCES

American Academy of Sleep Medicine. (2017). Clinical practice guideline for the pharmacologic treatment of chronic insomnia in adults: An American Academy of Sleep Medicine clinical practice guideline. Journal of Clinical Sleep Medicine, 13(2), 307–349. https://doi.org/10.5664/jcsm.6470

American College of Emergency Physicians. (2024). Clinical policy: Critical issues in the evaluation and management of adult out-of-hospital or emergency department patients presenting with severe agitation. Annals of Emergency Medicine, 83(1), e1–e30.

https://doi.org/10.1016/j.annemergmed.2023.09.010
American College of Obstetricians and Gynecologists. (2023). Treatment and management of mental health conditions during pregnancy and postpartum: ACOG clinical practice guideline No. 5. Obstetrics & Gynecology, 141(6), 1262–1288. https://doi.org/10.1097/AOG.0000000000005202
American Geriatrics Society Beers Criteria® Update Expert Panel. (2023). American Geriatrics Society 2023 updated AGS Beers Criteria® for potentially inappropriate medication use in older adults. Journal of the American Geriatrics Society, 71(7), 2052–2081. https://doi.org/10.1111/jgs.18372
American Psychiatric Association. (2020). The American Psychiatric Association practice guideline for the treatment of patients with schizophrenia (3rd ed.). American Psychiatric Association Publishing
Yatham, L. N., Kennedy, S. H., Parikh, S. V., et al. (2018). Canadian Network for Mood and Anxiety Treatments (CANMAT) and International Society for Bipolar Disorders (ISBD) 2018 guidelines for the management of patients with bipolar disorder. Bipolar Disorders, 20(2), 97–170. https://doi.org/10.1111/bdi.12609
Fineberg, N. A., Hollander, E., Pallanti, S., Walitza, S., Grünblatt, E., Dell'Osso, B., & Stein, D. J. (2020). Clinical advances in obsessive-compulsive disorder: A position statement by the International College of Obsessive-Compulsive Spectrum Disorders. International Clinical Psychopharmacology, 35(4), 173–193. https://doi.org/10.1097/YIC.0000000000000314
National Institute for Health and Care Excellence. (2018). Attention deficit hyperactivity disorder: Diagnosis and management. NICE
National Institute for Health and Care Excellence. (2018). Dementia: Assessment, management and support for people living with dementia and their carers. NICE
National Institute for Health and Care Excellence. (2022). Alcohol-use disorders: Diagnosis, assessment and management of harmful drinking and alcohol dependence. NICE
National Institute for Health and Care Excellence. (2022). Depression in adults: Treatment and management. NICE
National Institute for Health and Care Excellence. (2022). Psychosis and schizophrenia in adults: Prevention and management. NICE
Substance Abuse and Mental Health Services Administration. (2021). TIP 63: Medications for opioid use disorder. SAMHSA
U.S. Food and Drug Administration. (2002, updated 2023). Abilify (aripiprazole) prescribing information. https://www.accessdata.fda.gov/drugsatfda_docs/label/2023/021436s046lbl.pdf
U.S. Food and Drug Administration. (2003, updated 2021). Clozaril (clozapine) prescribing information. https://www.accessdata.fda.gov/drugsatfda_docs/label/2021/019758s092lbl.pdf
U.S. Food and Drug Administration. (2004, updated 2023). Cymbalta (duloxetine) prescribing information. https://www.accessdata.fda.gov/drugsatfda_docs/label/2023/021427s060lbl.pdf

U.S. Food and Drug Administration. (1983, updated 2022). Depakote (divalproex sodium) prescribing information. https://www.accessdata.fda.gov/drugsatfda_docs/label/2022/018723s060lbl.pdf
U.S. Food and Drug Administration. (2023). Exxua (gepirone hydrochloride extended-release tablets) prescribing information.
U.S. Food and Drug Administration. (1994, updated 2023). Lamictal (lamotrigine) prescribing information. https://www.accessdata.fda.gov/drugsatfda_docs/label/2023/020241s055lbl.pdf
U.S. Food and Drug Administration. (2010, updated 2023). Latuda (lurasidone hydrochloride) prescribing information. https://www.accessdata.fda.gov/drugsatfda_docs/label/2023/200603s036lbl.pdf
U.S. Food and Drug Administration. (1970, updated 2023). Lithobid (lithium carbonate) prescribing information. https://www.accessdata.fda.gov/drugsatfda_docs/label/2023/018557s110lbl.pdf
U.S. Food and Drug Administration. (2022). Qelbree (viloxazine extended-release) prescribing information. Supernus Pharmaceuticals. https://www.accessdata.fda.gov
U.S. Food and Drug Administration. (2022). Quviviq (daridorexant) prescribing information. Idorsia Pharmaceuticals. https://www.accessdata.fda.gov
U.S. Food and Drug Administration. (1993, updated 2023). Risperdal (risperidone) prescribing information. https://www.accessdata.fda.gov/drugsatfda_docs/label/2023/020272s090lbl.pdf
U.S. Food and Drug Administration. (2017, updated 2023). Sublocade (buprenorphine extended-release) prescribing information. https://www.accessdata.fda.gov/drugsatfda_docs/label/2023/209819s012lbl.pdf
U.S. Food and Drug Administration. (2025). Uzedy (risperidone extended-release injectable suspension for subcutaneous use) prescribing information.
U.S. Food and Drug Administration. (2010, updated 2023). Vivitrol (naltrexone for extended-release injectable suspension) prescribing information. https://www.accessdata.fda.gov/drugsatfda_docs/label/2023/021897s049lbl.pdf
U.S. Food and Drug Administration. (2008, updated 2023). Vyvanse (lisdexamfetamine dimesylate) prescribing information. https://www.accessdata.fda.gov/drugsatfda_docs/label/2023/021977s059lbl.pdf
U.S. Food and Drug Administration. (2003, updated 2023). Wellbutrin XL (bupropion hydrochloride extended-release) prescribing information. https://www.accessdata.fda.gov/drugsatfda_docs/label/2023/021515s037lbl.pdf
U.S. Food and Drug Administration. (1991, updated 2023). Zoloft (sertraline hydrochloride) prescribing information. https://www.accessdata.fda.gov/drugsatfda_docs/label/2023/019839s104lbl.pdf
Wilson, M. P., Pepper, D., Currier, G. W., Holloman, G. H., Jr., & Feifel, D. (2012). The psychopharmacology of agitation: Consensus statement of the American Association for Emergency Psychiatry Project BETA Psychopharmacology Workgroup. Western Journal of Emergency Medicine, 13(1), 26–34. https://doi.org/10.5811/westjem.2011.9.6866

XVII: CLINICAL PSYCHIATRIC EMERGENCIES

SECTION INTRODUCTION

Psychiatric emergencies represent acute disturbances in behavior, cognition, mood, perception, or physiologic stability that require immediate clinical assessment and timely intervention to reduce risk of harm to the patient or others. These situations may involve suicidality, severe agitation, psychosis, intoxication, withdrawal syndromes, medication toxicity, violent behavior, delirium, catatonia, serotonin syndrome, neuroleptic malignant syndrome, overdose, or rapidly deteriorating psychiatric and medical conditions. Early recognition and structured emergency management are essential to reduce morbidity, mortality, hospitalization complications, and long-term functional deterioration.

This section provides structured rapid-recognition and management protocols for psychiatric, behavioral, toxicologic, and psychopharmacologic emergencies encountered in outpatient and acute-care psychiatric practice. When a potentially life-threatening condition is suspected, clinicians should initiate appropriate stabilization measures immediately and activate emergency medical services (EMS) or higher levels of medical care without delay when clinically indicated.

Recommendations are aligned with major evidence-based clinical guidelines, emergency psychiatry frameworks, toxicology recommendations, and expert consensus sources, including the American Psychiatric Association (APA) Practice Guidelines, Project BETA (Best Practices in Evaluation and Treatment of Agitation), the American College of Emergency Physicians (ACEP), the American College of Medical Toxicology (ACMT), the EXTRIP Workgroup (Extracorporeal Treatments in Poisoning), and the American Society of Addiction Medicine (ASAM).

Medication doses included in this section represent typical adult emergency dosing ranges and should be individualized based on patient age, medical comorbidity, organ function, concurrent medications, intoxication status, physiologic stability, and institutional protocols. Clinical judgment and emergency medical evaluation remain essential in all high-risk situations.

Psychiatric emergencies are frequently encountered across outpatient clinics, emergency departments, inpatient psychiatric settings, urgent care environments, and telepsychiatry encounters. Patients may present with acute emotional distress, behavioral dysregulation, altered mental status, severe impulsivity, autonomic instability, confusion, aggression, or impaired reality testing. Because psychiatric symptoms may reflect underlying medical or neurologic pathology, clinicians must maintain a broad differential diagnosis and remain vigilant for potentially life-threatening medical contributors to psychiatric presentation.

Suicide-related emergencies remain among the most critical situations within psychiatric practice. Suicidal ideation, recent suicide attempts, severe hopelessness, psychosis, intoxication, impulsivity, mixed mood states, and access to lethal means substantially increase acute safety risk and may require urgent escalation of care. Comprehensive suicide risk assessment, safety planning, means-restriction counseling, collateral information gathering, and determination of the least restrictive safe level of care are fundamental components of emergency psychiatric evaluation.

Agitation and behavioral dysregulation represent additional high-risk clinical scenarios that may rapidly escalate into violence, self-injury, medical compromise, or emergency restraint situations. Agitation may result from psychosis, mania, delirium, intoxication, withdrawal, personality pathology, trauma-related disorders, neurologic illness, or severe anxiety. Initial management should prioritize verbal de-escalation, environmental safety, reduction of external stimuli, and trauma-informed communication whenever possible before progressing to pharmacologic or restrictive interventions.

Substance intoxication and withdrawal syndromes are major contributors to psychiatric emergencies and may produce severe autonomic instability, psychosis, seizures, delirium, aggression, respiratory compromise, or cardiovascular complications. Alcohol withdrawal, benzodiazepine withdrawal, opioid overdose, stimulant intoxication, serotonin toxicity, and polysubstance ingestion require rapid recognition and evidence-based stabilization because delays in treatment may lead to significant morbidity or death.

Psychotropic medication-related emergencies also require immediate clinical attention. Neuroleptic malignant syndrome (NMS), serotonin syndrome, lithium toxicity, clozapine complications, severe extrapyramidal symptoms, hypertensive crisis associated with monoamine oxidase inhibitors (MAOIs), and medication overdose may progress rapidly and require emergency medical management, intensive monitoring, or hospitalization. Clinicians should therefore remain familiar with early warning signs, diagnostic criteria, and acute treatment protocols for major psychopharmacologic emergencies.

Patients experiencing psychiatric emergencies frequently require coordination across multiple systems of care, including emergency medicine, inpatient psychiatry, toxicology, neurology, primary care, law enforcement, crisis intervention teams, social work, and family or caregiver support systems. Legal and ethical considerations—including involuntary evaluation, emergency detention statutes, decisional capacity, duty to protect, and emergency consent issues—may also become relevant during crisis management depending on jurisdiction and clinical severity.

Effective management of psychiatric emergencies requires rapid assessment, structured clinical reasoning, patient and staff safety prioritization, interdisciplinary collaboration, and careful documentation. Although stabilization of acute symptoms is essential, clinicians should also evaluate underlying psychiatric illness, substance use, psychosocial stressors, medication adherence, medical contributors, and longitudinal relapse risk in order to support continuity of care following emergency intervention.

The following sections provide a structured, evidence-informed framework for the recognition, assessment, stabilization, and management of psychiatric emergencies within outpatient and acute-care psychiatric practice. Recommendations are intended to support safe, clinically individualized, and timely emergency intervention while recognizing the importance of medical evaluation, trauma-informed care, interdisciplinary coordination, and professional clinical judgment during high-risk clinical situations.

1. ACUTE AGITATION / VIOLENT BEHAVIOR

Acute agitation is a behavioral emergency that may escalate to violence or medical instability. Management should prioritize safety, rapid evaluation, and controlled behavioral calming while avoiding excessive sedation.

Recognition

Common signs include:

- Severe psychomotor agitation
- Threatening or violent behavior
- Inability to follow instructions
- Verbal aggression or escalating hostility
- Severe anxiety, paranoia, or disorganized thinking

Patients may pose an immediate risk to themselves or others.

A. Common Causes

Category	Examples	Clinical Notes	Evidence Source
Psychiatric	Acute psychosis, bipolar mania, severe anxiety	Most common in psychiatric settings; always assess risk of violence	Project BETA (2012); ACEP (2024)
Substance-Related	Stimulant intoxication, alcohol intoxication, withdrawal states	Always rule out intoxication vs withdrawal before sedation	ACEP (2024)
Medical	Delirium, hypoglycemia, hypoxia, infection	Must rule out BEFORE labeling as psychiatric	ACMT (2023); ACEP (2024)

Always evaluate for medical causes of agitation before assuming a psychiatric etiology.

B. Stepwise Management Algorithm (Project BETA)

Step	Intervention	Key Actions	Clinical Notes	Evidence Source
1	Ensure Safety	Remove hazards, call assistance	Safety > diagnosis	Project BETA (2012)
2	Verbal De-escalation	Calm tone, reduce stimuli	First-line ALWAYS	Project BETA (2012)
3	Oral Medication	Preferred if cooperative	Avoid IM if possible	ACEP (2024)
4	IM Medication	If refusal or danger	Use lowest effective dose	ACEP (2024)
5	Monitoring	Reassess every 15–30 min	Watch airway, sedation	ACEP (2024)

C. Oral Medication Options

Medication	Typical Dose	Notes	Clinical Notes	Evidence Source
Olanzapine ODT	5–10 mg PO	Rapid dissolve	Preferred oral agent	Project BETA (2012)
Risperidone	1–2 mg PO	May combine with lorazepam	Good balance efficacy/tolerability	NICE CG178 (2014)
Lorazepam	1–2 mg PO	Useful in stimulant intoxication	Avoid if respiratory risk	ACEP (2024)

Reassess within 20–30 minutes.

D. Intramuscular Medications / First-Generation Antipsychotics

Drug	Dose	Onset	Key Considerations	Clinical Notes	Evidence Source
Haloperidol	2.5–10 mg IM	20–30 min	EPS, QT prolongation	Gold standard; combine with benzo if needed	FDA (2024); Project BETA (2012)
Chlorpromazine	25–50 mg IM	15–30 min	Hypotension, sedation	Less used due to side effects	FDA labeling; ACEP (2024)

E. Intramuscular Medications / Second-Generation Antipsychotics

Drug	Dose	Onset	Key Considerations	Clinical Notes	Evidence Source
Olanzapine IM	5–10 mg	15–30 min	Avoid benzo within 1 hr — combined IM olanzapine and parenteral benzodiazepines carry an FDA-labeled risk of severe cardiorespiratory depression, hypotension, and death; if a benzodiazepine is required, separate administration and monitor closely	First-line IM option	FDA (2023); Project BETA (2012)
Ziprasidone IM	10–20 mg	15–30 min	QT risk	Good metabolic profile	FDA (2023); Project BETA (2012)

Drug	Dose	Onset	Key Considerations	Clinical Notes	Evidence Source
Aripiprazole IM	5.25–15 mg	45–60 min	Slower onset	Use if sedation not desired	FDA (2024)

F. Emergency Medication Combinations

Combination	Dose	Clinical Use	Clinical Notes	Evidence Source
Haloperidol + Lorazepam	5 mg + 2 mg IM	Synergistic sedation; monitor for respiratory depression and ensure monitoring capacity before outpatient use	Reduces EPS risk	Project BETA (2012)
B52 Regimen	Haldol 5 + Lorazepam 2 + Diphenhydramine 50	Severe agitation	High sedation burden	ACEP (2024)

G. Rapid IM Sedation Comparison

Agent	Dose	Onset	Major Risk	Clinical Notes	Evidence Source
Haloperidol	2.5–10 mg	20–30 min	EPS	Widely used	FDA (2024)
Olanzapine	5–10 mg	15–30 min	Avoid benzo	Best balance	FDA (2023)
Ziprasidone	10–20 mg	15–30 min	QT	Lower metabolic risk	FDA (2023)
Aripiprazole	5.25–15 mg	45–60 min	Slow onset	Less sedating	FDA (2024)

H. Monitoring After Sedation

Parameter	Frequency	Clinical Notes	Evidence Source
Vital signs	Every 15 min initially	Monitor airway	ACEP (2024)
Respiratory status	Continuous if high risk	Especially with benzos	ACEP (2024)

Parameter	Frequency	Clinical Notes	Evidence Source
QT interval	If risk factors present	Obtain a baseline ECG for parenteral or high-dose haloperidol and when QT risk factors are present. Parenteral rapid tranquilization (including the B52 regimen) requires a setting with continuous pulse oximetry, airway and resuscitation capability, and a defined disposition plan; it should not be administered in an unequipped outpatient office	FDA (2024)

Goal of Treatment

Achieve rapid calming without excessive sedation, allowing safe psychiatric and medical evaluation.

2. DELIRIUM

A. OVERVIEW

Aspect	Clinical Notes	Evidence Source
Definition	Acute disturbance in attention, awareness, and cognition with fluctuating course	DSM-5-TR (APA, 2022)
Core features	Inattention, disorientation, fluctuating mental status, altered consciousness, sleep-wake disturbance	DSM-5-TR (APA, 2022)
Clinical importance	Medical emergency associated with increased morbidity and mortality	Inouye et al. (2014); DSM-5-TR (APA, 2022)
Common settings	Hospitalization, infection, polypharmacy, withdrawal states, medically frail older adults	Inouye et al. (2014); Clinical consensus

Aspect	Clinical Notes	Evidence Source
Outpatient relevance	Early delirium may first appear during psychiatric follow-up or medication evaluations	Clinical consensus

B. Diagnostic Considerations

Clinical Consideration	Clinical Notes	Evidence Source
Acute onset	Symptoms typically develop over hours to days	DSM-5-TR (APA, 2022)
Fluctuating course	Mental status often varies throughout the day	DSM-5-TR (APA, 2022)
Inattention	Impaired attention is a core diagnostic feature	DSM-5-TR (APA, 2022)
Altered consciousness	Reduced alertness or excessive somnolence may occur	Clinical consensus
Visual hallucinations	Visual perceptual disturbances are common, especially in severe cases	Clinical consensus
Sleep-wake disruption	Day-night reversal and fragmented sleep are common	Clinical consensus
Medical etiology search	Always evaluate for underlying medical, neurologic, infectious, metabolic, or substance-related causes	Inouye et al. (2014); Clinical consensus
DSM-5-TR diagnostic threshold	Acute, fluctuating disturbance of attention and awareness with an additional cognitive change, judged to be a direct physiological consequence of a medical condition, substance intoxication or withdrawal, or a medication.	DSM-5-TR (APA, 2022)

C. Differential Diagnosis

Condition	Distinguishing Features	Evidence Source
Dementia	Chronic progressive decline rather than acute fluctuating change	DSM-5-TR (APA, 2022)
Psychotic disorder	Attention and orientation are often relatively preserved	Clinical consensus
Mania	Increased energy and goal-directed behavior predominate rather than impaired awareness	DSM-5-TR (APA, 2022)
Substance intoxication	Temporal relationship to substance exposure may clarify diagnosis	DSM-5-TR (APA, 2022)
Withdrawal syndromes	Alcohol or benzodiazepine withdrawal may closely mimic delirium	Clinical consensus
Catatonia	Motor findings predominate; overlap may occur in severe illness	Clinical consensus

D. Common Medication-Related Contributors

Medication / Class	Clinical Notes	Evidence Source
Anticholinergic medications	Strong anticholinergic burden increases delirium risk, especially in older adults	AGS Beers Criteria (2023)
Benzodiazepines	May worsen confusion, sedation, and falls in vulnerable populations	AGS Beers Criteria (2023); Clinical consensus
Opioids	Sedation and cognitive impairment may precipitate delirium	Clinical consensus
Corticosteroids	May contribute to agitation, psychosis, or delirium	Clinical consensus
Polypharmacy	Multiple CNS-active medications substantially increase risk	AGS Beers Criteria (2023)

E. Initial Outpatient Response

Clinical Scenario	Recommended Action	Clinical Notes	Evidence Source
Suspected delirium without agitation	Arrange urgent same-day medical evaluation	Medical causes must be excluded promptly	Clinical consensus
Delirium with severe agitation or psychosis	Emergency department referral or hospitalization	Safety and medical stabilization may be required	Clinical consensus
Medication-related concern	Review recent medication changes and anticholinergic burden	Abrupt medication changes commonly contribute	Clinical consensus
Possible intoxication or withdrawal	Assess substance use history immediately	Withdrawal syndromes may become life-threatening	Clinical consensus
Older adult with abrupt confusion	Treat as potential medical emergency until proven otherwise	Delirium is frequently underrecognized in geriatric patients	Inouye et al. (2014)

F. Avoid / Use with Caution

Practice / Medication	Clinical Notes	Evidence Source
Routine outpatient-only management of severe delirium	Severe cases generally require emergency or inpatient evaluation	Clinical consensus
Excessive sedative use	May worsen confusion and respiratory compromise	Clinical consensus
Anticholinergic medications	May exacerbate delirium severity	AGS Beers Criteria (2023)
Polypharmacy escalation during active delirium	Additional medications may worsen diagnostic clarity and instability	Clinical consensus

Practice / Medication	Clinical Notes	Evidence Source
Delayed medical referral	Underlying medical illness may rapidly worsen without treatment	Inouye et al. (2014)

3. ACUTE DYSTONIA / OCULOGYRIC CRISIS

Medication	Dose	Route	Clinical Notes	Evidence Source
Benztropine	1–2 mg	IM/IV	First-line	FDA (2023)
Diphenhydramine	25–50 mg	IM/IV	Alternative	FDA (2023)

Repeat once after 20 minutes if needed. Continue benztropine 1–2 mg PO twice daily for 48–72 hours.

4. SEROTONIN SYNDROME

Recognition (Hunter Criteria)

- Spontaneous clonus
- Inducible clonus with agitation or diaphoresis
- Ocular clonus with agitation or diaphoresis
- Tremor with hyperreflexia
- Hypertonia with temperature above 38°C and ocular or inducible clonus
- In a patient who has taken a serotonergic agent, any one of these findings satisfies the Hunter criteria; the classic triad below is descriptive, whereas the Hunter criteria are the validated diagnostic decision rule.

Classic Triad

- Mental status changes
- Autonomic instability
- Neuromuscular abnormalities

Management

- Discontinue serotonergic agents
- Supportive care with IV fluids
- Benzodiazepines for agitation

Medication	Dose	Clinical Notes	Evidence Source
Lorazepam	1–2 mg IV q5–10 min	Control agitation	ACEP (2024)

Medication	Dose	Clinical Notes	Evidence Source
Cyproheptadine	12 mg, then 2 mg q2h; maintenance 8 mg q6h after stabilization (max 32 mg/24 h)	Oral only	Toxicology guidelines (ACMT 2023)

5. NEUROLEPTIC MALIGNANT SYNDROME (NMS)

Recognition

- Fever >38°C
- Severe rigidity
- Autonomic instability
- Altered mental status
- Elevated Creatine phosphokinase (CPK)

Management

- Stop antipsychotics
- ICU admission
- Aggressive hydration and cooling

Medication	Dose	Clinical Notes	Evidence Source
Dantrolene	1–2.5 mg/kg IV	First-line severe	ACMT (2023)
Bromocriptine	2.5–10 mg TID	Dopamine agonist	ACMT (2023)

6. LITHIUM TOXICITY

Severity	Serum Level (mEq/L)	Symptoms	Clinical Notes	Evidence Source
Mild	1.5 - 2.5	Nausea, vomiting, tremor, fatigue	Hold lithium; oral/IV hydration; monitor levels every 6–12 hours	Decker et al. (2015); FDA labeling (2023)
Moderate	2.5 - 3.5	Ataxia, dysarthria, confusion, coarse tremor	Hospital admission; IV fluids; serial lithium levels; monitor renal function	Decker et al. (2015)

Severity	Serum Level (mEq/L)	Symptoms	Clinical Notes	Evidence Source
Severe	>3.5 (or ≥2.5 with severe symptoms)	Delirium, seizures, coma	ICU management. Extracorporeal treatment (ECTR) is recommended when lithium is >4.0 mEq/L with impaired renal function, and for decreased consciousness, seizures, or life-threatening dysrhythmias regardless of concentration; ECTR is suggested when lithium is >5.0 mEq/L. Interpret serum levels together with clinical findings, toxicity type, and renal function; obtain urgent toxicology/nephrology consultation	Decker et al. (2015)

Clinical status overrides serum level.

Severe neurologic symptoms (e.g., seizures, coma) warrant dialysis regardless of lithium level.

7. VALPROATE TOXICITY TREATMENT

Clinical Features

- CNS depression
- Vomiting
- Hyperammonemia
- Hepatotoxicity
- Pancreatitis

Agent	Phase	Dose	Clinical Notes	Evidence Source
L-carnitine	Loading	100 mg/kg IV (max 6 g)	Indicated for severe valproate toxicity with hyperammonemia or hepatotoxicity	ACMT (2023)
L-carnitine	Maintenance	50 mg/kg q8h	Continue until improvement	ACMT (2023)

Clinical note

L-carnitine is the primary antidote for severe valproate toxicity. Supportive care including bowel decontamination and hemodialysis may be required in severe cases. ACMT (2023).

8. CLOZAPINE EMERGENCIES

Emergency	Findings	Management	Clinical Notes	Evidence Source
Agranulocytosis	ANC <500	Stop drug	Hematology consult	FDA labeling; FDA (2025)
Myocarditis	Chest pain	Cardiology	Early detection critical	FDA labeling; FDA (2025)
Ileus	Severe constipation	Urgent treatment	Can be fatal	FDA labeling; FDA (2025)

9. SEVERE AKATHISIA TREATMENT

Recognition

- Intense inner restlessness
- Pacing
- Severe distress

Treatment

Medication	Dose	Route	Clinical Notes	Evidence Source
Propranolol	20–40 mg	PO BID	First-line	NICE CG178 (2014)
Lorazepam	0.5–2 mg	PO/IM	Adjunct	NICE CG178 (2014)
Mirtazapine	15 mg	PO	Alternative	Clinical consensus

10. MAOI HYPERTENSIVE CRISIS

Recognition

- Severe headache
- Hypertension
- Neck stiffness

Emergency Management

Medication	Dose	Route	Clinical Notes	Evidence Source
Phentolamine	5 mg	IV	First-line	ACMT (2023)
Nitroprusside	0.3–10 mcg/kg/min	IV	ICU only	ACMT (2023)

11. SEROTONIN SYNDROME vs NMS vs ANTICHOLINERGIC TOXICITY

Feature	Serotonin Syndrome	Neuroleptic Malignant Syndrome (NMS)	Anticholinergic Toxicity	Evidence Source
Onset	Hours	Days	Hours	ACMT (2023)
Neuromuscular	Clonus	Rigidity (lead-pipe)	None	ACMT (2023)
Skin	Sweaty	Sweaty	Dry	ACMT (2023)
Key Sign	Hyperreflexia	Lead-pipe rigidity	Dry skin	ACMT (2023)

12. WITHDRAWAL SEIZURES (Alcohol / Benzodiazepines)

Abrupt discontinuation of alcohol or benzodiazepines can cause withdrawal seizures, a medical emergency potentially progressing to delirium tremens.

Recognition

- Generalized tonic-clonic seizures
- Typically 6–48 hours after last alcohol intake
- May be preceded by autonomic symptoms (tremor, tachycardia, diaphoresis)

Clinical Monitoring

Use CIWA-Ar scale (Clinical Institute Withdrawal Assessment for Alcohol, Revised)

CIWA Score	Severity	Recommended Action	Clinical Notes	Evidence Source
<8	Mild	Observation	No benzodiazepines required; reassess every 1–4 hours; consider outpatient management if stable	ASAM (2020)
8–15	Moderate	Benzodiazepine treatment	Initiate symptom-triggered therapy (e.g., lorazepam, diazepam); monitor vitals closely	ASAM (2020)
≥15	Severe	Aggressive treatment and monitoring	High risk of seizures and delirium tremens; consider IV benzodiazepines, continuous monitoring, possible ICU admission	ASAM (2020)

Assess every 1–4 hours depending on severity.

Immediate Management

- Stabilize airway, breathing, circulation
- Administer benzodiazepines

Category	Medication	Dose	Clinical Notes	Evidence Source
Benzodiazepine	Lorazepam	2–4 mg IV	Preferred in hepatic impairment; repeat every 15–20 min as needed	ASAM (2020)
Benzodiazepine	Diazepam	5–10 mg IV	Rapid onset; longer half-life; useful in severe withdrawal	ASAM (2020)
Supportive Care	Thiamine	100 mg IV	Prevents Wernicke encephalopathy; always give before glucose	ASAM (2020)
Supportive Care	Electrolyte correction	—	Correct magnesium and potassium abnormalities	ASAM (2020)

Clinical note

Hospital admission is recommended for seizures or severe withdrawal.

13. OVERDOSE (POLYPHARMACY / INTENTIONAL)

Recognition

- Altered mental status
- Respiratory depression
- Arrhythmias

Overdose Antidotes

Drug	Dose	Notes	Clinical Notes	Evidence Source
Naloxone	0.4–2 mg	Opioid OD	Repeat dosing	FDA (2023)
Flumazenil	0.2 mg IV	Benzo OD	Use cautiously; not for routine reversal. Avoid in chronic benzodiazepine dependence, suspected TCA or proconvulsant co-ingestion, and known seizure disorder (precipitates seizures and acute withdrawal)	ACMT (2023)
Physostigmine	0.5–2 mg IV	Anticholinergic	Specialist use; obtain an ECG first and avoid with TCA toxicity or QRS widening (risk of asystole, bradycardia, and seizures)	ACMT (2023)
Glucagon	3–5 mg IV	Beta-blocker OD	ICU setting	ACMT (2023)

14. Emergency Contact Numbers

Resource	Contact	Clinical Notes
Poison Control	1-800-222-1222	24/7
EMS	911	Immediate
Clozapine information	https://www.fda.gov/drugs/postmarket-drug-safety-information-patients-and-providers/information-clozapine	REMS eliminated June 13, 2025; ANC monitoring still recommended per FDA prescribing information
Suicide Lifeline	988	Crisis support

REFERENCES

American College of Emergency Physicians. (2024). Clinical policy: Critical issues in the evaluation and management of adult out-of-hospital or emergency department patients presenting with severe agitation. *Annals of Emergency Medicine*, *83*(1), e1–e30. https://doi.org/10.1016/j.annemergmed.2023.09.010

American Geriatrics Society Beers Criteria® Update Expert Panel. (2023). American Geriatrics Society 2023 updated AGS Beers Criteria® for potentially inappropriate medication use in older adults. Journal of the American Geriatrics Society, 71(7), 2052–2081. https://doi.org/10.1111/jgs.18372

American Psychiatric Association. (2022). *Diagnostic and statistical manual of mental disorders* (5th ed., text rev.; DSM-5-TR). American Psychiatric Publishing. https://doi.org/10.1176/appi.books.9780890425787

American College of Medical Toxicology. (2023). *Toxicology treatment recommendations and supportive management principles.* ACMT.

American Psychiatric Association. (2020). *The American Psychiatric Association practice guideline for the treatment of patients with schizophrenia* (3rd ed.). American Psychiatric Association Publishing. https://doi.org/10.1176/appi.books.9780890424841

American Society of Addiction Medicine. (2020). *The ASAM clinical practice guideline on alcohol withdrawal management.* ASAM.

Decker, B. S., Goldfarb, D. S., Dargan, P. I., Friesen, M., Gosselin, S., Hoffman, R. S., Lavergne, V., Nolin, T. D., Ghannoum, M., & EXTRIP Workgroup. (2015). Extracorporeal treatment for lithium poisoning: Systematic review and recommendations from the EXTRIP Workgroup. *Clinical Journal of the American Society of Nephrology*, *10*(5), 875–887. https://doi.org/10.2215/CJN.10021014

Inouye, S. K., Westendorp, R. G. J., & Saczynski, J. S. (2014). Delirium in elderly people. The Lancet, 383(9920), 911–922. https://doi.org/10.1016/S0140-6736(13)60688-1

National Institute for Health and Care Excellence. (2014). *Psychosis and schizophrenia in adults: prevention and management (Clinical Guideline CG178).* https://www.nice.org.uk/guidance/cg178

U.S. Food and Drug Administration. (2023). *Zyprexa (olanzapine) prescribing information.* https://www.accessdata.fda.gov

U.S. Food and Drug Administration. (2024). *Haldol (haloperidol) prescribing information.* https://www.accessdata.fda.gov

U.S. Food and Drug Administration. (2024). *Abilify (aripiprazole) prescribing information.* https://www.accessdata.fda.gov

U.S. Food and Drug Administration. (2025). *FDA removes risk evaluation and mitigation strategy (REMS) program for clozapine.* https://www.fda.gov/drugs/drug-safety-communications/fda-removes-risk-evaluation-and-mitigation-strategy-rems-program-antipsychotic-drug-clozapine

Zeller, S. L., Citrome, L., & Nordstrom, K. (2012). *Project BETA: Best practices in the evaluation and treatment of agitation. Western Journal of Emergency Medicine, 13*(1), 1–14.

XVIII: CLINICAL SCALES APPENDIX

SECTION INTRODUCTION

This appendix presents standardized psychiatric rating scales and structured clinical instruments commonly utilized within outpatient psychiatric practice to support diagnostic clarification, symptom quantification, longitudinal monitoring, and evidence-informed clinical decision-making. These instruments are widely used across clinical, academic, research, quality-improvement, and training settings and may assist clinicians in improving diagnostic consistency, treatment monitoring, functional assessment, and outcome measurement.

Standardized psychiatric scales may serve multiple clinical purposes, including quantifying symptom severity, monitoring treatment response over time, identifying relapse or clinical deterioration, supporting diagnostic evaluation, assessing functional impairment, and facilitating communication across providers and levels of care. Measurement-based care has become increasingly emphasized within modern psychiatric practice because structured symptom tracking may improve clinical monitoring, treatment adjustment, and patient engagement during longitudinal care.

The scales included in this appendix span multiple psychiatric domains, including depression, anxiety, suicidality, bipolar disorder, psychosis, obsessive-compulsive symptoms, ADHD, cognitive impairment, substance use disorders, sleep disturbance, trauma-related symptoms, movement disorders, and medication adverse effects. Some instruments are primarily clinician-administered, while others are designed for patient self-report or structured screening purposes. Selection of scales should remain individualized based on clinical presentation, diagnostic question, treatment setting, patient literacy, cognitive functioning, and time constraints.

Although standardized scales may significantly enhance clinical assessment, these instruments should complement—not replace—comprehensive psychiatric evaluation and professional clinical judgment. Scale scores must always be interpreted within the broader context of patient history, mental status examination, psychosocial factors, cultural considerations, medical comorbidity, collateral information, and longitudinal clinical presentation. Elevated or reduced scores should not be interpreted in isolation without appropriate clinical correlation.

Measurement-based care may be particularly valuable in patients with chronic psychiatric illness, treatment-resistant conditions, high relapse risk, substance use disorders, suicidality, neurocognitive disorders, and complex psychopharmacologic treatment regimens. Routine use of structured rating scales may also improve documentation quality, facilitate interdisciplinary communication, support insurance and regulatory requirements, and assist with clinical outcome tracking in institutional practice settings.

Clinicians should remain aware of the limitations of psychiatric rating instruments. Cultural factors, educational background, cognitive impairment, language barriers, malingering, symptom minimization, emotional distress, and variability in patient insight may influence scale performance and interpretation. Some instruments are validated primarily for screening rather than formal diagnosis, while others may require formal training or structured administration procedures to ensure reliability.

The following sections provide a structured collection of commonly utilized psychiatric scales and clinical assessment tools intended to support evidence-informed outpatient psychiatric practice. These instruments are included as adjunctive clinical resources to enhance symptom assessment, longitudinal monitoring, treatment evaluation, and standardized documentation within comprehensive psychiatric care.

1. DEPRESSION SCALES

1.1 Hamilton Depression Rating Scale (HAM-D)

A. OVERVIEW

Component	Detail	Clinical Notes	Evidence Source
Purpose	Measures the severity of depressive symptoms in major depressive disorder	Research gold standard; may overemphasize somatic symptoms	Hamilton (1960); NICE (2022)
Administration	Clinician-rated; typically 17-item version; 15–20 minutes	Requires a trained interviewer	Hamilton (1960); NICE (2022)
Scoring	Items scored 0–2 or 0–4; total range 0–52	Commonly used for baseline severity and treatment response	Hamilton (1960); NICE (2022)

B. Interpretation

Score	Severity	Clinical Action	Evidence Source
0–7	Normal / remission	No acute treatment change; continue monitoring if indicated	Hamilton (1960); NICE (2022)
8–16	Mild depression	Consider psychotherapy and close follow-up	NICE (2022)
17–23	Moderate depression	Pharmacotherapy and/or psychotherapy indicated	NICE (2022)
≥24	Severe depression	Consider combination treatment and higher level of care if warranted	NICE (2022)

1.2 Montgomery–Asberg Depression Rating Scale (MADRS)

A. OVERVIEW

Component	Detail	Clinical Notes	Evidence Source
Purpose	Measures severity of depressive symptoms; especially sensitive to change	Preferred in many treatment trials	Montgomery & Åsberg (1979); NICE (2022)
Administration	Clinician-rated; 10 items; about 10–15 minutes	Faster than HAM-D	Montgomery & Åsberg (1979); NICE (2022)

Component	Detail	Clinical Notes	Evidence Source
Scoring	Items scored 0–6; total range 0–60	Useful for monitoring response longitudinally	Montgomery & Åsberg (1979); NICE (2022)

B. Interpretation

Score	Severity	Clinical Action	Evidence Source
0–6	No depression / remission	Continue monitoring	Montgomery & Åsberg (1979); NICE (2022)
7–19	Mild depression	Consider psychotherapy; monitor response	NICE (2022)
20–34	Moderate depression	Initiate or adjust pharmacotherapy and/or psychotherapy	NICE (2022)
≥35	Severe depression	Aggressive treatment indicated; consider combination treatment	NICE (2022)

1.3 Patient Health Questionnaire-9 (PHQ-9)

A. OVERVIEW

Component	Detail	Clinical Notes	Evidence Source
Purpose	Depression screening and monitoring	Most widely used outpatient self-report depression scale	Kroenke et al. (2001); NICE (2022)
Administration	Self-report; 9 items; about 5–10 minutes	Easy to repeat at follow-up visits	Kroenke et al. (2001); NICE (2022)
Scoring	Items scored 0–3; total range 0–27	Item 9 requires clinical suicide follow-up	Kroenke et al. (2001); NICE (2022)

B. Interpretation

Score	Severity	Clinical Action	Evidence Source
0–4	Minimal	No treatment indicated; monitor as needed	Kroenke et al. (2001); NICE (2022)
5–9	Mild	Watchful waiting and/or psychotherapy	NICE (2022)
10–14	Moderate	Treatment indicated	NICE (2022)
15–19	Moderately severe	Active treatment and closer monitoring indicated	NICE (2022)
20–27	Severe	Evaluate suicidality; consider psychiatry referral/intensive treatment	NICE (2022)

2 ANXIETY SCALES

2.1 Generalized Anxiety Disorder-7 (GAD-7)

A. OVERVIEW

Component	Detail	Clinical Notes	Evidence Source
Purpose	Measures generalized anxiety severity	Validated in primary care and commonly used in psychiatry	Spitzer et al. (2006); NICE CG113
Administration	Self-report; 7 items; about 5 minutes	Useful for repeated monitoring	Spitzer et al. (2006); NICE CG113
Scoring	Items scored 0–3; total range 0–21	Also correlates with functional impairment	Spitzer et al. (2006); NICE CG113

B. Interpretation

Score	Severity	Clinical Action	Evidence Source
0–4	Minimal	No treatment indicated; monitor if clinically needed	Spitzer et al. (2006); NICE CG113
5–9	Mild	Monitor; consider psychoeducation/therapy	NICE CG113
10–14	Moderate	Initiate treatment	NICE CG113
15–21	Severe	Active treatment indicated; consider specialty referral if impaired	NICE CG113

3. PSYCHOSIS SCALES

3.1 Positive and Negative Syndrome Scale (PANSS)

A. OVERVIEW

Component	Detail	Clinical Notes	Evidence Source
Purpose	Measures positive, negative, and general psychopathology in schizophrenia	Research gold standard for psychosis severity	Kay et al. (1987); APA (2020)
Administration	Clinician-rated; 30 items; about 30–45 minutes	Requires trained rater	Kay et al. (1987); APA (2020)
Scoring	Items scored 1–7; total range 30–210	Primarily used for longitudinal change	Kay et al. (1987); APA (2020)

B. Interpretation

Score	Severity	Clinical Action	Evidence Source
30–58	Mild	Outpatient management and monitoring if clinically stable	Kay et al. (1987); APA (2020)
59–75	Moderate	Active treatment required; consider medication adjustment	APA (2020)
76–95	Moderately severe	Intensive treatment; consider higher-level services	APA (2020)
≥96	Severe	Consider hospitalization or intensive psychiatric management	APA (2020)

3.2 Brief Psychiatric Rating Scale (BPRS)

A. OVERVIEW

Component	Detail	Clinical Notes	Evidence Source
Purpose	Rapid assessment of psychotic and affective symptoms	More practical than PANSS in many clinical settings	Overall & Gorham (1962); APA (2020)
Administration	Clinician-rated; commonly 18-item version; about 10–20 minutes	Shorter than PANSS	Overall & Gorham (1962); APA (2020)

Component	Detail	Clinical Notes	Evidence Source
Scoring	18-item version scored 1–7; total range 18–126	Version dependent; 16-, 18-, and 24-item forms exist	Overall & Gorham (1962); APA (2020)

B. Interpretation

Score	Severity	Clinical Action	Evidence Source
<31	Mild	Monitor and continue outpatient treatment if otherwise stable	Overall & Gorham (1962); APA (2020)
31–40	Moderate	Active treatment indicated; consider medication adjustment	APA (2020)
>40	Severe	Consider intensive intervention/hospitalization depending on risk	APA (2020)

4. OBSESSIVE-COMPULSIVE DISORDER SCALES

4.1 Yale-Brown Obsessive Compulsive Scale (Y-BOCS)

A. OVERVIEW

Component	Detail	Clinical Notes	Evidence Source
Purpose	Measures the severity of obsessive-compulsive symptoms	Gold standard clinician-rated OCD scale	Goodman et al. (1989); NICE CG31; Fineberg et al. (2020)
Administration	Clinician-rated; 10 items; about 30 minutes	Rates the severity of obsessions and compulsions separately	Goodman et al. (1989); NICE CG31

B. Interpretation

Score	Severity	Clinical Action	Evidence Source
0–7	Subclinical	No treatment indicated	Goodman et al. (1989); NICE CG31
8–15	Mild	Cognitive behavioral therapy (CBT) with exposure and response prevention (ERP) first-line	NICE CG31; Fineberg et al. (2020)
16–23	Moderate	SSRI indicated; consider combined treatment	NICE CG31; Fineberg et al. (2020)
24–31	Severe	Combination therapy indicated	NICE CG31; Fineberg et al. (2020)
32–40	Extreme	Specialist care; consider augmentation strategies	NICE CG31; Fineberg et al. (2020)

5. BIPOLAR/MANIA SCALES

5.1 Young Mania Rating Scale (YMRS)

A. OVERVIEW

Component	Detail	Clinical Notes	Evidence Source
Purpose	Assesses the severity of manic symptoms	Standard clinician-rated mania scale	Young et al. (1978); NICE CG185 (2014)
Administration	Clinician-rated; 11 items; about 10–15 minutes	Widely used in acute mania assessment	Young et al. (1978); NICE CG185 (2014)
Scoring	Total range 0–60; four items weighted double	Useful during acute episodes and titration	Young et al. (1978); NICE CG185 (2014)

B. Interpretation

Score	Severity	Clinical Action	Evidence Source
0–12	Remission/euthymia	Continue maintenance monitoring	Young et al. (1978); NICE CG185 (2014)
13–19	Mild mania	Consider medication adjustment; closer monitoring	NICE CG185 (2014)
20–25	Moderate mania	Pharmacotherapy indicated	NICE CG185 (2014)
≥26	Severe mania	Consider hospitalization / urgent stabilization	NICE CG185 (2014)

6. SUICIDE RISK ASSESSMENT SCALE

6.1 Columbia Suicide Severity Rating Scale (C-SSRS)

A. OVERVIEW

Component	Detail	Clinical Notes	Evidence Source
Purpose	Standardized assessment of suicidal ideation and suicidal behavior	Used across outpatient, inpatient, ED, and crisis settings	Posner et al. (2011); APA (2003)
Administration	Clinician-administered; brief (2–5 min) or full (10–15 min) versions	Brief version for screening; full version for detailed risk assessment	Posner et al. (2011); APA (2003)
Domains	Ideation severity, intensity, suicidal behavior, lethality	Includes preparatory behavior and past attempts	Posner et al. (2011); APA (2003)

B. Interpretation

Finding	Interpretation	Clinical Action	Evidence Source
Passive ideation	Wish to be dead without an active plan	Monitor and reassess risk factors	APA (2003)
Active ideation	Active suicidal thoughts	Safety planning; assess intent, plan, and access to means	APA (2003)
Suicidal behavior (any)	Attempt, interrupted or aborted attempt, or preparatory behavior	Immediate intervention; ED referral or hospitalization as indicated	APA (2003)

7. COGNITIVE ASSESSMENT SCALE

7.1 Mini-Mental State Examination (MMSE)

A. OVERVIEW

Component	Detail	Clinical Notes	Evidence Source
Purpose	Screens for cognitive impairment	Less sensitive for mild cognitive impairment than MoCA	Folstein et al. (1975); NICE NG97 (2018)
Administration	Clinician-administered; about 5–10 minutes	Widely used but influenced by education and language	Folstein et al. (1975); NICE NG97 (2018)
Scoring	30-point scale	Copyright/licensing restrictions may apply	Folstein et al. (1975); NICE NG97 (2018)

B. Interpretation

Score	Interpretation	Clinical Action	Evidence Source
24–30	Normal	Monitor if concerns persist; consider MoCA if subtle deficits are suspected	Folstein et al. (1975); NICE NG97 (2018)
18–23	Mild impairment	Further evaluation indicated	NICE NG97 (2018)
0–17	Severe impairment	Dementia workup/safety assessment indicated	NICE NG97 (2018)

7.2 Montreal Cognitive Assessment (MoCA)

A. OVERVIEW

Component	Detail	Clinical Notes	Evidence Source
Purpose	Screens for mild cognitive impairment	More sensitive than MMSE for early deficits	Nasreddine et al. (2005); NICE NG97 (2018))
Administration	Clinician-administered; about 10–15 minutes	Official use requires training/certification	Nasreddine et al. (2005); NICE NG97 (2018)
Scoring	30-point scale; add 1 point if education ≤12 years	Education adjustment must be documented	Nasreddine et al. (2005); NICE NG97 (2018)

B. Interpretation

Score	Interpretation	Clinical Action	Evidence Source
≥26	Normal	Repeat annually or earlier if decline is suspected	Nasreddine et al. (2005); NICE NG97 (2018)
<26	Cognitive impairment	Further neurocognitive evaluation indicated	Nasreddine et al. (2005); NICE NG97 (2018)

8. MOVEMENT DISORDER MONITORING SCALES

8.1 Abnormal Involuntary Movement Scale (AIMS)

A. OVERVIEW

Component	Detail	Clinical Notes	Evidence Source
Purpose	Detects and monitors tardive dyskinesia	Required in patients treated with antipsychotics	Guy (1976); APA (2020)
Administration	Clinician-rated; 12 items; about 10–15 minutes	Evaluates face, extremities, trunk, and global severity	Guy (1976); APA (2020)
Scoring	Items 1–10 are scored 0–4 (items 1–7 rate abnormal movements; items 8–10 cover global severity and awareness); items 11–12 assess dental status and are answered yes/no	Longitudinal monitoring is essential	Guy (1976); APA (2020)

B. Interpretation / Monitoring

Finding / Risk Level	Interpretation	Clinical Action	Evidence Source
≥2 in ≥2 areas OR ≥3 in 1 area	Possible tardive dyskinesia	Evaluate clinically; consider dose reduction, switch, or VMAT2 treatment as appropriate	Guy (1976); APA (2020)
Standard risk	Routine monitoring	Repeat every 6 months	APA (2020)
High-risk patients	Increased TD risk	Repeat every 3 months	APA (2020)

9. SUBSTANCE WITHDRAWAL SCALES

9.1 Clinical Institute Withdrawal Assessment for Alcohol, Revised (CIWA-Ar)

A. OVERVIEW

Component	Detail	Clinical Notes	Evidence Source
Purpose	Measures alcohol withdrawal severity	Guides symptom-triggered benzodiazepine treatment	Sullivan et al. (1989); ASAM (2020)
Administration	Clinician-rated; 10 items; about 5–10 minutes	Requires patient cooperation and repeated reassessment	Sullivan et al. (1989); ASAM (2020)
Scoring	Total range 0–67	Best used in medically appropriate, cooperative patients	Sullivan et al. (1989); ASAM (2020)

B. Interpretation

Score	Severity	Clinical Action	Evidence Source
<10	Mild	Observation/supportive care; benzodiazepines usually not required	ASAM (2020); Sullivan et al. (1989)
10–18	Moderate	Initiate symptom-triggered benzodiazepines	ASAM (2020)
>18	Severe	Aggressive treatment; consider ICU / higher-acuity monitoring	ASAM (2020)

9.2 Clinical Opiate Withdrawal Scale (COWS)

A. OVERVIEW

Component	Detail	Clinical Notes	Evidence Source
Purpose	Measures opioid withdrawal severity; guides buprenorphine induction	Standard bedside withdrawal scale	Wesson & Ling (2003); SAMHSA TIP 63 (2021)
Administration	Clinician-rated; 11 items; about 5–10 minutes	Reassess during induction	Wesson & Ling (2003); SAMHSA TIP 63 (2021)
Scoring	Total range 0–48	Used to avoid precipitated withdrawal	Wesson & Ling (2003); SAMHSA TIP 63 (2021)

B. Interpretation

Score	Severity	Clinical Action	Evidence Source
5–12	Mild	Monitor; provide comfort measures	Wesson & Ling (2003); SAMHSA TIP 63 (2021)
13–24	Moderate	Start treatment; buprenorphine is often appropriate if COWS ≥8 and timing is appropriate	SAMHSA TIP 63 (2021)
25–36	Moderately severe	Aggressive management; close monitoring	SAMHSA TIP 63 (2021)
>36	Severe	Consider inpatient / high-acuity withdrawal management	SAMHSA TIP 63 (2021)

Clinical note

Buprenorphine is typically initiated at COWS ≥8

10. SUBSTANCE USE SCREENING SCALES

10.1 Alcohol Use Disorders Identification Test (AUDIT)

A. OVERVIEW

Component	Detail	Clinical Notes	Evidence Source
Purpose	Screens for hazardous or harmful alcohol use	First-line alcohol screening tool	Saunders et al. (1993); NICE CG115
Administration	Self- or clinician-administered; 10 items	Can be used in primary care and psychiatry	Saunders et al. (1993); NICE CG115
Scoring	Items scored 0–4; total range 0–40	Higher score indicates greater alcohol-related risk	Saunders et al. (1993); NICE CG115

B. Interpretation

Score	Interpretation	Clinical Action	Evidence Source
0–7	Low risk	Education / routine monitoring	Saunders et al. (1993); NICE CG115
8–15	Hazardous drinking	Brief intervention	NICE CG115
16–19	Harmful use	Structured intervention; consider referral	NICE CG115
≥20	Possible alcohol dependence	Specialty referral / AUD evaluation	NICE CG115

11. Summary Table: Recommended Scales by Clinical Context

Clinical Context	Primary Scale	Suggested Frequency	Clinical Notes	Evidence Source
Depression screening	PHQ-9	Baseline + each visit	Item 9 requires suicide follow-up	Kroenke et al. (2001); NICE (2022)
Depression severity	MADRS (preferred) / HAM-D	Baseline + every 4–8 weeks during treatment	MADRS preferred for response tracking	Montgomery & Åsberg (1979); NICE (2022)
Anxiety	GAD-7	Baseline + each visit	Useful for monitoring relapse/response	Spitzer et al. (2006); NICE CG113
Bipolar mania	YMRS	Baseline + each visit during acute episode	Use for medication adjustment and stabilization	Young et al. (1978); NICE CG185 (2014)
Suicide risk	C-SSRS	Baseline + any clinical change	Any suicidal behavior requires immediate intervention	Posner et al. (2011); APA (2003)
Psychosis	BPRS (clinical) / PANSS (research)	Inpatient every 1–2 weeks; outpatient every 4–8 weeks	BPRS faster clinically; PANSS more detailed	Overall & Gorham (1962); APA (2020)
OCD	Y-BOCS	Baseline + every 4–6 weeks	Guides SSRI titration and augmentation	Goodman et al. (1989); NICE CG31; Fineberg et al. (2020)
Cognitive impairment	MoCA (preferred) / MMSE	Baseline + annually	MoCA more sensitive for early decline	Nasreddine et al. (2005); NICE NG97 (2018)
Tardive dyskinesia	AIMS	Every 6 months; every 3 months if high-risk	Required for antipsychotic monitoring	Guy (1976); APA (2020)
Alcohol withdrawal	CIWA-Ar	Every 1–4 hours during acute withdrawal	Guides symptom-triggered benzodiazepines	Sullivan et al. (1989); ASAM (2020)
Opioid withdrawal	COWS	During induction / withdrawal	Buprenorphine commonly started at COWS ≥8 when appropriate	Wesson & Ling (2003); SAMHSA TIP 63 (2021)
Alcohol misuse screening	AUDIT	Baseline + annually or as indicated	Useful for outpatient screening	Saunders et al. (1993); NICE CG115

REFERENCES

American Psychiatric Association. (2003). Practice guideline for the assessment and treatment of patients with suicidal behaviors. American Psychiatric Association Publishing. https://doi.org/10.1176/appi.books.9780890423363.56008

American Psychiatric Association. (2020). *The American Psychiatric Association practice guideline for the treatment of patients with schizophrenia* (3rd ed.).

American Psychiatric Association. (2022). *Diagnostic and statistical manual of mental disorders* (5th ed., text rev.).

American Society of Addiction Medicine. (2020). *The ASAM clinical practice guideline on alcohol withdrawal management. Journal of Addiction Medicine, 14*(3S Suppl. 1), 1–72. https://doi.org/10.1097/ADM.0000000000000668

Folstein, M. F., Folstein, S. E., & McHugh, P. R. (1975). "Mini-mental state": A practical method for grading the cognitive state of patients for the clinician. *Journal of Psychiatric Research, 12*(3), 189–198.

Guy, W. (1976). *ECDEU assessment manual for psychopharmacology* (Rev. ed.). U.S. Department of Health, Education, and Welfare.

Hamilton, M. (1960). A rating scale for depression. *Journal of Neurology, Neurosurgery, and Psychiatry, 23*(1), 56–62. https://doi.org/10.1136/jnnp.23.1.56

Kay, S. R., Fiszbein, A., & Opler, L. A. (1987). The Positive and Negative Syndrome Scale (PANSS) for schizophrenia. *Schizophrenia Bulletin, 13*(2), 261–276.

Kroenke, K., Spitzer, R. L., & Williams, J. B. W. (2001). The PHQ-9: Validity of a brief depression severity measure. *Journal of General Internal Medicine, 16*(9), 606–613.

Montgomery, S. A., & Åsberg, M. (1979). A new depression scale designed to be sensitive to change. *British Journal of Psychiatry, 134*(4), 382–389.

Nasreddine, Z. S., Phillips, N. A., Bédirian, V., Charbonneau, S., Whitehead, V., Collin, I., Cummings, J. L., & Chertkow, H. (2005). The Montreal Cognitive Assessment, MoCA: A brief screening tool for mild cognitive impairment. *Journal of the American Geriatrics Society, 53*(4), 695–699.

National Institute for Health and Care Excellence. (2005, updated 2022). *NICE Guideline CG31: Obsessive-compulsive disorder and body dysmorphic disorder.*

National Institute for Health and Care Excellence. (2011). *NICE Guideline CG113: Generalized anxiety disorder and panic disorder in adults.*

National Institute for Health and Care Excellence. (2011). *NICE Guideline CG115: Alcohol-use disorders: Diagnosis, assessment and management of harmful drinking and alcohol dependence.*

National Institute for Health and Care Excellence. (2014). *NICE Guideline CG185: Bipolar disorder assessment and management.*

National Institute for Health and Care Excellence. (2018). *NICE Guideline NG97: Dementia assessment, management and support for people living with dementia and their carers.*

National Institute for Health and Care Excellence. (2022). *NICE Guideline NG222: Depression in adults.*

Overall, J. E., & Gorham, D. R. (1962). The Brief Psychiatric Rating Scale. *Psychological Reports, 10*(3), 799–812.

Posner, K., Brown, G. K., Stanley, B., Brent, D. A., Yershova, K. V., Oquendo, M. A., Currier, G. W., Melvin, G. A., Greenhill, L., Shen, S., & Mann, J. J. (2011). The Columbia-Suicide Severity Rating Scale: Initial validity and internal consistency findings from three multisite studies with adolescents and adults. *American Journal of Psychiatry, 168*(12), 1266–1277.

Saunders, J. B., Aasland, O. G., Babor, T. F., de la Fuente, J. R., & Grant, M. (1993). Development of the Alcohol Use Disorders Identification Test (AUDIT): WHO Collaborative Project on Early Detection of Persons with Harmful Alcohol Consumption-II. *Addiction, 88*(6), 791–804.

Spitzer, R. L., Kroenke, K., Williams, J. B. W., & Löwe, B. (2006). A brief measure for assessing generalized anxiety disorder: The GAD-7. *Archives of Internal Medicine, 166*(10), 1092–1097.

Sullivan, J. T., Sykora, K., Schneiderman, J., Naranjo, C. A., & Sellers, E. M. (1989). Assessment of alcohol withdrawal: The revised Clinical Institute Withdrawal Assessment for Alcohol (CIWA-Ar). *Addiction, 84*(11), 1353–1357. https://doi.org/10.1111/j.1360-0443.1989.tb00737

Substance Abuse and Mental Health Services Administration. (2021). *Medications for opioid use disorder (Treatment Improvement Protocol TIP 63).* https://store.samhsa.gov/product/TIP-63-Medications-for-Opioid-Use-Disorder/PEP21-02-01-002

Wesson, D. R., & Ling, W. (2003). The Clinical Opiate Withdrawal Scale (COWS). *Journal of Psychoactive Drugs, 35*(2), 253–259.

Young, R. C., Biggs, J. T., Ziegler, V. E., & Meyer, D. A. (1978). A rating scale for mania: Reliability, validity and sensitivity. *British Journal of Psychiatry, 133*(5), 429–435.

XIX: APPENDICES

SECTION INTRODUCTION

This appendix section provides supplemental psychopharmacology and clinical reference materials intended to support safe, practical, and standardized outpatient psychiatric practice. The appendices included throughout this section are designed as rapid-access clinical tools that complement the core chapters of the manual and assist clinicians with medication management, psychopharmacologic decision-making, emergency preparedness, patient education, and longitudinal treatment planning.

The materials included in this section focus primarily on high-yield operational resources frequently utilized in daily psychiatric practice, including antipsychotic equivalency tables, benzodiazepine conversion guides, oral-to-long-acting injectable (LAI) antipsychotic conversion strategies, monoamine oxidase inhibitor (MAOI) dietary restriction guidance, naloxone prescribing recommendations, overdose education, and other clinically relevant psychopharmacology support tools. These appendices are intended to facilitate safer prescribing, reduce medication-related errors, improve continuity of care, and support evidence-informed clinical decision-making across a wide range of psychiatric settings.

Several appendices contain approximate medication equivalency tables and conversion recommendations intended for clinical reference purposes only. Individual patient response, pharmacokinetic variability, prior treatment exposure, medical comorbidity, substance use, age, organ function, and medication tolerability may substantially influence dose equivalency and treatment outcomes. Medication conversions should therefore never be applied rigidly or mechanically without individualized clinical assessment, careful monitoring, and professional judgment.

Special attention is also given to medication safety, overdose prevention, withdrawal management, and patient education. Appendices addressing benzodiazepine tapering, MAOI interactions, opioid overdose response, and naloxone administration are intended to support both clinician guidance and patient-facing education within routine psychiatric practice. Many of these resources may also assist with interdisciplinary coordination, emergency planning, and risk-reduction strategies in medically and psychiatrically complex populations.

Long-acting injectable antipsychotic conversion tools and psychopharmacology reference tables are included to support continuity of treatment, adherence optimization, relapse prevention, and safer transitions between formulations and levels of care. Because institutional protocols, FDA labeling, and manufacturer recommendations may evolve over time, clinicians should always verify current prescribing information and local policy requirements when utilizing these materials in clinical practice.

The appendices included in this section are intended to function as practical clinical support resources rather than rigid treatment algorithms or substitutes for comprehensive psychiatric evaluation. Clinical recommendations and conversion guidelines must always be interpreted within the broader context of patient-specific factors, longitudinal reassessment, medical comorbidity, concurrent medications, and evolving clinical presentation. Safe psychiatric practice ultimately requires ongoing clinical judgment, interdisciplinary collaboration, individualized treatment planning, and careful patient monitoring throughout the course of care.

APPENDIX A: ANTIPSYCHOTIC EQUIVALENCY TABLE

Approximate Dose Equivalents (Clinical Practice Guide)

Antipsychotic	Approximate Equivalent Dose	Notes
Risperidone	2 mg	• 2 mg Risperidone ≈ 2 mg haloperidol • Dose-dependent EPS >6 mg
Paliperidone	3 mg	• Active metabolite of Risperidone • 3 mg Paliperidone ≈ 2 mg Risperidone
Olanzapine	5 mg	• High metabolic risk • Smoking significantly reduces olanzapine plasma levels (CYP1A2 induction)
Quetiapine	100 mg	• Lowest EPS risk • Highly variable individual response
Ziprasidone	60 mg	• Must take with food (~500 kcal) • Lowest metabolic risk
Aripiprazole	10 mg	• Partial agonist • Low metabolic risk
Haloperidol	2 mg	• High EPS risk • Gold standard for potency reference
Fluphenazine	2 mg	• Similar to haloperidol potency
Perphenazine	8 mg	• Intermediate potency
Chlorpromazine	100 mg	• 100 mg CPZ = 2 mg haloperidol (historical reference)
Lurasidone	40 mg	• Must take with food (≥350 kcal) • Different mechanism
Cariprazine	3 mg	• Active metabolites have prolonged half-life
Asenapine	10 mg	• Sublingual administration • BID dosing
Iloperidone	8 mg	• Slow titration required

Antipsychotic	Approximate Equivalent Dose	Notes
Milsaperidone	8 mg	• Active metabolite of iloperidone • Titrate to reduce orthostasis
Clozapine	100 mg	• Gold standard for TRS • Not equivalent in efficacy
Lumateperone	42 mg	• Fixed dose, no titration

IMPORTANT NOTE

These are approximate clinical guidelines only. Individual patient response varies. Always titrate based on clinical response and tolerability. Do not switch doses rigidly based on these tables alone.

APPENDIX B: BENZODIAZEPINE EQUIVALENCY TABLE

Approximate Dose Equivalents (Benzodiazepine Conversion)

Benzodiazepine	Approximate Equivalent Dose (mg)	Half-Life (hours)	Onset	Notes
Diazepam (Valium)	10 mg	20 – 100 (long)	Fast	Gold standard for equivalence
Chlordiazepoxide (Librium)	25 mg	24 – 48 (long)	Intermediate	Preferred for alcohol withdrawal
Clonazepam (Klonopin)	0.5 mg	20 – 80 (long)	Intermediate	Long half-life, less rebound
Lorazepam (Ativan)	1 mg	10 – 20 (intermediate)	Intermediate	No CYP metabolism; Preferred in hepatic impairment (minimal CYP metabolism)
Alprazolam (Xanax)	0.5 mg	6 – 12 (intermediate)	Fast	High abuse potential, rebound anxiety
Oxazepam (Serax)	20 mg	5 – 15 (short)	Slow	Minimal/no CYP metabolism (glucuronidated); slow onset
Temazepam (Restoril)	20 mg	8 – 20 (intermediate)	Intermediate	For insomnia, not anxiety
Triazolam (Halcion)	0.5 mg	1.5 – 5 (short)	Fast	Ultra-short, for sleep-onset insomnia

Conversion Rules of Thumb

Diazepam 10 mg = Lorazepam 1 mg = Clonazepam 0.5 mg = Alprazolam 0.5 mg

Converting to Diazepam	Multiply by:
Chlordiazepoxide	0.4 (25 mg Librium = 10 mg diazepam)

Converting to Diazepam	Multiply by:
Clonazepam	20 (0.5 mg Klonopin = 10 mg diazepam)
Lorazepam	10 (1 mg Ativan = 10 mg diazepam)
Alprazolam	20 (0.5 mg Xanax = 10 mg diazepam)
Oxazepam	0.5 (20 mg Serax = 10 mg diazepam)
Temazepam	0.5 (20 mg Restoril = 10 mg diazepam)

CRITICAL: When tapering benzodiazepines, reduce by 10 – 25% every 1 – 2 weeks based on tolerance and withdrawal symptoms. Slower for long-term, high-dose users.

APPENDIX C: ORAL TO LAI CONVERSION GUIDE

Switching from Oral Antipsychotics to Long-Acting Injectables

LAI	Oral Form	Conversion Strategy	Initiation Requirements	Notes
Risperdal Consta (Risperidone IM)	Risperidone oral	12.5 – 50 mg IM q2 weeks	Continue oral for 3 weeks after first injection	3-week release lag
Uzedy (Risperidone SQ)	Risperidone oral	50 – 250 mg SQ monthly/q2 months	Establish oral tolerance first	Newer SQ formulation; bipolar I maintenance uses the once-monthly regimen only (50–100 mg)
Invega Sustenna (Paliperidone 1m)	Paliperidone oral	39 – 234 mg monthly	No oral overlap; start with deltoid injections	Day 1: 234 mg, Day 8: 156 mg
Invega Trinza (Paliperidone 3m)	Invega Sustenna	273 – 819 mg q3 months	Stable on monthly for ≥4 months	Must use same dose range
Invega Hafyera (Paliperidone 6m)	Invega Sustenna	1092 – 1560 mg q6 months	Stable on Invega Sustenna monthly for ≥4 months, or after at least one Invega Trinza (3-month) cycle	Longest-acting LAI
Abilify Maintena (Aripiprazole)	Aripiprazole oral	300 – 400 mg monthly	Oral overlap ×14 days	First dose 400 mg

LAI	Oral Form	Conversion Strategy	Initiation Requirements	Notes
Abilify Asimtufii (Aripiprazole 2-month) †	Abilify Maintena (LAI) †	960 mg q2 months (720 mg if indicated)	After stabilization on Abilify Maintena 400 mg, give 960 mg in place of the next scheduled Maintena dose; no oral overlap.	If not on Maintena, use labeled oral-initiation regimen.
Aristada (aripiprazole Lauroxil)	Aripiprazole oral	441 – 1064 mg q4 – 8 weeks	Establish oral tolerability first. Initiate with Aristada Initio 675 mg + oral aripiprazole 30 mg with first Aristada, or 21 days oral overlap.	Multiple intervals
Zyprexa Relprevv (Olanzapine)	Olanzapine oral	150 – 405 mg q2 – 4 weeks	Establish oral olanzapine tolerability first; no routine oral overlap.	PDSS: restricted program + 3-hour post-injection observation.

† Abilify Asimtufii may be initiated from oral aripiprazole (with 14 days of oral overlap) or from established Abilify Maintena (administered in place of the next scheduled dose, with no oral overlap); prior Abilify Maintena stabilization is not required.

Oral to LAI Conversion Formulas:

Note: The following conversion formulas apply only to LAIs initiated directly from an oral antipsychotic. Agents such as Invega Trinza and Invega Hafyera are not converted from oral — they require prior stabilization on their respective monthly or shorter-acting LAI formulation (see table above).

LAI	Conversion Rule
Risperdal Consta	If oral Risperidone ≤3 mg → 25 mg IM q2 weeks If oral Risperidone 4 – 6 mg → 37.5 – 50 mg IM q2 weeks
Invega Sustenna	If oral Paliperidone 3 mg → 39 – 78 mg monthly If oral Paliperidone 6 mg → 117 mg monthly If oral Paliperidone 9 mg → 156 mg monthly If oral Paliperidone 12 mg → 234 mg monthly
Abilify Maintena	Oral aripiprazole 10 – 20 mg → 400 mg monthly Oral aripiprazole >20 mg → consider 400 mg monthly (clinical judgment)
Aristada	Use Aristada dose calculator (based on oral Aripiprazole dose and desired interval)

IMPORTANT: Always consult full prescribing information and institutional protocols. Dosing may vary based on individual patient factors and prior response.

APPENDIX D: MAOI DIETARY RESTRICTIONS (PATIENT HANDOUT)

Foods to Avoid While Taking MAOIs

HIGH TYRAMINE — ABSOLUTELY AVOID

Food Category	Examples
Aged Cheeses	Cheddar, blue cheese, brie, camembert, parmesan, Swiss, Gouda
Cured Meats	Pepperoni, salami, sausage, prosciutto, aged ham, dried fish
Fermented Foods	Sauerkraut, kimchi, pickles (fermented), tofu (fermented), tempeh
Sauces	Soy sauce, teriyaki sauce, fish sauce, oyster sauce, miso
Meat/Fish Extracts	Marmite, Vegemite, bouillon cubes, concentrated broths
Alcohol	Tap beer (unpasteurized), red wine (especially Chianti), sherry, vermouth
Overripe Fruits	Avocado (overripe), banana (overripe), figs (canned or overripe), raisins
Fava Beans	Broad beans, fava beans

LOW TYRAMINE — USE CAUTION (small amounts)

Food Category	Examples
Cheese	Cottage cheese, cream cheese, ricotta (fresh)
Alcohol	Bottled/canned beer (limit 1 – 2), white wine (limit 1 glass)
Fruits	Fresh banana (1 per day), avocado (fresh, not overripe)
Chocolate	Small amounts (contains phenylethylamine)
Caffeine	Limit coffee, tea, cola (excess can interact)

SAFE FOODS

Food Category	Examples
Fresh dairy	Milk, yogurt, ice cream, fresh cheeses
Fresh meats	Fresh chicken, turkey, beef, pork (not aged/cured)
Fresh fish	Fresh or frozen fish (not dried/pickled)
Vegetables	Most fresh vegetables (except fava beans, sauerkraut)
Grains	Bread, rice, pasta, cereal

Food Category	Examples
Fruits	Most fresh fruits (except overripe)

MEDICATIONS TO AVOID WITH MAOIs

- Decongestants (pseudoephedrine, phenylephrine)
- Cough suppressants (dextromethorphan — risk of serotonin syndrome)
- Stimulants (amphetamines, methylphenidate)
- Avoid serotonergic antidepressants unless an appropriate washout is completed (at least 14 days for most serotonergic agents; at least 5 weeks after fluoxetine before starting an MAOI)
- St. John's Wort
- Meperidine (Demerol) — fatal interaction
- Tramadol, methadone (serotonin syndrome risk)
- Linezolid (antibiotic) — risk of serotonin syndrome
- Intravenous methylene blue — risk of serotonin syndrome

WARNING SIGNS OF HYPERTENSIVE CRISIS

Seek Emergency Care Immediately

- Severe headache (usually occipital)
- Palpitations, chest pain
- Nausea, vomiting
- Neck stiffness
- Sweating, fever
- Confusion
- Call 911 or go to the nearest emergency room — this is a medical emergency.

APPENDIX E: NALOXONE PRESCRIBING AND PATIENT EDUCATION

When to Prescribe Naloxone (Narcan)

Risk Factor	Indication
Opioid use disorder	ALL patients (active or in recovery)
High-dose opioids	≥50 MME/day (morphine milligram equivalents)
Concurrent benzodiazepines	Any opioid + benzodiazepine prescription
Concurrent alcohol use	Any opioid + alcohol use
Respiratory conditions	COPD, sleep apnea, respiratory disease
Renal/hepatic impairment	Reduced opioid clearance
History of overdose	Prior opioid overdose

Risk Factor	Indication
Household members	Children, elderly, or other opioid users in home

PATIENT EDUCATION: HOW TO USE NALOXONE (NARCAN NASAL SPRAY)

1. **RECOGNIZE OVERDOSE**
   - Not waking up, not breathing
   - Deep snoring/gurgling sounds (death rattle)
   - Blue/gray lips or fingertips
   - Tiny pupils
2. **CALL 911**
   - Say: "Someone is not breathing and not waking up."
   - Give exact address/location
   - Follow dispatcher instructions
3. **GIVE NALOXONE**
   - Place the patient on their back
   - Insert the nozzle into one nostril
   - Press plunger firmly to spray entire dose
   - No need to prime or test spray
4. **START RESCUE BREATHING**
   - Tilt head back, lift chin
   - Pinch the nose shut
   - Follow current EMS/BLS guidance for rescue breathing
   - Continue until the patient breathes on their own or EMS arrives
5. **WATCH AND REPEAT IF NEEDED**
   - Naloxone wears off in 30 – 90 minutes
   - If the patient stops breathing again, give another dose
   - Repeat every 2 – 3 minutes until EMS arrives
6. **STAY WITH PATIENT**
   - Even if they wake up, they may lapse back into overdose
   - Do not leave them alone
   - EMS must evaluate all overdose patients

Naloxone Storage Instructions

Do	Don't
Store at room temperature (59 – 77°F)	Do not freeze
Keep in original packaging	Do not expose to direct sunlight
Check expiration date regularly	Do not use after expiration date

Do	Don't
Keep accessible (not locked away)	Do not store in car (heat/cold damage)
Tell family/caregivers where it is	Do not hide where others can't find

REFERENCES

American Psychiatric Association. (2020). *The American Psychiatric Association practice guideline for the treatment of patients with schizophrenia* (3rd ed.). https://doi.org/10.1176/appi.books.9780890424841

American Society of Addiction Medicine. (2020). *The ASAM clinical practice guideline on alcohol withdrawal management.* Journal of Addiction Medicine, 14(3S), 1–72.

Substance Abuse and Mental Health Services Administration. (2021). *TIP 63: Medications for opioid use disorder.* U.S. Department of Health and Human Services.

Taylor, D., Barnes, T. R. E., & Young, A. H. (2021). *The Maudsley prescribing guidelines in psychiatry* (14th ed.). Wiley-Blackwell. (particularly relevant for antipsychotic equivalency and LAI conversion)

U.S. Food and Drug Administration. (n.d.). *Drugs@FDA: FDA-approved drug products.* https://www.accessdata.fda.gov

ABOUT THE AUTHOR

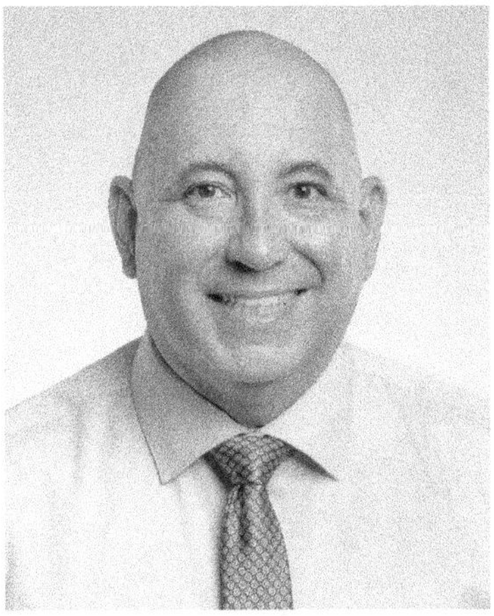

Marco Rabines, MD, is a board-certified psychiatrist and diplomate of the American Board of Psychiatry and Neurology, with advanced training in Psychiatry and Anesthesiology. He trained at Ponce Health Sciences University (formerly Ponce School of Medicine) in Ponce, Puerto Rico, and has practiced in Peru, Puerto Rico, and Florida.

A longtime educator of medical students and residents, he is the founder of NeuroSpark Press and the author of *NeuroSpark: From Atoms to Thoughts*. He developed the *Clinical Treatment Manual for Outpatient Psychiatry* to give clinicians concise, evidence-based, guideline-concordant guidance for everyday outpatient practice.

www.ingramcontent.com/pod-product-compliance
Lightning Source LLC
LaVergne TN
LVHW060023210926
848481LV00013B/3780